Let's Talk Vaccines

A Clinician's Guide to Addressing Vaccine Hesitancy and Saving Lives

Let's Talk Vaccines

A Clinician's Guide to Addressing Vaccine Hesitancy and Saving Lives

Gretchen LaSalle, MD

Family Physician, MultiCare Rockwood Clinic
Clinical Preceptor, University of Washington MEDEX program and
The Washington State University Elson S. Floyd College of Medicine
Spokane, Washington

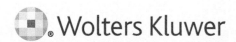 Wolters Kluwer

Philadelphia • Baltimore • New York • London
Buenos Aires • Hong Kong • Sydney • Tokyo

Acquisitions Editor: Sharon Zinner
Development Editor: Sean McGuire
Editorial Coordinator: Jolene Carr
Senior Production Project Manager: Alicia Jackson
Design Coordinator: Holly McLaughlin
Senior Manufacturing Coordinator: Beth Welsh
Prepress Vendor: TNQ Technologies

9 8 7 6 5 4 3 2

Printed in th United States of America

Library of Congress Cataloging-in-Publication Data

ISBN-13:978-1-975136-33-8

Cataloging in Publication data available on request from publisher.

---

shop.lww.com

To my husband,

whose unwavering love and support

give me roots and wings.

Reviews for
Let's Talk Vaccines

"As more parents are choosing not to vaccinate their children—and more children are suffering outbreaks of preventable infections—clinicians and public health advocates have become desperate to find a way to convince parents that their fears of vaccines are ill founded. Enter Dr. Gretchen LaSalle, who has provided the first book designed to help. Full of wonderful information ranging from the science of vaccine safety to the psychology of risk communication, this book couldn't have come at a better time."

—**Paul A. Offit, MD**
Division of Infectious Diseases
The Children's Hospital of Philadelphia
Author of Bad Advice: Or Why Celebrities, Politicians, and Activists
Aren't Your Best Source of Health Information

"An essential text for the clinician looking to discuss vaccination in a patient-centered and empathetic way. Dr. LaSalle thoroughly examines the issues underlying vaccine hesitancy, including many common questions that vaccine-hesitant patients have. A must-read for any primary care provider, this book provides thoughtful, evidence-based techniques to help patients understand vaccines in a meaningful way."

—**Max Cohen, ND**
Scientific Advisory Board, Boost Oregon
Contributing author, ndsforvaccines.com

"Finally—the answers we need, right at our fingertips! As family physicians, we know how important vaccines are and we trust the science, but we need a practical resource to help us fully dispel the myths and fears that plague our patients, friends, and family members. Anyone caring for patients and communities needs a copy of this book!"

—**Jill Grimes, MD, FAAFP**
Author of Seductive Delusions: how everyday people catch STIs
Editor-in-chief: Sexually Transmitted Disease:
An Encyclopedia of Diseases, Prevention, Treatment and Issues
University of Texas at Austin Student Health Services
UMASS Medical School Clinical Instructor

"With the increase in misinformation and skepticism about vaccines, we as physicians often face the challenge of educating our patients on the importance of these life-saving interventions. This can be a difficult conversation, and many physicians feel frustrated that our patients do not understand the importance of vaccines not only for themselves, but for those more vulnerable in their communities. Let's Talk Vaccines is an excellent primer for physicians on how to approach these discussions with evidence and with a communication style that allows us to continue working with our patients as a team, as is our ultimate goal."

—Shikha Jain, MD, FACP
Assistant Professor of Medicine
Division of Hematology, Oncology & Cell Therapy
Physician Director of Media Relations Rush University Cancer Center

"This much-needed book combines an engaging, accessible discussion with a wealth of information and practical tools that physicians can use to discuss vaccines with patients and help families through their concerns. It makes a compelling case for the need of physicians to step up and confront vaccine hesitancy."

—Dorit Reiss, LLB, PhD
Professor of Law at UC Hastings College of the Law
Member of the Parent Advisory Board of Voices for Vaccines

"Up-to-date information with real life examples and full of facts, Let's Talk Vaccines is a must read for all pediatricians, family physicians, and other vaccine advocates! I wish this book had been available when I first started practicing pediatrics—it encompasses much of what I've learned over the past 22 years and would have been a very handy teaching tool to have had from the start!"

—Christina Dewey, MD, FAAP
All About Children Pediatrics
Eden Prairie, MN

"'I want to know why' begins this amazing book for clinicians on how to respond to a patient's refusal of vaccines. Dr. LaSalle takes us from the horror of infectious disease, through vaccine development, the dark 'lie that started it all,' and then offers concrete methods to educate our patients. By understanding their apprehension, we can improve the health of each patient and the community at large. Let's Talk Vaccines is the book to help you help your patients."

—Frank J. Domino, MD
Professor
Editor: 5 Minute Clinical Consult
Department of Family Medicine & Community Health
University of Massachusetts Medical School

Acknowledgments

This book would not have been possible without the constant support of my family and friends. Thank you to my amazing husband, Sean, and to our sons, Jeremy and Charlie, for their encouragement and pride in my work and for the many loads of laundry, piles of dishes, and meals made while I was camped out on my computer. To my parents, for always believing in me and encouraging me to follow my dreams. Thank you for challenging me to step outside of my comfort zone and teaching me that I can do whatever I set my mind to if I'm willing to work for it. To my sister and best friend, for being a constant source of love and support. A big thank you to Dr. Paul Offit, Dr. Peter Hotez, Dorit Reiss, and many others who have been fighting for the health of our children and communities long before I got here. Their feedback and advice have been invaluable. Thank you to Dr. Jill Grimes, my mentor and friend, whose belief in my vision got me started on this journey. Thank you to Rebecca at Wolters Kluwer for taking a chance on me. Thank you to Kristin, Liz, and the rest of my editorial team for helping bring my vision to life. Thank you to my patients who inspire me on a daily basis and make me want to do better and be better. And, finally, a huge heartfelt thank you to the amazing woman who inspired my love of writing and literature and my annoying passion for proper grammar—my high school English teacher, Mrs. Jaye Rudolph. This one's for you!

Foreword

Since 2017, we have seen a disturbing public health trend, namely the return of childhood infectious diseases once thought to have mostly disappeared. The first sign of trouble was the return of measles. Europe has experienced tens of thousands of cases, with Italy, France, Germany, and some of the Eastern European countries the worst affected. By some estimates, there were 80,000 European measles cases in 2018. There have also been large measles outbreaks in America, notably in Minnesota in 2017; Missouri, New York, and New Jersey in 2018; and a significant epidemic in the Pacific Northwest in 2019, with measles cases now also popping up in Texas. Beyond measles, we are seeing a significant number of pediatric deaths from influenza among unvaccinated children.

A major reason for the return of measles (actually eliminated from the United States in the year 2000) and the mounting pediatric flu deaths is a decline in vaccine coverage, especially in focal areas of the United States and selected European nations. Moreover, while there might be several explanations for this, overwhelmingly, it is the result of growing vaccine hesitancy among parents. More than ever before parents are choosing not to immunize their children.

The modern anti-vaccine movement began in the late 1990s but has since grown into a small media empire. Some estimates indicate that there are literally now hundreds of anti-vaccine misinformation websites, whose information is amplified on several forms of social media, including Facebook. There are also widely distributed anti-vaccine documentaries and books and now even political action committees (PACs) lobbying state legislatures to make it easy for parents to exempt their kids from vaccines.

An end result of this impressive but almost diabolical misinformation campaign is that much of the vaccine information that parents now receive online is false or at least highly misleading. As pediatricians, family medicine physicians, and nurse practitioners know all too well, on any given day a parent will bring their child for a clinic visit armed with misinformation downloaded from the internet or with a dog-eared or yellow-highlighted anti-vaccine book in tow.

While there is good vaccine educational information available on reputable websites, including the CDC.gov site, it is often not easy to retrieve the information most relevant to a patient's or parent's immediate concern, especially during an office visit.

Dr. Gretchen LaSalle specifically wrote her book, *Let's Talk Vaccines: A Clinician's Guide to Addressing Vaccine Hesitancy and Saving Lives*, for the busy medical practitioner in order to provide timely, easily retrievable, and accurate information about vaccines and immunization. One of the important features of the book is that it specifically addresses common concerns that parents often raise during clinic visits. It directly targets the anti-vaccine movement's phony assertions about autism, autoimmune illnesses and allergies, toxic ingredients, overwhelming the immune system, conspiracies, and more. While no one book can address all the concerns raised by parents (indeed, there seems to be a constantly shifting array of claims to contend with), by reading Dr. LaSalle's book and becoming familiar with the most common issues and tested approaches to the vaccine discussion, her hope is that physicians and other medical providers will continue to be seen as knowledgeable and caring partners in their patients' care and will see greater successes in their vaccination efforts.

The anti-vaccine lobby is aggressive and adept at employing the Internet and social media. It also adapts itself to shifting trends and local political environments. *Let's Talk Vaccines* represents a bold step toward defusing a growing trend now affecting the health of children in America and Europe and possibly spreading globally down the road. The book provides detailed and up-to-date information on the latest anti-vaccine trends and strategies for refuting the most common parental objections to vaccination. It represents an important and much needed contribution to the canon of pro-vaccine books.

Peter Hotez, MD, PhD, is a professor of pediatrics at Baylor College of Medicine and Texas Children's Hospital where he is also dean of the National School of Tropical Medicine and codirector of the Texas Children's Center for Vaccine Development. He is the author of Vaccines Did Not Cause Rachel's Autism: My Journey as a Vaccine Scientist, Pediatrician, and Autism Dad (Johns Hopkins Press).

Introduction

It was the middle of flu season, and I was trying to convince one of my patients—we'll call her Anne—to take the flu shot. Like many of my partners in primary care, flu season found me experiencing more than the usual amount of frustration. We know that the flu shot and other vaccines have the potential to spare people significant morbidity and to save hundreds of thousands of lives. We have all had patients or have known people who have lost someone to the flu or to pneumonia. We've had patients suffer the terrible consequences of cervical cancer and throat cancer. We have patients who remember the scourge of polio, some of whom are now dealing with postpolio syndrome. For most of us in medicine, vaccines are a no-brainer. Why *wouldn't* we want to protect ourselves and our loved ones and others in the community? It is difficult for us to comprehend why some patients do not immediately get on board with our vaccination recommendations.

That's why, for the past several years, I don't allow the conversation with patients and their caregivers to stop at "No, thanks," when I offer vaccines. I want to know why. I owe it to my patients and to the health of the community to clarify and educate so that my patients can base their decisions on facts and not "fake news." So, when Anne said "No, thanks," I dug a little deeper.

"Tell me what worries you about the flu shot," I said.

"Well, I've heard that vaccines can cause cancer and almost everyone in my family died from some form of cancer. I don't want to do anything that would increase my chances."

A-ha! It made total sense. Obviously, if you heard that getting vaccinated would cause you to suffer a fate from which your entire family had died, you might have some doubts. Fear is what was driving Anne's hesitation, and fear is the motivating force behind many of our vaccine-hesitant patients' concerns.

This interaction was a turning point for me in how I viewed the vaccine discussion with my questioning patients. Instead of being defensive, I could approach the conversation with empathy. Vaccine-hesitant patients are not setting out to cause us angst. They are just trying to make the best decisions they can for themselves and for their loved ones with the information they are given. It is our responsibility, as health care providers, to make sure that they are given the correct information.

However, this book is not geared toward the patient. There are plenty of wonderful books out there that speak to parents about vaccine-preventable diseases, the importance of vaccination, and the dangers of the anti-vaccine movement. This book is for you, the "boots-on-the-ground" health care professional. Physicians and other medical providers frequently voice frustration in dealing with questioning patients. We feel overwhelmed by the amount of research it takes to counter the multitude of anti-vaccine assertions that our patients bring to the discussion. We feel handcuffed by the clock, barely having enough time to get through all our patients' active medical issues, let alone having the time to educate and counsel patients about vaccines. We are measured on our successes in getting patients vaccinated but oftentimes fall short of our goals.

This situation has prompted some clinicians to refuse care to nonvaccinating families, an approach that is hotly debated by professional medical societies, such as the American Academy of Pediatrics and the American Academy of Family Physicians. Still other health care providers have given up trying, allowing the conversation to end at "no," but then harboring resentment toward patients who won't vaccinate their children or themselves. As a family physician, I know that this can be a large burden to bare.

My goal in writing *Let's Talk Vaccines: A Clinician's Guide to Addressing Vaccine Hesitancy and Saving Lives* is to help you educate your patients with proven data so that they are more likely to accept your recommendation to vaccinate. I also hope that this book will help decrease the anger and frustration that you may experience in dealing with your vaccine-hesitant patients. My aim is to help you feel like you are, again, working side-by-side in partnership with your patients to discover the truth about vaccines and to prevent disease, instead of facing off in an unrewarding adversarial relationship.

Let's Talk Vaccines looks at the history of vaccine-preventable disease, vaccines, and vaccine hesitancy. It explores the psychology of the anti-vaccine movement and how fallacy and bias allow people to continue to believe information that has been proven wrong time and again. The book also discusses the issues of those who have been on the other side—people who were originally in the anti-vaccine camp who changed their minds—and will look at how the anti-vaccine movement shaped their views, how interactions with medical providers affected their choices, and how a healthy relationship with science helped bring them around. It then explores the development of vaccines and implementation of vaccination programs, so that we may understand the lengthy and rigorous testing that vaccines undergo before being released to market as well as the oversight that exists to ensure their safety and efficacy. Next, *Let's Talk Vaccines* highlights proven approaches to the vaccine discussion that will leave you with the ability to educate and encourage vaccination while allowing patients to come away feeling that their concerns and opinions have been heard and respected. It takes every anti-vaccine assertion that you've heard and provides point-by-point, data-supported arguments against them so that you will feel confident in providing your patients with factual and accurate information. We then explore organizational efficiencies that can help you find greater success in vaccinating as many of your patients as possible. Finally, the role that social media plays, pro and con, in the vaccine discussion is examined, encouraging you to become a vocal advocate for science and facts. Patients are going to get medical information from the media and the Internet whether we like it or not. Shouldn't physicians and other health care providers be the voices they are hearing?

At the end of the book, I offer simple talking points that you can use as quick educational material for your patients or staff, as well as handouts with descriptions of the many diseases, some no longer commonly seen, against which we vaccinate. You will also find lists of journal articles and educational videos for patients or staff who want to learn more about the science behind vaccines. My goal is to provide a comprehensive and easy-to-use resource that facilitates your discussion of vaccines with questioning patients so that you feel good about your interactions and achieve your greatest immunization successes. I hope that you enjoy *Let's Talk Vaccines*. Now, let's get out there and save some lives!

Your partner in care,
Gretchen LaSalle, MD

Table of Contents

1 Through the Lens of History: A Look at Vaccine-Preventable Disease and the Origin of Vaccines   *1*

2 What's Old Is New Again: Genesis of the Anti-vaccine Movement   *13*

3 Psychology of the Anti-vaccine Movement   *25*

4 There and Back Again: How Anti-vaxxers Change Their Minds   *35*

5 Who's Minding the Shop? Ensuring Vaccine Safety and Efficacy   *51*

6 Catching Flies: Approach Matters   *67*

7 A Risk Worth Taking   *79*

8 The Lie That Started It All   *91*

9 Addressing Your Patients' Vaccine Doubts: Point-Counterpoint, Part 1   *99*

10 Vaccine Concerns in Specific Populations: Point-Counterpoint, Part 2   *115*

11 Influenza and HPV: A Closer Look at Two "Controversial" Vaccines— Point-Counterpoint, Part 3   *133*

12 Vaccine Ingredients—What Is All That Stuff Anyway?   *149*

13 It's a Jungle Out There: Navigating Vaccine Advice in the News and on the World Wide Web   *159*

14 Making Your Clinic a Lean, Mean, Vaccinating Machine   *175*

15 A Call to Action   *183*

Appendix A: Vaccine-Preventable Diseases Information   *187*

Appendix B: Fast Facts About Vaccines for Patients and Clinic Staff   *219*

Appendix C: Vaccine Topics Explained (Videos)   *225*

Appendix D: Evaluating Graphical Data   *227*

Appendix E: Journal Articles Addressing Specific Vaccine Concerns   *243*

Appendix F: Navigating Information on the Internet and Social Media   *247*

Index   *249*

Through the Lens of History: A Look at Vaccine-Preventable Disease and the Origin of Vaccines

In 1736 I lost one of my sons, a fine boy of four years old, by the smallpox taken in the common way.
I long regretted bitterly and still regret that I had not given it to him by inoculation.

—BENJAMIN FRANKLIN

Vaccination and vaccine-preventable disease have a long and storied past. Vaccine-preventable diseases have toppled empires and changed the face of history. (**Box 1.1**) It wasn't until Edward Jenner's (**Figure 1.1**) discovery of the first vaccine against smallpox in 1796 that we had some hope of fighting back against these devastating illnesses. The development of vaccines has been one of the greatest scientific advances in history, saving more lives than almost anything else we do in modern medicine. Thanks to vaccines, smallpox has been eradicated from the planet; today's children no longer need immunization against smallpox as their grandparents did. Polio is no longer present in the United States and only occurs (and exceedingly rarely at that) in a few countries, with the hope of eradication in the near future. Many of today's physicians have never seen a case of tetanus. Whether it is completely causally related or not, we have not had an influenza pandemic like the Spanish Flu of 1918, during which one-third of the world's population was infected and an estimated 50 million people died (more than the number of people who died in all of World War I), since the introduction of the first influenza vaccine in 1938. The burden of vaccine-preventable disease has been reduced by 92% to 100% (depending on the disease in question)[2] since the advent of vaccination. As a result, the world is a safer and healthier place to live.

However, more than 220 years since Jenner's groundbreaking discovery, vaccine-preventable diseases are again on the rise. We are seeing tens of thousands of cases of measles in countries across Europe. In 2018, Queensland, Australia, saw its first death from diphtheria since 2011.[3] In the United States, we have had measles outbreaks affecting hundreds of people in California, Ohio, Minnesota, New York, Washington, Oregon, and Texas, among others. In 2017, mumps returned to the Pacific Northwest, with 891 cases in Washington state alone.[4] As of August of 2018, pertussis has sickened 260 people in Idaho, compared with just 32 cases for all of 2017.[5] As it so happens, vaccines have become a victim of their own success. Our collective memory, at least when it comes to the devastation caused by vaccine-preventable disease throughout world history, is short. We are victims of an "out of sight, out of

Box 1.1 Did You Know?

Did you know that quite a number of influential people in history were either themselves afflicted or lost loved ones to vaccine-preventable disease? You may be aware that President Franklin Delano Roosevelt was diagnosed with polio at the age of 39 years, but did you know that his son would later die in infancy of influenza? Presidents Lincoln, Garfield, and Cleveland all lost children to diphtheria before there was a vaccination for the illness. President Garfield also lost a child to pertussis. Abraham Lincoln himself contracted smallpox a few days before delivering the Gettysburg Address. Andrew Jackson and his brother William Jackson both contracted smallpox during the Revolutionary War. Unlike his brother, Andrew Jackson survived the illness. Eleanor Roosevelt died of complications of the now vaccine-preventable disease tuberculosis, which she acquired as a child. John Roebling, chief engineer of the Brooklyn Bridge, died of tetanus that he acquired while inspecting progress on the bridge. Lewis Carroll, author of *Alice in Wonderland*, died of influenza. Roald Dahl, author of *Charlie and the Chocolate Factory*, lost his daughter, Olivia, to measles. To die of a vaccine-preventable disease or to lose a child to one used to be relatively commonplace. The preservation of life and health as a result of vaccination is one of science's crowning achievements.[1]

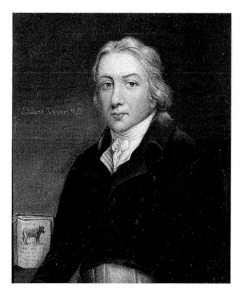

FIGURE 1.1 Edward Jenner is credited with developing the first vaccine. Jenner inoculated his first test subject with exudate from a cowpox lesion from the hand of a milkmaid, effectively protecting his subject against subsequent infection with smallpox. (Courtesy of Wellcome Library, London. Wellcome Images. Edward Jenner. Oil painting. https://wellcomecollection.org/works/ca86xk2y. CC BY 4.0)

mind" phenomenon. As a community, we no longer see these illnesses affecting our loved ones, so they no longer seem like an ever-present danger. Certain segments of our population have become complacent about immunizing, or turned away from it intentionally, and we are beginning to see a return of these vaccine-preventable illnesses in unvaccinated or undervaccinated communities as a result.

Recalling the history of vaccines and vaccine-preventable disease is, therefore, exceedingly important to maintaining our vigilance around immunization. Our history informs our present and our future. If we don't have a clear knowledge of that history, we risk repeating our past, an outcome that could prove deadly. This chapter offers a brief overview—thousands of years of history condensed into a few pages—of the history of vaccines and vaccine-preventable diseases. We will look at devastating historical illnesses like smallpox, polio, and influenza. We will review a timeline of the discovery of vaccines through our modern-day immunization campaigns. We will recall the darker side of vaccination through history and how this has potentially colored people's views of vaccines and of government involvement with immunization recommendations. Finally, this chapter will bring us to present day and to the illnesses that are resurfacing in our communities, thanks to decreasing rates of vaccination.

SMALLPOX, VARIOLATION, AND THE FIRST VACCINE

Smallpox, named for the numerous pus-filled blisters (or pocks) that it caused on those infected with the disease, was one of the greatest scourges in human history. The earliest evidence of its devastation is seen on mummified remains from the Egyptian dynasties (1570-1085 BC). Chinese writings from 1122 BC and Sanskrit texts from India are some of the earliest written recordings of the illness.[6] Smallpox traveled with settlers and merchants and made its way to Europe sometime around the fifth to seventh centuries. It was epidemic at various points throughout the Middle Ages and played an important role in the development of Western civilization. The Plague of Antonine killed nearly 7 million people and coincided with the beginnings of the fall of the Roman Empire. When Spanish and Portuguese conquistadores came to the New World, they brought smallpox with them, an introduction that was instrumental in the destruction of the great Aztec and Incan empires. Settlers on the eastern coast of North America introduced the native population to smallpox. It was later used as one of the first examples of biological warfare when the British used smallpox to kill off the "hostile" American Indian population during the French and Indian War.

The earliest efforts at inoculation against this deadly disease were first documented in China and the Middle East in the 15th century. Writings describe a process later named "variolation," whereby scabs from a person infected with smallpox (*variola virus*) were dried and powdered then introduced to a healthy person via nasal insufflation (blowing the powdered pox into the nose) or during which pustular matter was taken from an infected person and introduced to a healthy individual via scratches in the skin. Smallpox carried a 20% to 60% fatality rate. However, the process of variolation itself resulted in death for 1% to 2% of those on which it was used and had the potential to cause outbreaks if those infected spread the disease to others. This process was continued with varying success through the ages and across continents, finally making its way to England and North America with the slave trade in the 1700s.[7] However, as we still see today, albeit with much safer inoculation methods, the process of conferring immunity faced opposition. Injecting healthy people with a potentially fatal disease to induce a lesser case of illness and hopefully prevent more serious and deadly consequences was a hard pill to swallow **(Figure 1.2)**.

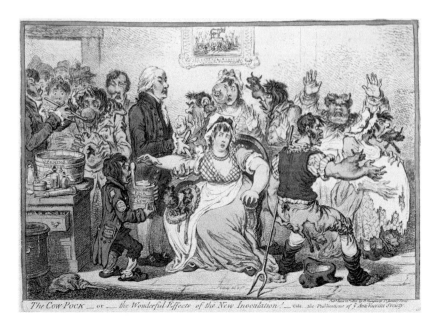

FIGURE 1.2 This illustrated cartoon from 1804 shows the unease and lack of understanding surrounding the smallpox vaccination. This sentiment still prevails today and hinders the deployment of effective vaccination programs. (Courtesy of the National Library of Medicine.)

It wasn't until the early to mid-1800s that variolation was largely abandoned in favor of a process termed "vaccination." The father of vaccination was an English physician scientist named Edward Jenner. Although he was not the first to observe that milkmaids infected with cowpox had immunity to smallpox, nor likely the first to test the observation, he was the first to disseminate results of his studies to the world and, thus, gains credit for the discovery. In 1796, to test his theory, Jenner used the matter from a milkmaid's cowpox lesion to infect his test subject, a boy named James Phipps. Cowpox is a member of the orthopoxvirus family, as is smallpox. However, cowpox is a much milder and generally nonfatal disease. Phipps came down with a mild illness but quickly recovered. Jenner then injected his subject with smallpox and found that Phipps never became ill. He repeated this exposure several times and Phipps remained immune. Thus was born the world's first vaccine, a term derived from the Latin word for cowpox (*vaccinia*),[6] a milestone that set us on the path to ultimate worldwide eradication of the virus in 1980, following a global immunization campaign led by the World Health Organization.

PANDEMICS IN RECENT HISTORY

More modern history recalls other deadly pandemics. In 1918, the world saw the greatest pandemic in centuries. The Spanish flu, so named for the reports of its particular devastation in Spain, a country not subject to the news blackouts that affected other countries during wartime, swept across the continents, killing 50 million people worldwide (with some estimates as high as 100 million). It killed even more people than died during World War I (which claimed an estimated 16 million lives). One-third of the world's population was infected. Most families were touched by loss, for some, many times over. The average life expectancy was diminished by 12 years during that one flu season as a result of this particularly virulent influenza strain.[8] Moreover, in an unusual fashion, the Spanish flu had a predilection for killing younger, healthier individuals sometimes within hours, their lungs filling with fluid and blood causing suffocation and death.

The influenza virus was not identified until 1933, and the first vaccine wasn't introduced until 1938. However, that initial vaccine and those soon to follow were only variably successful. The reasons for this, we ultimately discovered, were the multiple strains of influenza and the propensity of those influenza strains to mutate, changing their antigenic (infectious) properties as rapidly as from the time it takes to produce the vaccine to the time it is administered. Influenza can even mutate during the production phase, when it is being grown in its most common growth medium, the chicken egg. New methods of production, which are less prone to mutation, are in development, and we have hopes of a more universal flu vaccine in the future. However, for now, our current flu vaccine is the best way to decrease the chances of infection with influenza and its severe and potentially deadly consequences.

Even more recently, we may recall the polio epidemics that ravaged the United States and other parts of the world. Polio is a virus that is spread rapidly by close personal contact, through secretions from the mouth and nose, or by contact with contaminated feces. Although polio did not uniquely affect children, the name initially used to describe the condition (infantile paralysis) hints at its greater impact on the very young. Not everyone suffered so severely. In fact, nearly 95% of people had no symptoms of their infection at all. However, when the virus did impact the nervous system, resulting in a paralysis of the muscles including those muscles required for breathing, it caused devastating results. In a single year (1952), nearly 60,000 US children were infected with the polio-virus. Thousands were permanently paralyzed, and 3000 children died.[9] It's not difficult to find photographs from the United States in the 1950s that show children walking with braces, children with withered legs from the muscle atrophy that resulted from infection, and rows upon rows of iron lungs used to keep those whose breathing muscles had become paralyzed alive. Between 2% and 5% of children infected with the paralytic form of polio would ultimately die of their disease. Although fewer adults were affected, their prospects were even more dismal with up to 15% to 30% with paralytic polio dying of complications of their illness.[10]

In the 1900s, as vaccine science progressed, building upon the lessons learned from early immunization development, production, and large-scale vaccine deployment, the medical and lay worlds saw a growing number of available vaccines (**Table 1.1**). It is important to recognize here, and to be able to express to our questioning patients, that vaccinations are not produced for illnesses that are "not that severe," as those who oppose vaccines would claim. There are no vaccinations against the common cold or hand, foot and mouth disease, for example. That is because these infections very rarely cause illness severe enough to require hospitalization, leave permanent brain or other organ damage, or result in death. Immunizations are produced against those illnesses that have the propensity to cause significant risk to life. For example, in the United States, "in 1920, 469,924 measles cases were reported, and 7575 patients died; 147,991 diphtheria cases were reported, and 13,170 patients died. In 1922, 107,473 pertussis cases were reported, and 5099 patients died."[11] On a worldwide scale, this represents the loss of millions of lives. Immunizations are developed to fight against some of the greatest killers of children and others across the globe.

TABLE 1.1 Vaccine-Preventable Diseases by Year of Vaccine Development or Licensure in the United States (1798-2018)[11]

DISEASE	YEAR
Smallpox[a,d]	1798[b]
Rabies[d]	1885[b]
Typhoid[d]	1896[b]
Cholera[d]	1896[b]
Plague[d]	1897[b]
Diphtheria[a]	1923[b]
Pertussis[a]	1926[b]
Tetanus[a]	1927[b]
Tuberculosis[d]	1927[b]
Influenza • IIV[a] • LAIV[a]	 1945[c] 2003[c]
Yellow fever[d]	1953[c]
Poliomyelitis • IPV[d] • Enhanced-potency IPV[a] • OPV[d]	 1955[c] 1987[c] 1962[c]
Measles[a]	1963[c]
Mumps[a]	1967[c]
Rubella[a]	1969[c]
Anthrax[d]	1970[c]
Meningococcal disease • MPSV4[d] • MenACWY-D[a] • MenACWY-CRM[a] • MenB	 1974[c] 2005[c] 2010[c] 2014/15[c]

TABLE 1.1 Vaccine-Preventable Diseases by Year of Vaccine Development or Licensure in the United States (1798-2018)[11] (Continued)

DISEASE	YEAR
Pneumococcal disease	
• PPSV14[d]	1977[c]
• PPSV23	1983[c]
• PCV7[d]	2000[c]
• PCV13[a]	2010[c]
Adenovirus[d]	1980[c]
Hepatitis B[a]	1981[c]
Haemophilus influenza type b[a]	1985[c]
Japanese encephalitis[d]	1992[c]
Hepatitis A[a]	1995[c]
Varicella[a]	1995[c]
Lyme disease[d]	1998[c]
Rotavirus[a]	1998[c]
Human papillomavirus (HPV)	
• HPV4[d]	2006[c]
• HPV2[d]	2009
• HPV9[a]	2014[c]
Zoster (shingles)	
• Zostavax[d]	2006[c]
• Shingrix	2018[c]

[a] *Vaccine recommended for universal use in the US children.*
[b] *Vaccine developed (ie, first published results of vaccine usage).*
[c] *Vaccine licensed for use in United States.*
[d] *Either discontinued (for example, routine smallpox vaccination was discontinued in the United States in 1971) or not recommended for routine use in the United States.*

IIV, inactivated influenza vaccine; IPV, inactivated polio vaccine; LAIV, live attenuated influenza vaccine; MenACWY, meningococcal conjugate vaccine, strains A, C, W, and Y; MenB, meningococcal conjugate vaccine, strain B; MPSV, meningococcal polysaccharide vaccine; OPV, oral poliovirus vaccine; PCV, pneumococcal conjugate vaccine; PPSV, pneumococcal polysaccharide vaccine.

THE DARKER SIDE OF VACCINE HISTORY

Although vaccines have overwhelmingly been a positive advancement in medicine and public health, scientific research and vaccine production have had their dark moments. In the early 1900s, before we had the degree of regulation and oversight of vaccine manufacturing that we now enjoy, several events occurred that still color people's impressions of vaccine safety to this day. In 1901, 13 children died in St. Louis, Missouri, after accidentally receiving diphtheria antitoxin that had been produced from a horse that was infected with tetanus. Camden, New Jersey, saw the deaths of nine children from tetanus after they had been given contaminated smallpox vaccine. These incidences were traced back to errors in the vaccine production process. Consequently, the Biologics Control Act of 1902, which required governmental oversight of vaccine production, was enacted by Congress under President Theodore Roosevelt to help prevent such incidences in the future.[12]

Still other unfortunate occurrences in vaccination history have spurred further mistrust of vaccine manufacturers. In chapter 5, we will discuss the roles of our current regulatory bodies, the development of which were sometimes triggered by these events. The Cutter Incident is one of those blemishes on vaccine history in which vaccination ended up causing harm. In the mid-1950s, polio vaccine production was in full swing. The vaccine had been rigorously tested and offered a hope for protection against the devastating illness of polio, the threat of which terrorized communities in the 1940s and 1950s. During polio vaccine production at Cutter Laboratories, an error in manufacturing resulted in failure to completely inactivate the poliovirus. As a result, 40,000 children who received the Cutter vaccine were inadvertently infected with a live version of the virus and subsequently developed an active polio infection, leaving nearly "200 children with varying degrees of paralysis and killing 10."[13] In reaction to this event, oversight of vaccine manufacturers was significantly improved, and we have seen no further such incidents related to vaccine safety.

In the history of scientific investigation, one of the most damaging research studies conducted was the "Tuskegee Experiment." In 1932, the Public Health Service, in conjunction with the Tuskegee Institute, began a study to examine the natural history of syphilis. The research was titled the "Tuskegee Study of Untreated Syphilis in the Negro Male." Six hundred black men from rural Alabama were enrolled, 399 with syphilis and 201 without. They were told that they were being treated for "bad blood," a local term used to describe a variety of ailments including anemia, syphilis, and fatigue. They were offered free medical examinations, free meals, and burial insurance. The men were never provided information regarding the real purpose of the study and, even when penicillin became the treatment of choice for syphilis in 1947, study participants were never offered the treatment that would have cured their infection. Syphilis was knowingly allowed to progress and to spread untreated, resulting in 28 deaths from syphilis in the original 399 men studied, 100 deaths from related disease, the spread of disease to 40 of their wives, and the birth of 19 children with congenital syphilis.[14] These days, in our climate of more rigorous ethical standards for research, it is difficult to fathom such an immoral application of the scientific method. However, with history such as this, it is easy to see how a lack of trust in the scientific and medical communities and in governmental involvement in production and implementation of public health programs, including those involved with vaccination, might persist.

A FUTURE THREAT

Anti-vaccine sentiment was present long before Andrew Wakefield's assertion of a connection between the measles, mumps, and rubella (MMR) vaccine and development of autism (see chapter 8, The Lie That Started It All), but his impact in spurring on our modern-day anti-vaccine movement is undeniable. His assertions coincided with a time in our history when rapid advancement in Internet technology and the growing popularity of social media platforms, such as Facebook, Twitter, and Instagram, allowed for dissemination of information at a pace previously unknown. Anti-vaccine sentiment, pre-Internet, existed in isolated communities and was spread only by written correspondence and word of mouth. Now, with the ease of a few character strokes and the click of a button, anti-vaccine proponents can share their damaging messages with millions of people within seconds. Despite the fact that Wakefield's research has been debunked numerous times over and his ethical motivations have been called into question, the worry about a link between vaccines and autism continues to this day. Moreover, this is not the only concern voiced by the anti-vaccine movement. There seems to be a constantly shifting goalpost of claims that individuals against vaccines make, such as a belief that there are toxins in the immunizations, we are overwhelming our children's immune systems, and we are encouraging early sexual activity. Thanks to the Internet and social media, these assertions "go viral" and spread like the very diseases we are trying so hard to prevent. The anti-vaccine movement threatens our individual and public health in a very real way.

VICTIMS OF THEIR OWN SUCCESS

Many of us are familiar with the common ear infections and bronchitis that children suffer as a result of pneumococcal disease and *Haemophilus influenzae* type b. Less commonly do we encounter patients with invasive disease that can cause bacteremia, meningitis, or death—although these outcomes were all too common before the introduction of vaccinations against these infections. Many of today's medical graduates have never seen a case of measles, mumps, diphtheria, or tetanus. We learn about them in training, but when we are not faced with the frightening reality of these illnesses on a day-to-day basis, they can begin to seem a thing of the past, a remote risk that we need not worry about. It is easy to see how anti-vaccine propaganda telling parents that the risks of vaccines are greater than the risks of disease can be compelling. However, we are living in a global society, where travel between countries is common. Moreover, many of these countries, who are not blessed with the coordinated and well-run public health programs that we have in the United States or with a plentiful supply of vaccine, still see loss of countless lives to vaccine-preventable disease. While efforts from the World Health Organization and others have resulted in a worldwide reduction in measles deaths by 84% between 2000 and 2016 (saving an estimated 20.4 million lives), for example, there were still 89,780 deaths globally from measles in 2016, mostly in children younger than 5 years of age.[15] With intercontinental travel as easy as it is, we will all too quickly see the resurgence of illnesses heretofore thought to be eradicated from our country if we don't maintain vigilance around vaccination in the United States and around the world. When encouraging vaccinations, we not only have to think about protecting the individual, but we have to view our work as key to life-saving efforts both in our local and global communities.

Recent vaccine-preventable disease outbreaks demonstrate the very serious effects of falling prey to complacency and to the anti-vaccine agenda. As of December 6, 2018, New York City is seeing the largest measles outbreak in recent history with 89 cases documented. The outbreak began when travelers to Israel (which is seeing its own outbreak) became infected and then spread that infection to others upon return home to their unvaccinated or undervaccinated communities.[16] In 2017, Hennepin County, Minnesota, saw an outbreak of measles in its Somali-American community, whose rates of MMR vaccination had dropped from 92% in 2004 to a 45% vaccination rate by 2013, significantly below the rate required to maintain herd immunity. This decrease in vaccination resulted from a specific targeting of the population by anti-vaccine advocates after some Somali-American parents expressed concerns regarding the rates of autism that they were seeing in their children.[17] Of the 75 people (mostly children) who developed measles, 91% were unvaccinated.[18] In 2015, a multistate measles outbreak occurred which found its roots at the Disneyland amusement park in Anaheim, California. It likely spread from a traveler who had acquired the infection outside the country and then visited the park while still infectious. A total of 147 cases were identified, affecting people in seven states as well as Canada and Mexico. The Centers for Disease Control and Prevention notes that the large majority of these cases were unvaccinated or had undocumented vaccination status.[19] In 2014, 383 cases of measles occurred in an unvaccinated Amish community in Ohio. There are no religious rules against vaccinating in the Amish community, per se, but sentiments expressed by one member of the community in a National Public Radio interview during the outbreak sum up what likely is a common sentiment among people who live in tight-knit communities where disease is uncommon: "…there was no scare to us before… I guess we were too relaxed."[20]

HOW FAR WE'VE COME

Science has given us, and continues to develop and improve, the tools that we need to keep our patients healthy. We must recognize and celebrate our great successes—the elimination of smallpox from the earth and the huge reduction in mortality from measles and diphtheria that vaccination programs have brought about, for example. However, we must also acknowledge our very notable mistakes. Scientific investigation and advancement is an iterative process. We observe. We investigate. We test and retest. We implement. We observe again. We improve and perfect. Scientific study, by its very nature, holds itself accountable to the truth. If a study is not reproducible, it becomes invalidated. We must remember, and help our patients to understand, that we cannot look at individual studies to draw universal conclusions (for example, a 12-patient study proposing a link between the MMR vaccine and autism). We have to look at the body of evidence to determine when an intervention works or does not work. What I hope we will remember is that, although there have been some major missteps in our past in regard to scientific study and vaccine development, we have learned from those mistakes. We have improved the processes of monitoring and implementing our vaccination programs. We have set high ethical standards in the development of biological products, including vaccines, and have much stricter oversight than ever before. It is our responsibility as health care professionals to recall our medical roots, to remind our patients of how far we have come and of how much we have to lose if we go backward, and to put our energies and support behind encouraging immunization at the individual and community levels. If we do so, our future holds much promise for saving lives and minimizing suffering from vaccine-preventable disease, thus preserving our wonderful human potential.

Note: In Appendix A, you will find informational pages on each individual vaccine-preventable disease against which we have immunized in this country. There are images of what these illnesses look like, discussions of common signs and symptoms of each disease, and descriptions of complications of the disease. Details about the vaccines for each illness are provided, as is the impact of each illness in the pre-vaccine era and the reduction in illness that we have seen since introduction of vaccines. I encourage you to review these pages, to remind yourself of what our past used to look like in regard to vaccine-preventable disease and to rejoice in how far we have come in protecting life and health for every citizen of the world, especially those most vulnerable in our population.

References

1. Children's Hospital of Philadelphia. Just the Vax — Historical/Famous Figures and Vaccine-Preventable Diseases. Accessed February 5, 2019. https://www.chop.edu/centers-programs/vaccine-education-center/just-vax-historicalfamous-figures-and-vaccine-preventable-diseases.

2. Ventola CL. Immunization in the United States: recommendations, barriers, and measures to improve compliance: part 1: childhood vaccinations. *Pharm Ther*. 2016;41(7):426-436.

3. Rigby M. Diphtheria Death Shows Queensland is Failing to Properly Vaccinate, AMA Warns. Updated February 7, 2018. Accessed November 30, 2018. https://www.abc.net.au/news/2018-02-08/diptheria-death-shows-vaccination-failure-ama-says/9407920.

4. Washington State Department of Health. Mumps Outbreak 2017. Updated 2017. Accessed November 30, 2018. https://www.doh.wa.gov/YouandYourFamily/IllnessandDisease/Mumps/MumpsOutbreak.

5. Boone R. Whooping Cough Outbreak Worsens in Southwestern Idaho. U.S. News & World Report. Updated August 14, 2018. Accessed November 30, 2018. https://www.usnews.com/news/best-states/Idaho/articles/2018-08-14/whooping-cough-outbreak-worsens-in-southwestern-Idaho.

6. Riedel S. Edward Jenner and the history of smallpox vaccination. *Proc (Bayl Univ Med Cent)*. 2005;18(1):21-25.

7. U.S. National Library of Medicine. Variolation. In: Smallpox: A Great and Terrible Scourge. Updated July 30, 2013. Accessed November 30, 2018. https://www.nlm.nih.gov/exhibition/smallpox/sp_variolation.html.

8. National Archives and Records Administration. The Deadly Virus: The Influenza Epidemic of 1918. Accessed November 30, 2018. https://www.archives.gov/exhibits/influenza-epidemic/.

9. Beaubien J. Wiping Out Polio. How the U.S. Snuffed Out a Killer. Updated October 15, 2012. Accessed November 30, 2018. https://www.npr.org/sections/health-shots/2012/10/16/162670836/wiping-out-polio-how-the-u-s-snuffed-out-a-killer.

10. Poliomyelitis. In: Atkinson W, Wolfe S, Hamborsky J, McIntyre L, eds. *Centers for Disease Control and Prevention. Epidemiology and Prevention of Vaccine-Preventable Diseases*. 13th ed. Washington DC: Public Health Foundation; 2015. Updated April, 2015. Accessed January 25, 2018. https://www.cdc.gov/vaccines/pubs/pinkbook/downloads/polio.pdf.

11. National Immunization Program, CDC. Achievements in public health, 1990-1999 impact of vaccines universally recommended for children – United States, 1990-1998. *MMWR*. 1999;48(12):243-248. Accessed November 2018. https://www.cdc.gov/mmwr/preview/mmwrhtml/00056803.htm.

12. Center for Biologics Evaluation and Research History. The Road to the Biotech Revolution – Highlights of 100 Years of Biologics Regulation. Accessed November 12, 2018. https://www.fda.gov/downloads/AboutFDA/WhatWeDo/History/ProductRegulation/UCM593490.pdf.

13. Fitzpatrick M. The cutter incident: how America's first polio vaccine led to a growing vaccine crisis. *J R Soc Med*. 2006;99(3):156.

14. Centers for Disease Control and Prevention. The Tuskegee Timeline. Accessed December 19, 2018. https://www.cdc.gov/tuskegee/timeline.htm.

15. World Health Organization. Measles. Updated November 29, 2018. Accessed November 30, 2018. http://www.who.int/news-room/fact-sheets/detail/measles.

16. Goldblatt RL. Rockland Measles Outbreak: New Vaccine Clinic at Palisades Center, 91 Cases Reported. Lohud (USA Today). December 6, 2018. Accessed December 19, 2018. https://www.lohud.com/story/news/local/rockland/west-nyack/2018/12/06/rockland-measles-outbreak-new-vaccine-clinic-palisades-center/2225136002/.

17. Sohn E. Understanding the History Behind Communities' Vaccine Fears. Shots Health News from NPR. May 3, 2017. Accessed November 30, 2018. https://www.npr.org/sections/health-shots/2017/05/03/526595475/understanding-the-history-behind-communities-vaccine-fears.

18. Minnesota Department of Health, News Release. Health Officials Confirm Measles in Hennepin County Child. August 7, 2018. Accessed November 30, 2018. http://www.health.state.mn.us/news/pressrel/2018/measles080718.html.

19. Centers for Disease Control and Prevention. Year in Review: Measles Linked to Disneyland. December 2, 2015. Accessed December 19, 2018. https://blogs.cdc.gov/publichealthmatters/2015/12/year-in-review-measles-linked-to-disneyland/.

20. Tribble SJ. Measles Outbreak in Ohio Leads Amish to Reconsider Vaccines. Shots Health News from NPR. June 24, 2014. Accessed December 19, 2018. https://www.npr.org/sections/health-shots/2014/06/24/323702892/measles-outbreak-in-ohio-leads-amish-to-reconsider-vaccines.

2

What's Old Is New Again: Genesis of the Anti-vaccine Movement

If history repeats itself, and the unexpected always happens, how incapable must Man be of learning from experience.

—GEORGE BERNARD SHAW

Although it may feel like the anti-vaccine movement is only a recent plague upon our medical and public health efforts, anti-vaccine sentiment has been alive and well as long as there have been vaccines. Although the years have led to significant advances in science, technology, and health care, the concerns voiced and the tactics used by the modern-day anti-vaccine community are much the same as they were back in the 18th and 19th centuries, when Jenner first introduced the world to his vaccine against smallpox. In the age-old struggle that exists between anti-vaccine and pro-vaccine activists, it was said of that time that "Pro-inoculators tended to write in the cool and factual tones encouraged by the Royal Society, with frequent appeals to reason, the modern progress of science and the courtesy subsisting among gentlemen. Anti-inoculators purposely wrote like demagogues, using heated tones and lurid scare stories to promote paranoia."[1] Sound familiar? Not much has changed.

However, this should not necessarily instill within us a sense of hopelessness. We will likely never come to a universal consensus about immunizations, but in knowing our past and seeking to understand the reasons behind anti-vaccine concerns and the tactics used by anti-vaccinators then and now, we may hope to foster a better appreciation for the effectiveness and safety of vaccines in the future **(Box 2.1)**. Arguments against vaccination, whether in the 1800s or the 2010s, take many forms, but generally can be boiled down to the following: issues related to cleanliness or purity, concerns regarding infringement upon personal liberties, distrust in science and medicine, distrust of government and industry, and religious concerns. This chapter delves into each of these concerns **(Box 2.2)**, examining their origins and bringing us forward to our modern-day struggle. We will then look at the one major cultural and technological shift, the age of the Internet, which has allowed localized and isolated anti-vaccine entities to organize and spread their message worldwide.

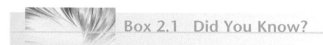

Box 2.1   Did You Know?

There is a lot of interesting research being done in the area of vaccines. The National Institute of Allergy and Infectious Disease is currently working on developing a more universal flu vaccine—one that would use part of the influenza virus that is less prone to mutation—which would make a yearly flu shot a thing of the past. To eliminate the need for that pesky poke, scientists are also working on vaccines delivered by alternate routes. Edible vaccines, using potatoes and bananas, for example, have shown promise in preliminary testing for delivering immunity to hepatitis B and norovirus. We are already familiar with the nasal flu vaccine, but researchers are looking into this formulation for other vaccines as well. Moreover, the use of a skin patch delivery system to trigger dendritic cells, the skin's immune cells, is being tested against illnesses, such as traveler's diarrhea, seasonal flu, anthrax, and others. And even more exciting is the research looking into the use of vaccines to treat existing diseases, such as cancers, HIV, and multiple sclerosis. Isn't science amazing?[2]

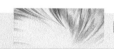

Box 2.2   Overview of Common Factors
Contributing to Vaccine-Hesitancy

- A desire to do things "naturally"
  - "Natural" immunity better than "artificial" immunity from vaccines
  - Concern that "toxins" in vaccines are harmful to health
- A desire to preserve individual freedoms
  - A parent should have control over what happens to their child
  - A person should have control over what happens to their body
- Distrust of organizations/industry
  - Distrust of the government's and pharmaceutical industry's role in health
  - Questioning the motivations of doctors and scientists
- Religious concerns
  - Ethical dilemmas about how vaccines are produced
  - Belief in noninterference with God's will
- Fear
  - Triggered by anecdotal stories of injury or sickness from vaccinations
  - Supported by misleading information about the safety of vaccines and their ingredients

CONCERNS WITH CLEANLINESS AND PURITY

The smallpox vaccine, first introduced by Jenner in 1796, was administered to subjects either through scoring the skin on a person's arm and injecting into it the pus from a cowpox blister or injecting lymph from a person who had been recently vaccinated. Issues concerning hygiene and contagion were not as well understood then as they are now, so it was not uncommon for persons to develop a secondary bacterial skin infection during the process. It was also possible for the recipient to come down with some other infectious disease being carried by the individual from whom the lymph was taken. This potential to develop sickness from the process of prevention was understandably worrisome to many and led people to view the vaccination process as unclean.

Today, we have much higher standards for the purity and safety of our vaccine supply and its administration, though these have come, in some cases, as a direct result of lessons learned from past mistakes. Chapter 1 discusses the deaths from tetanus that occurred in Camden, New Jersey, following vaccination with a contaminated small-pox vaccine and in St. Louis, Missouri, from contaminated diphtheria antitoxin. We learned about the Cutter incident in which the polio vaccine from Cutter Laboratories was incompletely inactivated and children were unintentionally injected with live polio virus. These are significant dark spots in vaccine history, but response to these tragedies resulted in the much more robust system of oversight, safety testing, and monitoring that we enjoy in our vaccine manufacturing process today.

Yet, concerns about the cleanliness and purity of vaccines still exist. In today's anti-vaccine climate, these commonly take shape in one of two ways; either in the form of the often faulty assumption that a vaccine can actually give you the disease against which it was meant to protect, or the concern over alleged toxins used in modern-day vaccines that are somehow going to poison us and cause sickness. We can counter the first assertion by explaining the difference between a killed virus and a live-attenuated virus vaccine and by cautioning patients about the normal revving up of their immune system that happens after vaccination, which can sometimes make them feel under the weather. We can also appropriately select patients to vaccinate with live-attenuated vaccines so that we aren't putting those with a suppressed immune system at unnecessary risk. The concern over "toxins" is a bit more difficult to tackle.

Thimerosal (containing ethyl mercury), as one example of a "toxin" frequently cited, was used for many years to prevent bacterial and fungal contamination of multidose vials of vaccine, ironically to help them stay more clean and pure. However, the thimerosal content of vaccines has been a concern for the anti-vaccine movement, specifically those who buy into the vaccines/autism link suggested by Wakefield. As a result of growing public concern, the Public Health Services agencies, the American Academy of Pediatrics, and vaccine manufacturers agreed to reduce or eliminate thimerosal in vaccines.[3] In 2001, thimerosal was removed from all but the multidose vial of influenza vaccines, not because of any reproducible evidence of harm, but just to take it off the table as an issue. However, in doing so, we have only contributed to the rising cost of vaccines, each dose of which now has to be individually packaged. And, when there were no significant safety problems with thimerosal to begin with, we have fed the suspicions of some anti-vaccine advocates that vaccines weren't safe from the start. See chapter 9 for discussion of other purported toxins in vaccines and why these are, in reality, *not* harmful to us in the concentrations present in vaccines.

INFRINGEMENT UPON PERSONAL LIBERTIES

In England, the Vaccination Act of 1853 made it mandatory for infants up to 3 months old to receive vaccination for smallpox. The Vaccination Act of 1867 expanded this to include all persons up to 14 years of age. Both acts penalized parents who refused vaccination. These mandates were felt by some to have violated their personal liberties to control their own bodies and the bodies of their children. Consequently, the first Anti-Vaccination leagues were founded, protests were held, and court battles ensued. The most memorable anti-vaccine protest was the Leicester Demonstration March of 1885 during which more than 80,000 people marched through the streets carrying children's coffins, banners, and a burning effigy of Edward Jenner. As a result of these and other similar demonstrations, a commission designed to study vaccination was formed. In 1896, the commission supported the recommendation for vaccination against small-pox, recognizing its protective benefit to the population, but suggested removing penalties. The Vaccination Act of 1898 then created a "conscientious objector" clause that allowed parents to apply for an exemption certificate if they desired not to vaccinate their children.[4]

The United States saw similar movements with the formation of the Anti-Vaccination Society of America in 1879 after a visit by the prominent British anti-vaccinationist William Tebb (more than 100 years later we would see a similar tour of the United States by anti-vaccinationist Andrew Wakefield). Other leagues, such as the New England Anti-Compulsory Vaccination League and the Anti-Vaccination League of New York sprang up. These organizations were active in trying to repeal vaccination mandates through the courts in California, Wisconsin, Illinois, and others.[4] The most important court case in the early battles over mandatory vaccination came in 1902 after an outbreak of smallpox in Cambridge, Massachusetts. The board of health ordered vac-cination of all residents of the city, and a man named Henning Jacobson refused on the grounds that it violated his right to control what happened to his body. The state filed criminal charges against him and he lost his local court battle. Jacobson appealed the decision to the US Supreme Court, making it the first and most famous Supreme Court case concerning the states' power in public health law. The Court found in the state's favor, granting that the state could enact mandatory laws to ensure protection of the public in the event of a communicable disease.[5] The Court's decision continues to be used today as a foundation against which states' rights versus individual rights claims can be judged. As stated by Justice John Harlan, Associate Justice presiding over *Jacobson v Massachusetts*:

> *[T]he liberty secured by the Constitution…does not import an absolute right in each person to be…wholly freed from restraint…. On any other basis organized society could not exist with safety to its members…. [The Massachusetts Constitution] laid down as fundamental…social compact that the whole people covenants with each citizen, and each citizen with the whole people, that all shall be governed by certain laws for the 'common good' and that government is instituted 'for the protection, safety, prosperity and happiness of the people, and not for the profit, honor or private interests of any one man…*[6]

DISTRUST IN SCIENCE AND MEDICINE

In the 19th century, at the time of the smallpox vaccine introduction and at the begin-ning of mandatory vaccination programs, the understanding of how disease spreads was in its infancy, with much debate among scientists and doctors about whether there was a specific etiology of disease (such as an infectious organism). Many at the time believed in an atmospheric theory of disease causation, suggesting that disease was pro-duced from "noxious emanations from decaying organic matter."[7] Jenner's vaccine, the existence of which was based upon the theory of a specific etiology of smallpox, ran counter to this commonly held belief about disease. It is no wonder that the average person was confused and fearful of Jenner's methods when even scientists and doctors were at odds about how this approach could work. Study of the anti-vaccine movement in the 19th century suggests that the movement was "part of a wider public distrust of scientific medicine and 'new science' and a cherishing of 'natural' methods of treatment and 'sanitary' methods of prevention."[8] Again, this feels familiar. Just as it was back then, the introduction of any new vaccine (or for that matter, any new treatment or medication) that is unknown or poorly understood can be confusing and frightening.

Our more modern distrust of science and medicine can find its origin, at least in part, in a groundbreaking book by Rachel Carson, published in 1962. *Silent Spring* put forth the idea that technological and scientific advancement, through the creation and use of chemicals in pesticides, was poisoning the Earth and its inhabitants. It triggered a growing concern for man's impact upon our Earth and birthed the environmental movement, which ultimately led to development of the Environmental Protection Agency. At the same time, however, it spawned a distrust of industry and science, which continues to impact us to this day.

There are "bad actors" in all parts of society—people motivated by greed, willing to advance at the expense of others—and science and medicine are not immune. In chapter 1 we discussed the Tuskegee Experiment. More recently, we have learned of researchers' use of what have become known as HeLa cells. The name HeLa is derived from a cervical cancer patient, Henrietta Lacks, from whom the cells were taken. She later succumbed to her disease. These cells have been used for over 60 years to propagate cell lines for use in scientific research, but without ever having received consent from Ms. Lacks.[9] Just within the last few months, *The New York Times* Health division made public the story of a well-respected Harvard researcher who reportedly "fabricated or falsified data in 31 published studies."[10] Our understanding of physicians as healers and of scientists as learned scholars working to advance the common good makes our knowledge of these unethical and immoral practices all the more disturbing. These stories create a strong emotional imprint upon our psyche and hold people's attentions to a significantly greater degree than the more typical stories of people helped by science and medicine and things gone well. If we are going to fight these misconceptions, we have to hold each other to a higher standard, promote transparency, and encourage science and medicine to become more approachable and accessible to the general public.

DISTRUST OF GOVERNMENT AND INDUSTRY

It is probably not difficult for you to think back over history and recall ways in which governments, not only US governments but governments around the world, have mistreated their people (look no further than Nazi Germany). In the United States, much of this mistreatment was set against a backdrop of racial discrimination. In the French and Indian Wars (1754-1763), the British used smallpox-infected blankets to spread disease in an attempt to wipe out the Native American population.[11] More modern history recalls the relocation and internment in concentration camps of citizens of Japanese descent during WWII. The entire history of blacks in America is one of common mistreatment at the hands of government (whether local or national) and its representatives. Still today, a history of severe governmental control in their native country plays a role in the decision to decline vaccinations made by some of our citizens of Russian descent. A recent article in *The Moscow Times* quotes a Russian pediatrician as saying "…doubt in any authority has been building up over many generations in Russians. If our government has been controlling people for many decades, here is one sphere of life where a person can stand in opposition."[12] Even in the United States, today's politicians are sometimes seen, whether fairly or not, as people motivated by benefit to self or party and not by what is best for their constituents. Given this history, we might understand why some people doubt the motivations of government when it mandates things such as vaccination for school entry.

When it comes to distrust of the pharmaceutical industry, we question the motivation of drug companies when we hear, for example, of Mylan's 400% price hike for the EpiPen, making it much harder for the average person to afford this life-saving drug. At the same time, the CEO's salary increased from nearly 2.5 million to almost 19 million dollars (a 671% increase) over the course of 8 years.[13] It is a challenge for everyone, even clinicians, to have confidence in the good intentions of drug companies and insurance companies when prices for essential medications continue to climb. The high cost of insulin, for example, forces as many as 25% of insulin-dependent patients to not take it as they should because they just can't afford to. This self-rationing leads to inadequate control with resulting higher rates of diabetic complications, such as blindness, kidney disease, or even death.[14] The cost in dollars and lives is enormous. Unfortunately, reports such as these cast a negative light, not just on government or big business, but on the medical industry as a whole. It makes all involved, even clinicians, appear to place priority on the dollar and not the patient.

RELIGIOUS CONCERNS REGARDING VACCINATION

Across centuries, the world's religions and their leaders have often been involved with both physical and spiritual healing. Buddhist nuns were some of the first to use variolation to try to protect against smallpox. Maimonides, a Sephardic Jewish philosopher and physician living during the 1100s, stated, "Anyone who is able to save a life, but fails to do so, violates 'You shall not stand idly by the blood of your neighbor,'" a teaching later interpreted by Jewish scholars to encourage smallpox vaccination.[15] Christian teachings promoting charity and caring for others led to the development of organized nursing and hospitals. The Catholic Health Ministry in the United States is the largest group of nonprofit health care providers in the nation today.[16] Moreover, the 14th Dalai Lama, himself, has been directly involved in promoting polio vaccination campaigns for his people.

Unfortunately, though religion and healing have been closely intertwined, religious arguments against vaccination are not uncommon. As vaccination was unknown in the formative days of the world's religions, original religious teachings on the subject do not exist. Therefore, to form religious consensus, doctrine requires interpretation, and sometimes reinterpretation, by modern-day scholars. Arguments against immunization in the context of religious beliefs are numerous and vary by religion. However, there are some general concerns that are common. Among these is the ethical dilemma associated with the use of human cells to produce vaccines, which is an issue for some of our Catholic patients who have strongly held anti-abortion beliefs. Also, the belief that the body is sacred and should not be tainted by chemicals or blood and tissue from animals can raise concerns for

Jews and Muslims, among others, who's teachings state that consuming pork (pork gelatin is used in the production process of making immunizations) is forbidden. Furthermore, some religious groups believe that we should not interfere with God's Divine Providence—that the body should be healed by God, if that is His will.[17] See chapter 10 for discussion of these individual beliefs and the faith teachings that counter these concerns.

In his in-depth exploration of religious teachings and how they apply to vaccinations and immunoglobulins, Grabenstein[15] finds that none of the world's major religions has fundamental doctrinal teachings that oppose vaccination. Only two groups (Christian Scientists and the Dutch Reformed Church) have shown a precedent of widely rejecting vaccinations.[18] Therefore, most "religious" exemptions, he argues, are truly philosophical exemptions in disguise. Moreover, some of what we might attribute to religious apprehensions raised by faith groups may more often be social or cultural concerns, sometimes based on suspicion and mistrust of the motivations behind vaccination programs.

With regard to the post-9/11 mistrust of vaccines by some in the Muslim community, for example, Ali Guda Takai, a World Health Organization doctor investigating polio in Kano, Nigeria, told *The Baltimore Sun*, "What is happening in the Middle East has aggravated the situation. If America is fighting people in the Middle East, the conclusion is that they are fighting Muslims."[19] The local Taliban in Southern Afghanistan have called polio vaccination campaigns an "American ploy to sterilize Muslim populations" and claim that they represent an attempt to avert Allah's will.[20] In Nigeria in 2003, religious leaders in three different Nigerian states urged their followers not to accept polio vaccination, claiming that "the vaccine could be contaminated with antifertility agents (estradiol hormone), HIV, and cancerous agents."[21] The war in the Middle East has eroded trust in the United States and in US-supported public health efforts, and trust is essential in promoting public health interventions, particularly vaccination programs, which target healthy people. However, work between public health experts and religious leaders can often help rebuild that trust. It can resolve objections and lead to a clearer understanding of the aims and safety of immunization efforts, thus allowing us to continue the work of keeping all people healthy.

Religious exemptions are on the rise. As many states are working to limit philosophical exemptions to vaccines to increase vaccination rates in school-age children, more people are claiming religious reasons for not vaccinating. In New Jersey, for example, the number of parents seeking exemption from vaccines on religious grounds rose from 1641 in 2005-2006 to 8977 in 2013-2014.[22] Other states are seeing similar trends. The only states currently not allowing religious exemptions to vaccination are California, Mississippi, and West Virginia. When laws are passed limiting nonmedical exemptions, we see a rise in the uptake of vaccination for school entry (**Figure 2.1**). Until other states can enact such laws, however, the issue with religious exemption persists. It is unlikely that we would have time for an in-depth discussion with each questioning patient regarding the tenets of their specific religion as they relate to vaccines. However it is helpful to have a basic understanding of commonly voiced religious beliefs and how these beliefs affect patients' medical decision-making. If we can acknowledge patients' concerns, pay respect to their religious principles, and then offer resources for further reading or make suggestions for discussion with faith leaders, we may be able to help allay our patients' faith-based worries and move them toward improved vaccine acceptance.

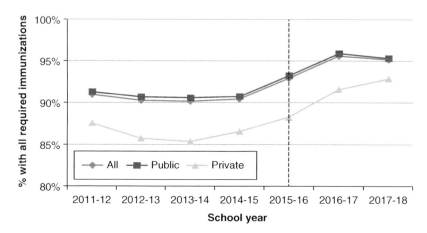

FIGURE 2.1 This graph shows vaccination rates among kindergartners in California from the years 2011-2012 through 2017-2018. Vaccination rates increased when Senate Bill No. 277 (SB277), banning nonmedical exemptions, was passed into law on June 30, 2015 (dashed line), following the Disneyland measles outbreak earlier that year. (Modified from California Department of Public Health. *2017-2018 Kindergarten Summary Report.* https://www.cdph.ca.gov/Programs/CID/DCDC/CDPH%20Document%20Library/Immunization/2017-2018KindergartenSummaryReport.pdf.)

WHY DOES IT SEEM LIKE ANTI-VACCINE SENTIMENT IS SO MUCH MORE COMMON?

The major difference between the anti-vaccine movement of old and that of current times is the existence of the Internet and social media. In the past, word of mouth and the printed word were how opponents of immunizations spread their message. Today, pro-immunization messages are drowned out by a vocal and prolific minority of anti-vaccine activists who utilize Internet search engine optimization tools and social media blitzes to proliferate their message to millions. Try googling any vaccine-related concern and you are likely to come across anti-vaccine propaganda near the top of the list of sources referenced. With strategic posts and tweets, they take advantage of the echo chamber that is social media, targeting people who are trying to get answers to their questions with an overload of unsubstantiated claims and fears. To a vaccine-hesitant person, it may therefore seem like the majority of data to be found cast doubt on immunization safety and effectiveness and may only solidify that person's concerns about vaccines. This attack strategy feeds biases and, with the click of a button, allows misinformation and pseudoscience to spread across the globe in a matter of seconds (See Appendix F: Navigating Information on the Internet and Social Media.).

Take, for example, the video series viewable on YouTube called "The Truth about Vaccines," hosted by Ty Bollinger, ex-bodybuilder and purveyor of cancer-fighting supplements. In the introduction, Bollinger claims that he seeks to offer truths about vaccines that will facilitate discussion, so that people can make informed decisions when it comes to vaccination. The series goes on to parade every vocal anti-vaccine activist (Joseph Mercola, DO; Sherri Tenpenny, DO; Barbara Loe Fisher, Andrew Wakefield, and others) across the screen without giving any time or attention to the opposing, factual point of view. It is a compelling video and appears, on the surface, to be promoting a science-based assessment of the harms of vaccines. However, in digging deeper, which many watching are unlikely to do, the video's assertions are full of holes and are often patently untrue. The popularity of such videos and other social media messaging is frightening. Just the first of Bollinger's seven videos has nearly 637,000 shares on Facebook alone. Whereas a counterpoint to this video titled "The Truth About Vaccines Episode 1: Top Ten lies debunked,"[23] though not listing the number of Facebook shares, has only a mere 393 comments, many of which are from the anti-vaccine point of view.

Not only do we have to be concerned with our home-grown anti-vaccinationists, we now also have to worry about strategic use by other countries of bots and trolls in sowing the seeds of discontent, not only in our elections, but in issues, such as vaccination, that remain divisive in our country. Linkedin.com defines an Internet bot as a "software application that runs automated tasks (scripts) over the Internet… at a much higher rate than would be possible for a human alone." Whereas an Internet troll is defined as "a person who sows discord on the Internet…with the intent of provoking readers into an emotional reaction."[24] A recent article in the *American Journal of Public Health* examined the effect of Twitter bots and Russian trolls in the online vaccine debate. The researchers "compared bots' to average users' rates of vaccine-relevant messages" and used "content analysis of a Twitter hashtag associated with Russian troll activity." The study reviewed data from July 2014 to September 2017[25] and found that bots were 75% more likely to share anti-vaccination messages than average Twitter users. It also revealed that trolls used more polarizing language (both pro- and anti-vaccine) "linking vaccination to controversial issues in American society, such as racial and economic disparities…using vaccination as a wedge issue"[26] and promoting conflict and division. For the unsuspecting Twitter user, the result is greater ideological divide and a false sense that there is increasing public concern and debate over the safety of vaccines.

The news media has also contributed, perhaps unwittingly, to the spread of unnecessary alarm regarding vaccines. In upholding the First Amendment and giving equal voice to all, television and news media outlets have served as a bullhorn for politicians, actors, actresses, and others well-known in popular culture to call into question the safety of vaccines. Scientists and physicians, themselves largely unknown, are at a significant disadvantage when trying to counter the claims of those whose fame draws a large audience. The mere fact that national news outlets choose to address anti-vaccine claims reinforces them and lends unwarranted credibility (see chapter 3, Psychology of the Anti-vaccine Movement.) How does the news media balance a responsibility to avoid spreading misinformation with a need to uphold freedom of speech? There is unlikely to be a simple answer to that question. However, perhaps we should be telling the story of the success of vaccines and not merely jumping on headlines when controversy arises (See chapter 13 for further discussion of the impact of media on the vaccine discussion).

Although the same issues raised and strategies employed by the anti-vaccine movement over 200 years ago are still in use today, the introduction of television news media and Internet technology has been a game changer for the ease with which misinformation can be disseminated. The anti-vaccine movement is more organized, well-funded, and they put out a slick and convincing product. If we are going to successfully fight the pseudoscience and fearmongering being spread by anti-vaccine proponents, the scientific and medical communities have to get more vocal about countering anti-vaccine claims and more proactive in our utilization of the news media and social media platforms to educate the public on a broader scale.

References

1. Iannelli V. History of the Anti-Vaccine Movement. Verywell Family. Updated October 14, 2018. Accessed December 17, 2018. https://www.verywellfamily.com/history-anti-vaccine-movement-4054321.

2. National Institute of Allergy and Infectious Diseases. Vaccines of the Future. Accessed February 7, 2019. https://www.niaid.nih.gov/research/vaccines-future.

3. Centers for Disease Control and Prevention. Thimerosal in Vaccines. Accessed December 17, 2018. https://www.cdc.gov/vaccinesafety/concerns/thimerosal/index.html.

4. The College of Physicians of Philadelphia. History of Anti-Vaccination Movements. The History of Vaccines. Updated January 10, 2018. Accessed December 17, 2018. https://www.historyofvaccines.org/content/articles/history-Anti-Vaccination-movements.

5. Gostin L. Jacobson v Massachusetts at 100 years: police power and civil liberties in tension. *Am J Public Health*. 2005;95(4):576-581.

6. *Jacobson V. Massachusetts, 197 U.S. 11*; 1905.

7. Browne C. Thomas Paine's theory of atmospheric contagion and his account of an experiment performed by George Washington upon the production of marsh gas. *J Chem Educ*. 1925;2(2):99.

8. Porter D, Porter R. The politics of prevention: anti-vaccinationism and public health in nineteenth-century England. *Med Hist*. 1988;32:231-252.

9. *HeLa cell*. In: *Encyclopædia Brittanica*. July 20, 1998. Accessed December 20, 2018. https://www.britannica.com/science/HeLa-cell.

10. Kolata G. *Harvard Calls for Retraction of Dozens of Studies by Noted Cardiac Researcher*. New York Times; October 15, 2018. Accessed January 15. 2019. https://www.nytimes.com/2018/10/15/health/piero-anversa-fraud-retractions.html.

11. Flight C. Silent Weapon: Smallpox and Biological Warfare. BBC. Updated February 17, 2011. Accessed December 17, 2018. www.bbc.co.uk/history/worldwars/coldwar/pox_weapon_01.shtml.

12. Gershkovich K. *Russia Has A Vaccination Problem*. Moscow Times; September 28, 2018. Accessed December 17, 2018. https://themoscowtimes.com/articles/russia-has-a-vaccine-problem-63017.

13. Popken B. *Mylan CEO's Pay Rose Over 600 Percent as EpiPen Price Rose 400 Percent*. NBC News; August 23, 2016. Accessed December 17, 2018. https://www.nbcnews.com/news/amp/ncna636591.

14. Campbell K. *Insulin Costs Are Skyrocketing. This Is Why*. U.S. News & World Reports; June 29, 2018. Accessed December 17, 2018. https://health.usnews.com/health-care/for-better/articles/2018-06-29/whats-behind-the-rising-costs-of-insulin.

15. Grabenstein J. What the world's religions teach, applied to vaccines and immune globulins. *Vaccine*. 2013;31(16):2011-2023.

16. Catholic Health Association of the United States. Facts -- Statistics: Catholic Health Care in the United States. Updated January 2018. Accessed December 17, 2018. https://www.chausa.org/about/about/facts-statistics.

17. The College of Physicians in Philadelphia. Cultural Perspectives on Vaccination. The History of Vaccines. Updated January 10, 2018. Accessed December 17, 2018. https://www.historyofvaccines.org/content/articles/cultural-perspectives-vaccination.

18. Blumberg A. *Here's Where Major Religions Actually Stand on Vaccines*. Life (HuffPost); March 31, 2017. Accessed December 17, 2018. https://www.huffpost.com/entry/heres-where-major-religions-actually-stand-on-vaccines_n_58dc3ef0e4b08194e3b71fc4/amp.

19. Murphy J. *Distrust of U.S. Foils Effort to Stop Crippling Disease*. Baltimore Sun; January 4, 2004. Accessed December 17, 2018. https://www.baltimoresun.com/news/bal-polio0104-story.html.

20. Warraich H. Religious opposition to polio vaccination. Centers for disease control and prevention. *Emerg Infect Dis*. 2009;15(6):978.

21. Jegede A. What led to the Nigerian boycott of the polio vaccination campaign? *PLoS Med*. 2007;4(3):e73.

22. Livio SK. *Nearly 9,000 N.J. School Children Skipped Vaccinations on Religious Grounds Last Year*. NJ.com; 2014. Updated August 25, 2015. Accessed December 17, 2018. https://www.nj.com/healthfit/index.ssf/2014/11/9000_nj_school_children_skipped_vaccinations_on_religious_grounds.html.

23. Bollinger T. *The Truth About Vaccines Episode 1: Top 10 Lies Debunked*; April 18, 2017. Accessed December 17, 2018. https://vaccinesworkblog.wordpress.com/tag/ty-bollinger/.

24. Potts J. *What Is the Difference Between a Troll and an Internet Bot*. LinkedIn; April 11, 2017. Accessed December 17, 2018. https://www.linkedin.com/pulse/what-difference-between-troll-internet-bot-jarrett-potts.

25. Broniatowski D, Jamison A, Qi S, et al. Weaponized health communication: twitter bots and Russian trolls amplify the vaccine debate. *Am J Public Health.* 2018;108(10):1378-1384.

26. George Washington University. *Bots and Russian Trolls Influenced Vaccine Discussion on Twitter, Research Finds: New Study Discovers Tactics Similar to Those Used During 2016 US Election.* Science Daily; August 23, 2018. Accessed December 17, 2018. https://www.sciencedaily.com/releases/2018/08/180823171035.htm.

3

Psychology of the Anti-vaccine Movement

The most common of all follies is to believe passionately in the palpably not true. It is the chief occupation of mankind.

—H. L. Mencken

Although it is disconcerting to believe, studies show that there is no reproducibly effective approach to the vaccine discussion with anti-vaccine patients, at least not that we've found so far. Particularly, attempts at education and correction of misinformation about vaccines rarely cause people opposed to immunization to change their minds and can actually cause their doubts to become more entrenched.[1-3] As tempting as it is to do, it turns out that throwing numbers and percentages at people may not be the most useful approach. This is not to suggest that education about vaccines isn't important, however. It is vital for medical providers to be able to easily discuss the facts, data, and science behind vaccines. Anti-vaccine people have often done hours of "research" to support their concerns, and, if we don't have the knowledge to speak to those concerns, we will lose their confidence and only fuel their belief that they are more educated on the subject of vaccines than we are (see chapters 9, 10, and 11 for detailed discussions about anti-vaccine concerns and their data-driven counterarguments). Likewise, if we don't acknowledge the very rare, but real, potential adverse effects of vaccines, we will lose patients' trust, and they may be less inclined to believe that we have their best interest, or that of their children, at heart.

The statistics about vaccines and vaccine-preventable disease are impressive to us as scientists and medical professionals, but some of our patients will more naturally gravitate to the "lies, damned lies, and statistics" view of such data. Science hasn't always given us correct information (for example, the now-corrected assertion that all fats are bad for you), and patients may not fully trust that these data or numbers should be believed or that they are applicable to their family's lives. As medical providers, we are often working against an inherent mistrust of the medical system as well as invisible enemies (family, friends, Facebook groups, Twitter campaigns) who play on the fears of our patients, particularly the fears of parents. So, what can we do to change people's views?

When we think about the anti-vaccine movement, a certain picture comes to mind. It conjures up images of hostile people shouting at their public representatives, individuals wielding signs at rallies that accuse doctors of being in bed with Big Pharma, and making claims that vaccines cause everything from seizures to multiple sclerosis to cancers and worse. We may recall uncomfortable encounters we have had with patients who absolutely refuse to hear our recommendations about vaccines and our explanations of safety and effectiveness. We may feel insulted and frustrated by people who seemingly don't trust our years of education and self-sacrifice to help and to heal. For a small minority of people, these images may be correct. However they are by no means representative of what all anti-vaccine people are like. We have a tendency to think of people who refuse vaccines as a homogenous group, but it turns out, as with everything else in life, there is a spectrum.

I would argue that we have found no one effective approach to the vaccine discussion with our anti-vaccine patients, because there is no one type of vaccine-resistant person. They are not a single-minded group. They are a group with varying concerns and motivations. Understanding those motivations and understanding the different belief systems at play in the anti-vaccine movement are vital to helping scientists and medical providers bridge the divide between reason and emotion that is so central to their line of thinking.

This chapter will look at the fascinating work that is currently underway examining the psychology of the anti-vaccine movement, trying to better understand what drives it. We will look at studies that try to find commonalities in belief, for example, by evaluating the socioeconomic breakdown of the anti-vaccine community and looking for patterns in the political leanings of the group's members. We will look at the field of social psychology, exploring cognitive bias and errors in logic and how they allow us to perpetuate and support beliefs that fit our preexisting views on a subject.[4] This very important research is, I believe, where we will find our most helpful guidance in tailoring our message. Then perhaps, going forward, our investigations into strategies for dealing with anti-vaccine sentiment will take the varying subgroups of belief into account. As we are learning, a one-size-fits-all approach to the vaccine discussion is not working.

ANTI-VACCINE VERSUS VACCINE-HESITANT

First, it is important to recognize the difference between a truly *anti-vaccine* patient and the merely *vaccine-hesitant* patient. The anti-vaccine patient is part of a vocal minority, those angry individuals that we initially envision, who organize and lobby and bring literature to their appointments to try to educate *us* about vaccines. These folks are so entrenched in their way of thinking that we are hardly going to be able to hold a civil conversation, let alone change their minds about vaccines. They are operating from a place, not of reason, but of emotion and paranoia. Attempting to convince them of a more reasoned way of thinking is only going to increase anger and frustration on both sides.

Not engaging in debate with anti-vaccine patients is easier said than done, particularly when it comes to the ill-informed decisions they make on behalf of their children, who are the innocent bystanders in the vaccine discussion. I'm not suggesting that we should discontinue offering vaccines to people who adamantly refuse. On the contrary, we should *continue* to offer vaccines to anti-vaccine patients even though they may have declined in the past, to show that we care about their health and well-being. There is always hope that something will change their minds. Moreover, with continued emphasis on the importance of immunization, particularly during well-child visits, we may provide further education to their children who will hopefully grow up knowing the value of vaccines and will eventually make their own more-reasoned, pro-vaccine decisions as adults.

The people on whom we should focus more attention are those that would be better classified as vaccine-hesitant or vaccine-questioning. These people are not conspiracy theorists. They don't think all doctors are shills. They generally trust our expertise and motivations. Some may have merely seen too many scary anti-vaccine claims come across their Facebook or Twitter feeds. Others may have been a part of parent groups where doing everything "naturally" to avoid "toxins" is promoted. Still others are afraid of frightening diagnoses, such as cancers and autoimmune diseases, that the anti-vaccine movement claims vaccines cause. Moreover, many merely need additional information to fill in gaps in their understanding of vaccines that will allow them to feel more confident in their decisions. These are patients who have had grains of doubt and fear introduced into their minds, but they are generally eager to find reassurance and confidence in the counsel of their trusted medical provider. Working with our vaccine-hesitant patients is where we will find our greatest successes.

THE SOCIOECONOMIC AND POLITICAL BREAKDOWN

So, who are these vaccine-hesitant individuals? Studies looking at this question have found that people who use philosophical exemptions from vaccination are more likely to be white, college educated, married, and with a higher family income. Unvaccinated nonwhites from lower-income groups are more likely to be so due to limited access to health care services or limited financial resources.[5] Unfortunately, it is also this population who would potentially see the greatest adverse impact should they or their child suffer from a vaccine-preventable disease. With a lack of job flexibility and security and the financial resources to support days to weeks off of work, potentially dealing with complications of illness that may require expensive medical visits, treatments, or hospitalizations, lower-income individuals and families have the most to lose. Reminders, flu clinics, and community outreach for vaccines, approaches that will decrease the cost and increase the convenience of getting immunized, may prove more effective in reaching our unvaccinated or under-vaccinated lower-income patients. Whereas, addressing vaccines with our middle- to upper-middle-class vaccine-hesitant patient population may require a more intensive and individualized focus.

These days, in the battle to lay blame at the feet of one group or another, it is also tempting to look for political affiliations that may be common to the nonvaccinating or vaccine-hesitant community. It turns out, however, that general anti-vaccine sentiment is not purely a conservative or liberal issue. It is more an issue of people with very strongly held beliefs, on both sides of the political spectrum. Charles McCoy, Assistant Professor of Sociology, SUNY Plattsburgh, has studied the political leanings of parents who refuse vaccination for their children, trying to understand any common motivations or concerns. Prior research on the topic of political affiliation and views on vaccination has been conflicting. However, McCoy's evaluation of recent surveys by the PEW Research Center shows that the more staunchly conservative or staunchly liberal someone is, the more likely they are to believe that vaccines are unsafe. In looking at the political divide regarding vaccination mandates, however, it *is* more often the conservatives who feel that vaccination should be primarily under the purview of parents and not mandated by the government. McCoy's research found that, as a group, conservatives are "twice as likely as moderates to think that [vaccination] should be a parent's choice" compared with liberals who "are 43.5% less likely" than moderates to think it should be a parent's choice.[6] Though we don't often delve into the political views of our patients unless they are voluntarily offered up, McCoy's research does give us interesting food for thought, regarding how we may approach the vaccine discussion differently, depending on the leanings of our patients. For example, it may be a greater motivator to conservatives to hear about how not achieving herd immunity can limit the freedoms of those children and adults who would desire to participate in their community without being at risk for serious illness and disease.

FALLACY AND THE ANTI-VACCINE MINDSET

Understanding the ways that errors in logic can impact our decision-making is important as we try to develop approaches to vaccine-hesitant patients that will bring them to a greater level of confidence in vaccines. As human beings, we have an innate tendency to want to draw connections between events in our lives. These connections satisfy an emotional need for reason and purpose. They also represent an adaptive measure that helps us learn from our mistakes and protects us from making them again in the future. For example, if I grab the hot handle of a pot on the stove and burn my hand, then I will think twice before reaching to pick up something hot again in the future. This logical association is protective. However, some of our associations represent faults in logic that have the potential, as in the case of erroneous thinking about vaccines, to put us at risk. These errors in logic are called fallacies and we often see them at work in arguments used by the anti-vaccine community **(Box 3.1)**. For the purposes of this book, we will examine a few of the most common.

A prime example is the fallacy in thinking that allows people to continue to draw a connection between the measles, mumps, and rubella (MMR) vaccination and autism, despite a large body of work showing no causal relationship. In this instance, we know that autism begins to show more overt signs and symptoms around the same age that the MMR vaccine series is administered (age 12 months to 4-6 years). Drawing the false conclusion that there is a causal relationship between the two because one event is followed by the other in time is a classic example of the *Post Hoc, Ergo Propter Hoc Fallacy* (Latin for "after this, therefore because of this").[7] We are, by nature, uncomfortable not knowing the reason behind events in our lives, particularly highly impactful events, such as when one of our children develops autism. "We can't tell you why your child developed autism" doesn't sit well with parents. We feel more settled with an erroneous explanation than with no explanation at all.

Some of the fallacies that are employed by the anti-vaccine movement could actually be used to our advantage. For example, the *Appeal to Authority Fallacy* happens when a statement is thought to be true just because someone in authority said it was true. We've seen this in the case of celebrities and politicians, such as Jenny McCarthy and Robert F. Kennedy, Jr, who claim, for example, that vaccinations cause autism or that the aluminum adjuvant in vaccines causes autoimmune disease.[7] Perhaps, if we can

 Box 3.1 Anti-vaccine Fallacies

For more reading on the multitude of fallacies employed by those opposed to vaccines, check out this article by the Vaccine Education Center at the Children's Hospital of Philadelphia:

- Children's Hospital of Philadelphia: Logical Fallacies and Vaccines—https://media.chop.edu/data/files/pdfs/vaccine-education-center-logical-fallacies.pdf

engage equally well-known individuals to speak publicly in support of vaccines and the science behind their safety and efficacy, we can gather more questioning people to the pro-vaccine side.

The *Appeal to Pity Fallacy* uses emotion to draw someone into a way of thinking to evade the discussion of facts.[7] We see this used by the anti-vaccine movement all the time—the heartbreaking stories of parents whose children suffered some significant adverse event (they believe) following vaccination. It is difficult not to feel empathy for these parents. Our hearts go out to them. We wouldn't begrudge them their suffering, and it is difficult for data to counter the pull of heartfelt emotional testimony. However, the emotions of sorrow and pity that we feel for someone whose child is struggling with a difficult condition have nothing to do with whether vaccines are safe. In an effort to appeal to the emotions of those who may be on the fence about vaccines, we too can use this approach. The impact of personal stories can be used to our advantage if we are able to offer testimony of how vaccine-preventable disease has impacted our patients or our loved ones.[8] Highlighting the plight of the family whose child developed seizures and loss of limb after meningococcal meningitis or of the wife whose husband, father to their young children, died from a flu-induced heart attack can make a strong emotional impact and can help reinforce the importance of personal and community vaccination.

The *Bandwagon Fallacy* is another common error in logic. It leads people to think that something is true just because it is a widely held belief.[7] We have all talked to those patients whose argument is: "If so many people have concerns about vaccines, there must be a real reason that we should be concerned." To start with, our impression of "so many people" is likely skewed. Just because we see it on Facebook, Twitter, and other media outlets does not mean that a large percentage of the population feels that way. As we've stated previously, the most vocal of the anti-vaccine group are, in fact, a small minority, so perhaps we can use this bandwagon fallacy to our advantage. After all, many out there will follow the crowd because of an assumption that the crowd knows more than they do, and if they believe that most people are following a particular action, then it must be the right thing to do. In this case, when the "action" is immunizing, it's true; it *is* the right thing to do. So, perhaps we should be sharing the fact that, despite all the anti-vaccine hubbub, the large majority of parents *do* vaccinate. In the United States during the 2016-2017 school year, for example, the kindergarten vaccination coverage for MMR; diphtheria, tetanus, and pertussis; and varicella approached 95% (though vaccination rates vary by state and by county).[9] Like the majority of US patients and parents, they also can choose to vaccinate, which is one of the best things they can do for their own personal health and for the health of the community (**Box 3.2**).

 Box 3.2   Did You Know?

The World Health Organization estimates that immunizations prevent approximately 2 to 3 million deaths each year worldwide. An estimated 1.5 million additional deaths could be prevented if vaccine coverage improved globally.[10] Economic analysis of 10 vaccines used in 94 low- to middle-income countries estimates that a $34 billion dollar investment in vaccination programs would produce a savings of $586 billion in costs of illness and $1.53 trillion in broader societal costs. Not only is vaccination best for preventing disease and keeping individuals healthy, it also helps to decrease the overall cost of health care.[11]

THE ROLE OF BIAS IN ANTI-VACCINE THINKING

Bias is defined in the *English Oxford Living Dictionaries* as prejudice "for or against one person or group, especially in a way considered to be unfair."[12] In science, it is extremely important to be aware of bias as it has the potential to impact and skew the outcomes (usually unintentionally) of our research. It also impacts how we take in and receive new information. As scientists, we need to be cognizant of our biases, but it is equally important for the lay person, in attempting to do research or reading about vaccination, to be aware of their own innate biases. One of the most prevalent forms of bias at play in anti-vaccine thinking is *Confirmation Bias*. Confirmation bias refers to the fact that we tend to gravitate toward information that supports our preexisting point of view.[13] Ego has a difficult time accepting information and ideas that run counter to its deeply held beliefs. It takes insight and tremendous strength of character to do so, as is evidenced by the individuals highlighted in our upcoming chapter interviewing former anti-vaccine people who now support vaccination. If we are truly going to be open to new information, we have to work hard to put confirmation bias aside and be objective in our investigation into a new or alternate idea.

Brendan Nyhan of Dartmouth and Jason Reifler of the University of Exeter have studied bias as it relates to everything from media and advertising to unsupported political beliefs to health-related issues, such as misinformation regarding vaccines. They discovered that, when attempting to correct misinformation by presenting data contrary to a person's preexisting points of view, many people dug in their heels and held on even tighter to their original beliefs.[14] This *Motivated Reasoning* is a type of confirmation bias taken to the extreme. It "drives people to develop elaborate rationalizations to justify holding beliefs that logic and evidence have shown to be wrong."[15] Chris Mooney, writing for *Mother Jones*, explains how this motivated reasoning might occur. The theory of motivated reasoning, he states, builds on the insight that "reasoning is actually suffused with emotion…. Not only are the two inseparable, but our positive or negative feelings about people, things, and ideas arise much more rapidly than our conscious thoughts, in a matter of milliseconds." Mooney attributes this type of reasoning to human evolution, which "required us to react very quickly to stimuli in our environment… We push threatening information away; we pull friendly information close. We apply fight-or-flight reflexes not only to predators, but to data itself."[16]

But how is it that people can believe even more firmly in an erroneous view after they have been given information that contradicts or debunks that view? Nyhan and Reifler found that repeating information, even to debunk it, often backfires. They call this, appropriately, the "backfire effect." One reason, they postulate, is that with greater repetition of a false concept comes an increased believability.[17] Additionally, discussing false information with someone who didn't originally have that particular concern can introduce a new doubt. Therefore, in our approach to the vaccine debate, we should work hard not to repeat erroneous facts in our discussions. I believe this to be particularly true when engaging in social media information campaigns, where large numbers of people have the potential to see our comments. Our focus should be on highlighting truths, not contradicting falsehoods. In doing so, we will also decrease the chances that our efforts accidently introduce a new doubt to someone who had not previously heard the concern.

Nyhan and Reifler then took their work a step further. They looked at various approaches to providing corrective information to see what might work best. More work specifically in the vaccine realm needs to be done, but, if we may apply their findings from studies of political misperceptions to those of vaccine misperceptions, we might find that similar approaches will work for our vaccine-hesitant patients. In their 2017 paper, "The Roles of Information Deficits and Identity Threat in the Prevalence of Misperceptions," they looked at two different approaches of interest. First, they evaluated an approach using self-affirmation, the theory that "rejection of uncomfortable facts is a form of defensive processing that protects one's self-identity" and that "when one's self-integrity is affirmed in some other domain, people may be less likely to respond defensively."[14] Next, they theorized that the prevalence of misperception might relate to the fact that people may not have encountered accurate information about a topic or that information is presented in a format that allows for easy counter argument. They specifically looked at how information presented in graphical form may be more effective at countering misinformation than information presented in equivalent text format. Interestingly, their findings regarding self-affirmation showed no statistical improvement in the ability to bring about point-of-view change. This contradicts the findings of other social psychology studies, they note. However their results regarding use of graphical data as compared with those of textual relaying of information do show a significant reduction in misperceptions.[14] (See Appendix D: Evaluating Graphical Data.)

In our approach to the vaccine-hesitant patient, I see no downside in approaching the conversation first with an affirmation that parents and patients seeking to educate themselves about their health and the health of their family is a wonderful thing. We applaud them for being proactive and informed. We should affirm our understanding that they are loving parents who are working hard to do what is best for themselves and for their child (this all fits nicely into the models of motivational interviewing described in chapter 6). It may also be helpful to then demonstrate information regarding vaccine effectiveness and safety in a graphical representation (For example, **Figure 3.1**). It is easy to get into a sparring match regarding vaccines, particularly on social media, where both parties are bashing the other's intelligence or motivations. It is much more difficult to argue with a graph. Moreover, graphical information provides the person the time and opportunity to read and interpret what is being presented, instead of reacting instinctively and emotionally to the spoken or written word.

Another bias that runs rampant in the vaccine-hesitant community is the *Omission Bias*. Omission bias has to do with the difference between bringing about an outcome by acting (commission) versus failing to act (omission). Omission bias leads to the "tendency to prefer inactive to active options even when inaction leads to worse outcomes or greater risks."[18] For certain patients, the low risks associated with vaccination seem more real and frightening than the much higher risk of contracting a vaccine-preventable illness and the potential complications that arise as a consequence of that illness. People tend to believe that they will feel a greater sense of responsibility and guilt about a negative outcome from vaccinating than they would about the negative outcomes that arise from the decision not to vaccinate. This is called the fear of *Anticipated Regret*.[18,19]

When patients rarely, if ever, experience vaccine-preventable disease affecting their personal lives, it is easy to see how they could interpret the potential small risk of adverse reactions to vaccines as greater than the real risk of the illness itself. When it comes to vaccines, and feeling conflicted or confused about the information that is out there, it is easy for the nonmedical person to become overwhelmed and default to a sense that inaction is safer than action. However, if we can turn the tables on omission bias, we may be able to use it to our advantage, making not vaccinating the omission. Using the bandwagon fallacy, if we can get patients to see vaccination as the norm (which it is), then choosing not to vaccinate or seeking exemptions from vaccination becomes the "act" and deferring to community standards becomes the "omission." Perhaps using

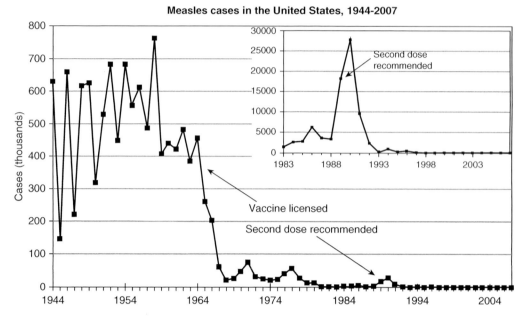

FIGURE 3.1 Graph showing reduction of measles cases after introduction of first measles vaccine in 1963 by John Enders and colleagues and then further reduction when improved measles vaccine was introduced by Maurice Hilleman and colleagues in 1968. In 1989, two doses of MMR were recommended, and since 2000, measles has been declared no longer endemic in the United States. (Courtesy of 2over0. From Wikipedia. https://en.wikipedia.org/wiki/File:Measles_US_1944-2007_inset.png. Data from the US Centers for Disease Control.)

ourselves as an example, we can then discuss the fear of anticipated regret to highlight how the parent might feel if they committed the act of refusing vaccines and their child suffered significant consequences of an illness they could have likely prevented through vaccination. For example, "Gosh, I can't imagine how I would feel if my child became severely ill and there was something I could have done about it but chose not to. I don't ever want to experience that guilt and I would hate for any of my patients or families to experience it either."

Another exciting area of research, using *Inoculation Theory* to address faulty or resistant health attitudes, is gaining interest in the vaccine community. This theory, proposed in 1961 by a social psychologist named William McGuire, suggests that "attitudes could be inoculated against persuasive attacks in much the same way that one's immune system can be inoculated against viral attacks." By exposing people to a "persuasive message that contains weakened arguments against an established attitude (eg, a two-sided message, or a message that presents both counterarguments and refutations of those counterarguments), individuals would develop resistance against stronger, future persuasive attacks."[20] Even though there are limited studies to date testing this type of persuasion, the theory offers promise. A study by Wong and Harrison published in the *Journal of Women's Health, Issues and Care* in 2014 examined the use of two different inoculation strategies to confer resistance to anti-vaccination messages about the HPV vaccine and the practice of childhood vaccination. They found that "inoculation messages about HPV vaccination promoted resistance to messages attacking the perceived safety and efficacy toward the HPV vaccine [and that] inoculation messages about vaccination in general promoted resistance to messages attacking the perceived safety of HPV vaccines, but not efficacy. Inoculation also promoted childhood vaccinations, measured by attitudes and behavioral intentions."[21]

What if, during family planning visits, we offered our patients early exposure to scientific data on vaccine safety and efficacy and then gave clear information about the techniques that the anti-vaccine movement uses to promote science denial and misinformation, thus inoculating them and providing immunity to future anti-vaccine arguments? As Marianna Baggio and Matteo Motterlini from the Università Vita-Salute San Raffaele suggest in their article titled "Could We Use 'Cognitive Vaccination' against 'Anti-Vaxx'?," this use of inoculation theory gently teaches "techniques to de-bias oneself in all science-related areas of public policy interest…and spreads across social networks, protecting also others and working just like herd immunity."[22]

There are a multitude of social and psychological factors that go into allowing people to believe, despite copious evidence to the contrary, that vaccines are unsafe or ineffective. Discovering those factors, trying to understand them, and learning ways to work with them, allowing us to use the logical fallacies employed by the anti-vaccine movement to our advantage, is no easy task. There is much work to be done. However, what we can say for certain is that blanket approaches to the vaccine discussion don't work and that we have to tailor our efforts to the individual patient or to the individual belief system. To do this, we must take the time to dig into the reasons behind patients' particular concerns. We must establish trust and listen without judgment. If we do so, we will have greater chances of success in convincing patients of the personal and community benefits of vaccination,[23] and we will hopefully make inroads into regaining the confidence of our patients and of a society who seems to have lost faith in our good will and altruistic motivations.

References

1. Briss P, Shefer A, Rodewald L. Improving vaccine coverage in communities and healthcare systems. No magic bullets. *Am J Prev Med.* 2002;23:70-71.
2. Nyhan B, Reifler J, Riches S, et al. Effective messages in vaccine promotion: a randomized trial. *Pediatrics.* 2014;133(4):e835-e842.
3. Hornsey MJ, Harris EA, Fielding KS. The psychological roots of anti-vaccination attitudes: a 24-nation investigation. *Health Psychol.* 2018;37(4):307-315.
4. Politi MC, Jones KM, Philpott SE. The role of patient engagement in addressing parents' perceptions about immunizations. *J Am Med Assoc.* 2017;318(3):237-238.
5. Smith PJ, Humiston SG, Marcuse EK, et al. Parental delay or refusal of vaccine doses. Childhood vaccination coverage at 24 months of age, and the health belief model. *Public Health Rep.* 2011;126(suppl 2):135-146.
6. McCoy C. *Anti-Vaccination Beliefs Don't Follow the Usual Political Polarization.* The Conversation; August 23, 2017. Accessed December 30, 2018. https://theconversation.com/anti-vaccination-beliefs-dont-follow-the-usual-political-polarization-81001.
7. *Logical Fallacies and Vaccines.* Vol 2. Children's Hospital of Philadelphia Vaccine Education Center; 2018.
8. Kempe A, Daley MF, McCauley MM, et al. Prevalence of parental concerns about childhood vaccines: the experience of primary care physicians. *Am J Prev Med.* 2011;40(5):548-555.
9. Seither R, Calhoun K, Street EJ, et al. Vaccination coverage for selected vaccines, exemption rates, and provisional enrollment among children in kindergarten — United States, 2016–17 school year. *MMWR.* 2017;66(40):1073-1080.
10. World Health Organization. 10 facts on Immunization. Updated March 2018. Accessed February 7, 2019. https://www.who.int/features/factfiles/immunization/en/.
11. Ozawa S, Clark S, Portnoy A, et al. Return on investment from childhood immunization in low- and middle-income countries, 2011-20. *Health Aff.* 2016;35(2):199-207.

12. Bias. In: English Oxford Living Dictionaries. Accessed January 4, 2019. https://en.oxforddictionaries.com/definition/bias.

13. Heshmat S. *What Is Confirmation Bias? Wishful Thinking.* Psychology Today; April 23, 2015. Accessed December 30, 2018. https://www.psychologytoday.com/us/blog/science-choice/201504/what-is-confirmation-bias.

14. Nyhan B, Reifler J. The roles of information deficits and identity threat in the prevalence of misperceptions. *J Elections, Public Opin Parties.* 2019;29:222-244. Accessed January 2, 2019. doi:10.1080/17457289.2018.1465061.

15. Motivated Reasoning. The Skeptic's Dictionary. Updated October 27, 2015. Accessed December 30, 2018. www.skepdic.com/motivatedreasoning.html.

16. Mooney C. *The Science of Why We Don't Believe Science: How Our Brains Fool Us on the Climate, Creationism, and the Vaccine-Autism Link.* Mother Jones; May/June, 2011.

17. Nyhan B, Reifler J. When corrections fail: the persistence of political misperceptions. *Polit Behav.* 2010;32(2):303-330.

18. Connolly T, Reb J. Omission bias in vaccination decisions: where's the "omission"? Where's the "bias"?. *Organ Behav Hum Decis Process.* 2003;91(2):186-202.

19. Lombrozo T. Psychological biases play a part in vaccination decisions. *Cosmos Cult NPR.* February 9, 2015. Accessed December 30, 2018. https://www.npr.org/sections/13.7/2015/02/09/384877284/psychological-biases-play-a-part-in-vaccination-decisions.

20. Compton J, Jackson B, Dimmock JA. Persuading others to avoid persuasion: inoculation theory and resistant health attitudes. *Front Psychol.* 2016;7:122.

21. Wong N, Harrison K. Nuances in inoculation: protecting positive attitudes toward the HPV vaccine and the practice of vaccinating children. *J Women's Health Issues Care.* 2014;3(6).

22. Baggio M, Motterlini M. *Could We Use "Cognitive Vaccination" Against "Anti-Vaxx"?* BPP Blog. October 16, 2017. Accessed December 30, 2018. https://bppblog.com/2017/10/16/could-we-use-cognitive-vaccination-against-anti-vaxx/.

23. Politi M. The Best Shot at Overcoming Vaccination Standoffs? Having Doctors Listen to – Not Shun – Reluctant Parents. The Conversation. Updated July 7, 2018. Accessed December 30, 2018. https://theconversation.com/the-best-shot-at-overcoming-vaccination-standoffs-having-doctors-listen-to-not-shun-reluctant-parents-81592.

There and Back Again: How Anti-vaxxers Change Their Minds

A man should never be ashamed to own he has been in the wrong, which is but saying, in other words, that he is wiser today than he was yesterday.

—ALEXANDER POPE

One of the challenges faced by medical providers in dealing with vaccine-hesitant patients is that many of us have lost hope. Perhaps we have tried to educate and to encourage and have been unsuccessful so many times that we no longer have confidence that we can make a difference. Or perhaps we have had such a negative or angry encounter with a patient or parent who is anti-vaccine that it has colored our view of these patients as unreasonable conspiracy theorists who will never change their minds. It is true that there are staunch anti-vaccine patients out there whose heels are dug in and are unlikely to be open to considering the other side. However, these are the minority of patients, and, as we will discover, these folks are likely to seek out providers who support their anti-vaccine sentiment and are unlikely to be coming to us anyway.

Most patients we work with fall into the vaccine-hesitant camp. They are people who were probably vaccinated themselves as children. They may understand the public health benefit that we have seen from vaccination efforts over the years. They want to do what is best for their personal health or for their child's health, but various claims that they have heard from friends, family, and social media about toxins in vaccines and increasing rates of autoimmune disease and better immunity from natural infection give them reason for doubt. These are the patients with whom we have the greatest ability to reach. These patients are eager for dialogue. They have faith in their providers but need to have their concerns addressed (in a respectful way) in order to move forward with vaccination. They don't doubt our motivations as a medical community. They are simply trying to make sure that their decisions are in the best interests of themselves or their child.

For those of us who have lost confidence that our efforts will pay off, this chapter should offer some glimmer of hope. In the pages to follow, we will talk to people who were initially in the anti-vaccine or vaccine-hesitant camp but who, for a variety of reasons, have changed their minds about vaccines and now speak up for the importance of immunization. We will look at how their initial anti-vaccine sentiment developed, the tactics and approaches used by the anti-vaccine community that fed their concerns, how a healthy relationship with the medical and scientific communities helped in their ideological shift, and recommendations they offer for providers who are working with vaccine-hesitant patients and families.

35

A special thanks goes out to Voices for Vaccines, a "parent-driven organization supported by scientists, doctors, and public health officials that provides parents clear, science-based information about vaccines and vaccine-preventable disease, as well as an opportunity to join the national discussion about the importance of on-time vaccination,[1]" for introducing me to the brave and insightful individuals who we will meet below. It takes a tremendous amount of courage to challenge your own beliefs, and I am eternally grateful to KO, LC, and CA for sharing their stories with us and offering us a light at the end of the vaccine-hesitant tunnel.

TELL ME ABOUT YOUR UPBRINGING IN REGARD TO VACCINES. WHAT DID YOUR PARENTS DO ABOUT VACCINES?

KO: I have two younger sisters. We were fully vaccinated according to the recommended schedule at the time. My mom has said that my middle sister screamed and cried inconsolably on the way home from the doctor after receiving vaccinations and came down with a fever. My mom wasn't vocally anti-vaccine while I was growing up, but she was always skeptical of modern medical practice. Both my younger sisters were born at home because my mom hated having me in the hospital in 1976. She felt like she wasn't in control of her body or her experience. Her legs were strapped into stirrups. She had an episiotomy and was not allowed to hold me after I was born because she had a slight fever in the hours after delivery. My mom joined La Leche League after my middle sister was born and I went to the meetings with her, surrounded by babies and breastfeeding moms and lots of talk about all things natural. It was definitely a non-mainstream, granola upbringing—especially for the time.

When I was pregnant with my first child and spoke with my mom about my concerns regarding vaccination, she said she shared those concerns. I don't think she would have tried to convince me not to vaccinate if I was leaning that way, but she was definitely supportive of my decision not to.

LC: My mom decided not to vaccinate my two sisters and I. We got the chickenpox and I'm not even sure if I knew at 12…that there was a vaccine to prevent it. My mom did tell me our family physician had been lax on vaccines and told her something like "the kids will be ok without them." I don't know why she thought they were bad, though.

CA: My parents were the textbook early '80s/'90s parents. They did everything they could that their doctor said to do in reference to me and my younger sister's health.

WAS THERE AN EVENT OR SERIES OF EVENTS/ENCOUNTERS THAT TRIGGERED DOUBTS FOR YOU ABOUT VACCINES?

KO: My upbringing primed me for having doubts about vaccines. As a young adult I grew increasingly interested in all things "natural," but probably had a bit of a skewed notion of what constitutes "natural." I think…I came to the topic of vaccination with an ingrained bias, though I'm not sure I would have called it such at the time. I framed it as skepticism, as a lack of trust in the medical and pharmaceutical industries and an assumption that those industries were motivated by profit rather than by an interest in public health and safety. In college, I took a graduate level course that examined the history of medical practice in America. We learned about the Tuskegee syphilis experiment and the intentional vilification of midwives as the push for hospital births grew….

On my own I read about Vioxx and other pharmaceutical mishaps and recalls including thalidomide and what it did to children in Britain. I read about the live polio vaccine causing paralysis. Science doesn't always get it right the first time, and I felt like vaccines might be another area where the kinks were still being worked out, with children as the guinea pigs.

LC: There was no particular incident. I joined a local mom's group on Facebook after meeting a few of them in person, and I think that's where the idea that [vaccines] were poisonous came from.

CA: The thing that actually triggered my doubts about vaccines was that I had gotten into this new-hippie/crunchy lifestyle that was all the rage…in young mothers. What really got me was that they were saying…that vaccines caused autism.

HOW DID YOU GET INVOLVED IN THE ANTI-VACCINE MOVEMENT? TO WHAT EXTENT WERE YOU INVOLVED?

KO: I do not consider myself to have been involved in The Movement. I'm an introvert and not a big joiner or vocal supporter of causes. I tend to just quietly read and think and analyze. Years ago, I hesitatingly posted a couple of mildly anti-vaccine links and comments on Facebook, but that was about the extent of it.

LC: I don't know that I'd say I was really involved in the movement as far as protesting or picketing or going to organized meet-ups…. But I did share bad articles on the topic on Facebook—pseudoscience explanations of vaccines' toxicity and anecdotal stories mostly.

CA: I was the prime example of an uneducated person just flocking with the herd. All of my friends were following the trends associated with being crunchy. They read what other people saw on the Internet and they did no research of their own, and neither did I…. Every time I got the chance to share some Internet graphic about the dangers of vaccines with my friend list, oh man did I. I brought it up at dinner, I brought it up with friends, and everywhere I went I was sharing my uneducated beliefs. I was young and easily influenced.

WERE YOU AND YOUR SPOUSE ON THE SAME PAGE REGARDING WHETHER OR NOT TO VACCINATE YOUR CHILDREN?

KO: He…left most of the work and decision-making to me. When the girls were infants and toddlers, he was caring for his elderly father, so he didn't have a lot of time or energy left at the end of the day. His mom and sisters were concerned that I hadn't vaccinated the girls, though, and they would question him, which in turn led him to question me. Initially, I was defensive about it, but as time went on and my own doubts began to grow, I considered his opinion in my decision to change course. He mentioned it in the midst of the Disneyland measles outbreak, and a time when I was already questioning my decision, so it was a timing issue as well.

LC: My husband remained skeptical of the anti-vax stuff but let me take care of doctor visits, and it was left up to me. Later, when I came around to the logical side of the topic, then we were in agreement that vaccines are necessary.

CA: The kids' dad was not into making choices like that. Everything was up to me and, whatever I decided to do, he would stand behind it.

WHEN DID YOU START TO HAVE DOUBTS ABOUT THE CLAIMS BEING MADE BY THE ANTI-VACCINE MOVEMENT?

KO: I don't think I was ever 100% secure in my position.... I spent a lot of my younger years agonizing over options in various areas of my life, and often ultimately made the passive choice not to do anything. I think that [behavior] was at play when I didn't vaccinate my children. Suppose I vaccinated my children and one or more of them were later diagnosed with autism spectrum disorder or some other condition that people frequently blame on vaccines? If that happened, then I would always feel some degree of guilt. On the other hand, if my children weren't vaccinated, then I'd be absolutely certain that vaccines were not the cause of their disorder or condition and my conscience would be clear. If I did vaccinate, there'd be no way for me to know for sure, and I was afraid that I would feel terribly guilty for the rest of my life. What I hadn't considered fully was the reverse: What would happen and how I would feel if my children contracted a vaccine-preventable disease? Now I see the cognitive dissonance there, but I don't think I did at the time.

The balance began to tip when several events converged in my mind. Over the course of a few months, the Disneyland measles outbreak made headlines, I had a conversation with a respected colleague who disagreed with my choice not to vaccinate, my husband had questioned me a couple of times about why we hadn't vaccinated the girls, and my family all contracted rotavirus. I still remember a moment of clarity that completely changed everything.... I had a sudden thought that I couldn't ignore: What if the people who were against vaccinating, the people whose words and arguments I had relied on to make my decision, were completely wrong? Almost immediately I grabbed my laptop and started looking at pro-vaccine websites and reading the information they contained... And when reading about some anti-vaccine claim or another (such as "The CDC admits vaccines cause autism!!!"), I began carefully following the links to the study or other cited evidence of the headline's claim. What I began finding concerned me: When I read the cited study, I never could find the smoking gun or evidence that the article writer claimed it contained. Often, I found the exact opposite to be the case.

LC: A friend of mine, who has a boy close in age to my boy, was skeptical of vaccines for a bit. She worked where my husband was finishing his bachelor's degree and I had some high regard for her. She eventually started talking about how she was duped by the same type of information I was reading and then shared articles that debunked them.

CA: I started having doubts when I had to lie to the school about my religious beliefs when enrolling my daughter in kindergarten.... I am proud of my beliefs and to say that vaccines were against my religion, I felt, was one of the worst ways that you could sin in the eyes of God.... My daughter went to a Christian school and...I looked them right in the eye and lied. Then I saw a video on social media of a baby coughing and hacking because they had contracted a virus that could have been prevented had someone gotten the vaccine. The sound of the mother crying in the background of the video touched my soul and I started thinking, "What if that had been me? What would I do in that moment?" After that, I started to actually do my own research.

DURING YOUR ANTI-VACCINE DAYS, HOW DID YOU RECONCILE PERSONAL CHOICE VERSUS THE CHOICE TO PROTECT THOSE IN THE COMMUNITY WHO COULD SEE HARM FROM DECREASING RATES OF VACCINATION?

KO: I don't think I ever reconciled that issue. I was aware of the concerns that lowered vaccination rates could lead to an increase in vaccine-preventable disease, and that herd immunity protected people in the community who could not be vaccinated. Ardent anti-vaxxers claim that herd immunity is actually a myth, and that it has never been demonstrated as a scientific fact. They claim that parents should not be compelled to vaccinate their children (or, as they put it, to inject their children full of harmful toxins) in order to protect other people from disease. They also argue that, since vaccines are "harmful and can actually cause health problems" and are not as effective as advertised, the whole argument about herd immunity offering protection to those who can't be vaccinated is just propaganda.

I also bought into the anti-vaccine idea that improved sanitation and advances in treatment were largely responsible for the decrease in communicable disease…. Clean drinking water, sanitation, improved nutrition, breastfeeding, and advanced medical care are the primary drivers of good health and a reduction in communicable disease. The idea is that an optimized, "uncompromised" immune system can effectively fight off disease if given the ideal conditions and environment.

LC: I wasn't aware of the consequences. Or rather, I didn't believe herd immunity was true, and I didn't really know the other benefits of mass vaccination.

CA: At the time I was told that herd immunity was not actually true and…I believed everything that I read and heard from the…anti-vaccine groups. I told myself that I was making the right choice because I was trying to protect my family and my family was more important than everyone else…. I also was so convinced that the government was out to get me. I didn't trust them at all. It wasn't until my Grandma got very sick that I really started doing research on herd immunity because it was dangerous for her to be around people who weren't vaccinated that could be a carrier. Her immune system was so fragile. I knew that if she contracted one of these things that she probably wouldn't make it through it. That scared me so much for her and for every other person that can't get vaccines, including newborn babies. There was a newborn baby in my area not long ago that died from exposure to something that could have been prevented if someone had vaccinated their children. These are just the constant reminders of why we need to increase herd immunity and why we need to vaccinate our children. You can never be too careful, and you need to help take care of the people who can't take care of themselves. Period.

FROM WITHIN THE MOVEMENT, WERE THERE CERTAIN APPROACHES OR TACTICS THAT WERE ENCOURAGED TO SWAY PEOPLES' OPINIONS ABOUT VACCINES?

KO: Fear is a powerful motivator, and when I was trying to find information about the safety of vaccines, I came across some pretty scary stories online about children who were allegedly injured by vaccines. We assume that parents know their children deeply, and when a parent claims their child changed drastically and immediately after a series of immunizations, I think our instinct is to believe that parent…. It is hard for a nonmedically trained person to put those testimonials aside and take a doctor's or drug company's word for it that vaccines are safe. It is hard not to see…those grieving parents as up against a Goliath…. Any attempt to question the parent, to ask for some evidence that vaccines were actually the cause, is met with swift and ferocious backlash. The general message is "How dare you question this parent after all they've been through!"

Other significant tactics focus on the insistence that even the government and pharmaceutical companies are aware of the dangers of vaccines. Package inserts are a frequent topic. If someone doesn't know how package inserts work, or what they are legally required to state, it's not easy to read that long list of possible side effects and not feel concerned about bringing their child in for immunizations. The general idea is that there is a great big conspiracy hiding in plain sight.

The other thing they do is talk about ingredients in vaccines and work on making a connection between the ingredients and the constellation of theorized harms that those ingredients can cause. I think many anti-vaxxers are also careful to state that they are not ideologically opposed to vaccines, but rather they just want to see "safer" vaccines. Unfortunately, the goal post for what constitutes "safer" always seems to be moving.

Finally, another big one is the National Vaccine Injury Compensation program and VAERS [Vaccine Adverse Events Reporting System]. People seem to misunderstand how these programs work, and their lack of understanding allows them to be easily manipulated into believing that the government knows that vaccines are unsafe and is quietly shelling out billions of dollars for scientifically proven and legitimate cases of vaccine injury.

LC: The fear aspect was used a lot. "Be fearful of the ingredients and the harm they could cause your kids." There were articles about lawsuits against the CDC…as if that was evidence that the vaccines indeed caused permanent injury to kids.

CA: The thing that I saw the most within the movement was people who would share articles written by one doctor with no real evidence of substantial quality speaking out about vaccines. People would cling to anything they could find about any adverse reaction or ingredient that might be slightly harmful and blow those things up out of proportion.

DO YOU THINK THAT THERE IS AN ORGANIZED MOVEMENT, OR IS THIS JUST INDIVIDUALS EXPRESSING THEIR OPINIONS IN A VOCAL MANNER?

KO: I think it's a little of both. A large segment of the movement circulates in and around the National Vaccine Information Center, Dr. Joseph Mercola, Generation Rescue and other anti-vaccine autism awareness groups, Natural News, Dr. Tenpenny, David Wolfe, Andrew Wakefield, anti-vaccine mommy bloggers, etc. The organizations and individuals generally preach to the choir, gathering and posting further "evidence" of the risks of vaccination, which are then shared widely over social media, where vaccine-hesitant and fence-sitting parents inevitably come across them. Some seem to like to portray themselves as selfless missionaries, out there spreading the truth despite persecution.

Other people are probably more like me, somewhere on the spectrum from quietly not vaccinating one's children to openly and loudly broadcasting one's opinions about the dangers of vaccinating, but within a smaller sphere of influence.

LC: Both. There's [famous people] who share so much misinformation and [have a] following. There's others like [author, entrepreneur, and spokesperson] David "Avocado" Wolfe [as well]. How organized [they are] I really don't know. I'm sure they're just trying to make money.

CA: I think that it is a bunch of people who are selfish and uneducated on the real facts. People are…quick to turn against anything that is mandated in today's society. I don't think it is organized very well, I just think that people are following in the hopes of fitting in and doing what everyone else in their circle of friends is doing. However, I do think the movement has grown…and more needs to be done about it.

(See chapter 13 for more information on the tactics used by anti-vaccine web sites.)

WHAT ULTIMATELY DROVE YOU TO CHANGE YOUR MIND ABOUT THE IMPORTANCE AND SAFETY OF VACCINES?

KO: There were many things that kind of came together at once in my mind, not least that my family contracted rotavirus…. After we were sick, I went back to Google with a specific, intentional mindset. I said to myself, "Let's pretend that I'm pro-vaccine and I'm looking for evidence to support my stance." It completely changed the way I viewed the information I came across. Something just clicked. It was a revelation. I knew I had been wrong **(See Table 4.1)**.

TABLE 4.1 Let's Imagine: Helping Your Patients See the Other Side of the Argument

Many patients seeking vaccine information using Google and other search engines usually only see one side of the vaccine discussion. When patients seek your professional advice, try proposing these what-if scenarios as a form of mental exercise that may stimulate vaccine-hesitant patients to look at the other side of the argument.	
SCENARIO	**PURPOSE**
Imagine that you are pro-vaccine. What evidence can you find to support your pro-vaccine stance?	• Helps patients recognize the echo chamber that social media provides
Imagine that you are the parent of a child with leukemia. How would you feel about others' decisions not to vaccinate if your child then comes down with a potentially deadly vaccine-preventable disease?	• Helps parents consider the benefit of herd/community immunity and our responsibility to protect those more vulnerable in our population
Imagine that your child came down with meningococcal meningitis and lost an arm and developed a life-long seizure disorder as a result. How would you feel? What emotions would you have to live with?	• Helps parents anticipate the regret of purposefully declining an intervention that could have saved their child a lifetime of suffering
Imagine how your daughter would feel if she developed cervical cancer in her 20s and had to have a hysterectomy, preventing her from having children? How do you think she would feel about the decision to decline the HPV vaccine?	• Also helps parents anticipate regret
Imagine that your child comes down with influenza and recovers but transmits the infection to his or her grandmother who dies from influenza-related pneumonia as a result. How would you and your child feel about this outcome?	• Another means of highlighting herd immunity and regret from unwanted outcomes

Continued

Imagine that you are head of a government entity charged with preserving the health of the entire US population, particularly those in underserved populations. How would vaccines play a role in your efforts?	• Helps patients see the public health reasons for vaccination recommendations
Imagine that your child grows up and wants to be a doctor. Would you discourage him or her because your opinion of doctors is that they are corrupt and just in it for the money? Can you imagine that your child might have only honest and benevolent motivations for wanting to help people? How does this change your view of others that enter the field of medicine?	• Helps patients acknowledge the good intentions of those in the medical field and hopefully helps rebuild trust

I also came to view parent testimonials claiming vaccine harm in a new way. While I still have a lot of empathy for these parents…I began to see some cracks in their stories. Well, giant chasms, actually. The only thing that connected these children's conditions to vaccines was the coincidence of timing. Even as a nondoctor, some things just seemed implausible on second thought, especially as I learned more about how vaccines work. The human brain is wired to look for connections and patterns. I think, in our efforts to solve a problem or settle a matter, we sometimes connect dots where there aren't any.

LC: Opening those articles about vaccine safety that specifically debunked what I thought was true. Then I met some credible people belonging to a Facebook group called Crunchy Skeptics. They hold a sort of database, saved documents, a ton of studies and articles about vaccine safety that are available to the group's members.

CA: In the end, what drove me to change my mind was the hours and days and weeks of endless research—reading medical reports and everything there was on vaccines. When all the research points one way, it probably means that it is true.

WHERE DO YOU GET YOUR INFORMATION ABOUT VACCINE SCIENCE/ RECOMMENDATIONS NOW AND WHAT RESOURCES DID YOU USE WHEN YOU WERE IN THE ANTI-VACCINE CAMP?

KO: Today I consider just about any mainstream, pro-vaccine source to be valuable in terms of giving predictably reliable information about the benefits of and science behind the safety and efficacy of vaccines. That's the great thing about science. No matter where you read about gravity, or evolution, or climate change, you're going to find a high degree of consistency among the sources that use proven scientific facts. I read a lot of Paul Offit's work. I absolutely loved Eula Bliss' *On Immunity*. Her words tapped into both my rational and emotional self at the same time. I think many parents who are hesitant about vaccines would appreciate her book.

Prior to vaccinating, I relied on the old anti-vaccine standbys which were mostly the result of Google searches. I also read *The Vaccine Book* by Dr. Sears and the *Vaccine Safety Manual* by Neil Z. Miller. I sought out information written by medical professionals and was able to rationalize that if even a small handful of actual physicians and medically trained people have concerns about vaccines, there must be some legitimacy to the argument that vaccines might not be safe.

LC: I like skepticalraptor.com, the CDC website, redwineandapplesauce.com whose blogger writes for a large News Corp I believe, and plumbed.com. I can't even remember where I'd gotten bad info. I think mostly mommy blogs.

CA: I have scoured the Internet for medical journals, observations, and tests over the years. I was in an anti-vaccine group on social media before and there was this one main leader who started the group who would post social media graphics. I would share those graphics on my page without actually doing the research behind the facts…. You must do your research before sharing information that can change people's lives.

WHAT ROLE, IF ANY, DO YOU THINK MEDIA/SOCIAL MEDIA PLAYED IN YOUR ORIGINAL ANTI-VACCINE VIEWS AND NOW IN YOUR CURRENT PRO-VACCINE STANCE?

KO: Parent testimonials about vaccine harm and injuries are widely circulated on social media and have tremendous emotional currency. In former times, alternative practitioners and so-called experts who spoke against vaccination would generally be limited in terms of the audience they could reach. Now, with a worldwide platform, these voices can have a much larger influence than before. The things people shared on social media definitely had a huge role to play in turning me against vaccines. But, conversely, social media also helped me change those views. I think one of the biggest life lessons I've learned throughout this experience is that…our own biases shape the way we receive information (**Box 4.1**). Once I became aware of my bias, I was able to take a more critical look and better separate emotion from fact.

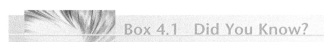

Box 4.1 Did You Know?

Numbers can be misleading. For example, examine your reaction to the following information. In the 2017-2018 flu season:
- 80,000 people died in the United States from influenza.
- The influenza death rate in the United States was 0.00024.
- The influenza death rate in the United States was 0.024%.
- The influenza death rate in the United States was 1 in 4084.

The number of deaths in the 2017-2018 flu season was indeed 80,000. However, if you divide 80,000 by 325.7 million (the US population in 2018), you get 0.00024. Multiply that by 100 and you have 0.024%. Divide 1 by 4084, and it also equals 0.00024. Multiply by 100 and you have 0.024%. Even though all of these numbers are equivalent, we likely have a different gut reaction to each value. When I look at these numbers, the rate of 0.00024 seems much smaller than 1 in 4084, yet they are exactly the same. When evaluating information online, we have to drill down and really look at the numbers being used. We need to ask ourselves how else the information could be presented, and how it might color our opinion of the facts.

LC: Facebook is where it was all shared and how I casually came across the info…. If I wasn't on social media when my kids were little, it's very possible I would have gone along with doctor recommendations and never stopped vaccinations for my kids.

CA: I think the social media role in this uprising is one of the biggest ways of spreading false information and untrue statistics.

WERE YOUR KIDS SCHOOL-AGE AT THE TIME THAT YOU WERE DECLINING VACCINES AND, IF SO, HOW DID YOU HANDLE THE REQUIREMENTS FOR YOUR STATE TO BE VACCINATED PRIOR TO ENTRY TO SCHOOL? DID YOU USE A RELIGIOUS OR PERSONAL EXEMPTION?

KO: My children were still young when I changed my mind. My twins were three and my oldest was five. For preschool, I wrote a religious/philosophical exemption, which was difficult for me, because while I have a lot of values that are consistent with Christian values, I don't consider myself to be religious. I was able to get my oldest up-to-date on what was required before she entered kindergarten.

CA: I started having doubts when I had to lie to the school about my religious beliefs when enrolling my daughter in kindergarten.

HOW ARE YOU INVOLVED IN THE PRO-VACCINE MOVEMENT AT THIS TIME?

KO: I contributed my story to Voices for Vaccines and, nearly 2 years later, people still reach out to request an interview or conversation. I've considered writing a follow-up piece because I have some thoughts about the anti-vaccine movement and how it responded to my story going viral. I'm a member of a few Facebook groups. I attended the Kansas Immunization Conference last June and spoke about my experiences. So, I guess I'm not actively involved in any strategic way, but I do what I can when people reach out to me.

LC: At the time I switched to pro-vaccine, I was vocal about that change on Facebook as well as shared articles/videos that broke down and debunked the myths. Today, I'm not sharing much. I did share my story with Voices for Vaccines and now this!

CA: I have written articles and always try to share any real medical articles with proven research with my peers.

HAVE YOU HAD ANY REPERCUSSIONS WITH FAMILY OR FRIENDS FROM YOUR DECISION TO SUPPORT VACCINATION EFFORTS?

KO: My decision greatly affected a close relationship. After months of awkwardness and some uncharacteristic arguing between us, [my friend] finally admitted that she couldn't get past my change of stance on vaccinating. We didn't communicate for over a year, but she resurfaced and we have hashed some things out. I had some long discussions with my mom and my maternal grandmother who also researches and embraces alternative health ideas and practices with gusto. My family is pretty live-and-let-live so they love and support me no matter what.

LC: My older sister is anti-vaccine so we've had arguments in the past.

CA: Of course I lost friends in my group when I stated that I was pro-vaccine and, when I wrote the article, the "holistic parents of mid Missouri" group on Facebook kicked me out. They shared my article and called me names and talked terribly about who I was as a person and as a mother, just because of one small article. Every person should be able to believe what they want or don't want to believe. That's the thing about this movement. You are either strongly for or strongly against and people are so mean to you if you are on the opposing side. There is no gray area.

WHAT KIND OF ENCOUNTERS WITH YOUR MEDICAL PROVIDERS AFFECTED YOUR OPINIONS ABOUT VACCINES, PRO OR CON?

KO: When my oldest was born…I quickly found [a] practice [whose] physicians did not vaccinate. When that practice closed, I went looking for a provider who wouldn't harass me about vaccinations. I made an appointment with a doctor my mom recommended but…after 15 minutes of lecturing and finger-wagging, I left flustered and shaking, feeling completely chastised and belittled. The encounter actually strengthened my resolve not to vaccinate, as I began to associate his condescension and lecturing as representative of a holier-than-thou, just shut up and vaccinate attitude among vaccine advocates. Not long after that, I found another clinic closer to my home [that did not vaccinate].

LC: Doctors did encourage vaccines but didn't push it if I said no.

CA: I have many people in the medical field in my family and when I was younger and on the nonvaccine side of things, they would always tell me that I was crazy and that I was putting my child's life in danger.

WHEN YOU HAD MORE OF AN ANTI-VACCINE SENTIMENT, DID YOU SEEK OUT PROVIDERS THAT FELT SIMILARLY, OR DID YOU JUST CONTINUE TO SEE A LONG-TERM TRUSTED PROVIDER?

KO: Yes, I specifically sought out providers who would be supportive of my decision not to vaccinate. When I was pregnant with my first daughter, I found a group of midwives who, while not vocally anti-vaccine, supported my choice and kind of treated it as a nonissue…. Being that I live in a metropolitan area, I think it was relatively easy for me to find practitioners who supported my position on vaccines.

LC: We had Medicaid for a few years and our options were limited, but I didn't search for a specific doctor sharing the same ideas.

CA: You cannot find any practitioners who have the sentiment that you should not give vaccines to your children. You just can't. That should be a large enough statement for most people, but most of the movement just ignores that fact or they go to a chiropractor instead of an actual doctor because…some chiropractors don't believe in vaccines.

HAVE YOU FOUND THAT YOU'VE BEEN ABLE TO DISCUSS YOUR CONCERNS ABOUT THE ANTI-VACCINE MOVEMENT WITH FRIENDS/FAMILY FROM THAT GROUP? HAVE YOU BEEN ABLE TO SWAY ANYONE TO SEEING YOUR SIDE OF THE STORY SINCE BECOMING PRO-VACCINE?

KO: After my story went viral, there was a lot of uproar and backlash among anti-vaxxers. Instead of refuting my story with facts, all they did was attempt to discredit me. Somebody cooked up a conspiracy theory, complete with images from my Facebook file and a handy little infographic, attempting to connect me with Big Pharma. People started sending me messages calling me a murderer with blood on my hands. I jumped in on a couple of discussions in an attempt to set the story straight, but I don't think I made serious headway with the anti-vaccine crowd. I think I might do a halfway decent job speaking to concerned, vaccine-hesitant parents, but the entrenched anti-vaxxers are dug in deep.

LC: I didn't get into conversations on the topic with that group. Because of moving further from town, I've lost touch with them except for one person. She actually stopped talking to me for 3 years after seeing my pro-vaccine posts on Facebook. She took offense. Once we reconnected, though, she seemed to be on the fence and more open to the idea that vaccines might be safe.

CA: My goal is not to sway people to change their minds but just to inform them of the facts.

WHAT MADE YOU WANT TO TELL YOUR STORY OF TRANSITION FROM ANTI-VACCINE TO PRO-VACCINE?

KO: I live a lot of my life in my head, and once I was firmly in favor of vaccination, I spent some time mentally working out how it all happened. I felt like writing about the experience would kind of close that chapter in my life. The testimonials on Voices for Vaccines, most especially those that chronicled a parent's transition from anti- to pro-vaccine were instrumental in helping change my mind and feel sure of my decision… Since the website had helped me, I figured I'd give back by sharing my story.

LC: I'd like to help. It's evident that the pockets of anti-vaccine communities are having terrible effects on others who can't get vaccinated and are causing outbreaks. It needs to stop.

CA: I just felt that there were probably people who were in my shoes and wanted them to know that it's ok to go against the crowd. You have to do what is right, and true friends would not stop being your friends for that.

WHAT ADVICE WOULD YOU GIVE MEDICAL PROVIDERS IN DISCUSSING VACCINATIONS WITH THEIR VACCINE-HESITANT PATIENTS?

KO: I would advise medical providers, above all else, to summon their empathy and try to put themselves in the shoes of parents who are nervous and unsure about vaccinating. Tread lightly. Give unbiased, factual information and remain calm and kind (**Box 4.2**). These parents, despite their misinformation and defenses, still love their children and want to do what's best for them.

 Box 4.2   Sample Vaccine Conversation

Doctor: "Because this is Emily's first-year well-visit, she's due for a few shots. This includes her final Hib and pneumococcal vaccines, hepatitis A, and her first MMR and chickenpox vaccines. And since it is October, she should also get her flu shot."

Mom: "I'm not sure I want her to get all of those shots."

Doctor: "Oh, really? Ok, let's talk it through. Tell me what worries you about these shots."

Mom: "Well, it's really just the MMR and chickenpox shots. I've heard that it's better to get these infections naturally. Also, I've heard that the MMR vaccine has toxic stuff in it that can cause autism."

Doctor: "I get it. This is a really confusing time to be a parent. There is so much conflicting information out there about vaccines that it can be hard to know what to believe."

Mom: "Right. I know that vaccines have really improved health and kept kids from getting some bad diseases, but we don't see these diseases anymore and the risks of the vaccines seem greater."

Doctor: "That's a common concern. But I firmly believe in the benefit of vaccines and have done many, many hours of research into the safety and effectiveness of vaccines, and I'd love to tell you my thoughts. Is that ok?"

Mom: "Sure!"

Doctor: "Thank you. First, it's important to recognize that we don't vaccinate against run-of-the-mill illnesses. Measles, mumps, rubella, chickenpox… historically, these have killed hundreds of thousands of children around the world each year. You might hear that measles, for example, is not that big of a deal. But did you know that 1 in 4 kids with measles will have to be hospitalized; 1 in 1000 will develop brain inflammation that can cause permanent brain damage; and 1 to 2 in 1000 will die from the disease?"

Mom: "No, that's a lot worse than I thought."

Doctor: "The reason we hardly see these illnesses anymore is *because* of vaccinations. Unfortunately, some people are now choosing not to vaccinate, so we are again seeing these deadly diseases show up in our communities. Recently, we have seen measles outbreaks in Minnesota and New York. Last year, there was a mumps outbreak in Washington. These preventable illnesses are on the rise again."

Continued

Mom: "I heard about those."

Doctor: "As for the MMR vaccine and the concerns voiced by some in the anti-vaccine community, none of our studies looking at hundreds of thousands of kids has shown any link to autism. In fact, since mercury was removed from all but the multidose flu vaccines in 2001, we have seen an *increase* in autism rates, not a decrease. And the "toxins" that people claim can cause harm are, in fact, naturally occurring substances. We are exposed to aluminum and formaldehyde in much greater quantity in our foods and in the products we use every day than we get in any series of vaccines. In the case of aluminum, babies get more aluminum in breast milk than they get in 6 months' worth of vaccines."

Mom: "I didn't realize that."

Doctor: "Not many people do, which is why I'm so glad we have the chance to talk about this before you make a choice against vaccinating. I strongly encourage my families to vaccinate because I truly believe it is the best thing we can do to protect the health and future of our loved ones. I fully vaccinate myself and my children and I wouldn't do that if I had any doubts whatsoever. Vaccines work and they are safe. I really appreciate you taking the time to listen and if you have any more questions, I'm happy to answer them or give you some resources for further reading. So, what do you say? Shall we get Emily vaccinated?"[b]

---

[a]Don't sell yourself short. You went to medical school (or years of other medical training) and you are reading this book. You have done your research!

---

[b]Of course, there are many turns that this conversation could take. This is just one example of dialogue that can happen that will both inform and leave the parent/patient feeling like their concerns have been heard and respected.

LC: Possibly start with genuine questions. "Why do you believe this? Do you know who your source is or their credentials?" I imagine one could start by telling them something like "We're happy you're here and taking good care of your kids. Can you please explain why you don't want them inoculated?"

CA: Show them the facts—the actual studies and evidence of the things that these diseases can do to children and the elderly who can't receive vaccines.

Although the journeys and backgrounds of KO, LC, and CA are varied, it is obvious that they share some similar experiences and there is much we can learn from their stories.

- Don't just follow the crowd: Sometimes anti-vaccine or vaccine-hesitant people are just following the crowd, trusting that the information that others in their same circles are sharing is true.

- Do your own research: Taking the time to do one's own personal research (using complete journal articles, not just snippets taken out of context, and referencing reputable sources) before making the very serious decision not to vaccinate is extremely important and is an obvious theme that emerges from the stories above. This is a message that we can help our patients to understand (See Appendix F: Navigating Information on the Internet and Social Media.).

- "Natural" doesn't have to mean anti-vaccine: There is a move in some segments of society to pursue a more "natural" lifestyle. However, there does not have to be a disconnect between pursuing this lifestyle and accepting vaccines. Arguments are made that aluminum and formaldehyde are unnatural "toxins" that are harmful to our bodies. What the majority of people don't understand, however, is that these substances are completely natural. Aluminum is found in Earth's crust (I can't think of anything more natural than the earth itself) and is common in our environment. To escape aluminum exposure, you would have to leave the planet. And formaldehyde is necessary for our bodies to function. It is actually produced by our bodies in concentrations much greater than we would get in a series of injections. To escape formaldehyde exposure, you'd have to leave your own body!

- Finger-wagging doesn't work: Who among us likes to feel chastised or belittled? When dealing with vaccine-hesitant patients, treating them like an insolent child or writing off their concerns may only serve to strengthen their anti-vaccine resolve.

- Fear is a powerful motivator: Much of the attraction of the parent testimonials about vaccine harm is that they tug at our heartstrings and they make us fearful that we might make a decision that would harm our children in a similar way. To move past fear and to understand the safety of vaccines, parents and patients need to be approached with empathy and without judgment. This is an important decision they are trying to make, and they need us to be on their side.

- Social media is a big player: It is certainly obvious that social media played a large role in each of the three stories above. It is an extremely easy way to share information across a wide audience and is being utilized quite well by the anti-vaccine movement. We, as purveyors of science and reason, need to have a wider voice on social media in order to drown out the misinformation that is so widely circulated (see chapter 13 for further discussion of this issue).

- If we are lax about encouraging vaccines, our patients will be lax about getting them: Studies show that provider support and encouragement of vaccination is the number one reason that patients choose to vaccinate. If we allow the conversation to stop at "No, thanks," we are doing a disservice to our patients, to our communities, and to ourselves.

Additional Resources

For patients seeking further information on vaccines:

- Centers for Disease Control and Prevention—Vaccines and Immunizations: www.cdc.gov/vaccines/index.html.
- American Academy of Pediatrics—HealthyChildren.org: www.healthychildren.org.
- Children's Hospital of Philadelphia—Vaccine Education Center: www.chop.edu/centers-programs/vaccine-education-center.

- Immunization Action Coalition: www.immunize.org.
- Voices for Vaccines: www.voicesforvaccines.com.
- Institute for Vaccine Safety: vaccinesafety.edu.
- Families Fighting Flu: www.familiesfightingflu.org.
- Vaccinate Your Family: www.vaccinateyourfamily.org.
- Skeptical Raptor: www.skepticalraptor.com.
- Facebook group: Crunchy Skeptics: https://www.facebook.com/groups/184944741680963/.
- Science-Based Medicine: sciencebasedmedicine.org.

Reference

1. Voices for Vaccines. Mission statement. https://www.voicesforvaccines.org/about/. Accessed January 5, 2019.

5

Who's Minding the Shop? Ensuring Vaccine Safety and Efficacy

The safety of the people shall be the highest law.

—Marcus Tullius Cicero

One of the most popular arguments used by the anti-vaccine movement is that vaccines are not studied or monitored thoroughly enough before coming to market. Some people opposed to vaccines will claim that they are "not against vaccines, per se." They just want them to be "safer." The reality is that vaccines are among the most thoroughly tested and monitored interventions that we offer in modern medicine. This chapter will review the evolution of vaccine safety regulations and the organizations that enforce them. It will also follow vaccines through their lifecycle, looking at the development of immunizations, their testing, and the postlicensure monitoring that provides highly effective checks and balances for these life-saving interventions.

The assertion is also made that, because pharmaceutical companies ("Big Pharma") are involved with vaccine production and because pharmaceutical companies are in business to make a profit, there is inherent corruption in the vaccine development process—that somehow vaccines are pushed through without proper regulation just to turn a profit for the "pharmaceutical fat cats." In the following pages, we will also look at the role that drug companies play in the development of immunizations and offer hope that they are not, after all, pushing through untested vaccines or bilking the medical establishment and patients out of billions of dollars.

We will next look at the alphabet soup of organizations that play a role in vaccine oversight and monitoring. We will gain a better understanding of the organizational structure of vaccine and public health-related governmental programs as well as those privately funded groups that aid their efforts. Finally, we will dive deeper into the Vaccine Adverse Events Reporting System (VAERS), its successes and limitations, and the misconceptions about this system that allow people to think that there is some national conspiracy to offer unsafe medical interventions.

HISTORY OF VACCINE REGULATION

Today, the US vaccine supply is among the safest in the world, thanks to the extensive oversight and regulation that exists to ensure efficacy and safety. However, this was not always the case. Certain unfortunate events in the history of vaccines spurred the development of the highly successful system of checks and balances that we use today. Let's look at a few of these events and the safety measures that were put in place as a result.

1902 Biologics Control Act

In 1901, 13 children in St. Louis, Missouri, died of tetanus after being treated for their diphtheria illnesses with a contaminated antitoxin. It was common at that time to use horse's blood to make antitoxin serum but the blood of a horse that died of tetanus was accidentally collected and used in production. A similar tragedy occurred in Camden, New Jersey, when nine children died from tetanus after being given contaminated smallpox vaccine. These products had been produced in local laboratories with no uniform controls in place to ensure purity and potency and had undergone no inspection or testing of the final product prior to use. This triggered Congress to pass the 1902 Biologics Control Act, which gave the government control over processes used to make biological products and responsibility to ensure their safety. Under this act, the Hygienic Laboratory of the Public Health and Marine Hospital Service mandated that manufacturers of biologics be licensed and that their facilities undergo inspection. Production of biologics had to be overseen by a qualified scientist, and products had to have clear labeling, showing the product name and expiration date. In 1930, the Hygienic Laboratory was renamed the National Institutes of Health (NIH), and oversight of biologics remained under its purview until 1972 when the Food and Drug Administration (FDA) assumed control. Today, the FDAs Center for Biologics Evaluation and Research regulates biological products.[1]

Polio and the Cutter Incident

In 1955, Jonas Salk's vaccine held significant promise for preventing the devastation of polio that was ripping across the United States. Salk's vaccine had been tested on 1.8 million subjects and proved safe and effective.[1] However, once in use, case reports of children contracting polio after being given the inoculation began showing up. It was determined that the affected individuals had received a vaccine that contained live polio virus, which had survived the inactivation process during production at Cutter Laboratories in Berkeley, CA. In what came to be known as the Cutter Incident, more than 40,000 cases of polio were attributed to immunization with the Cutter vaccine, resulting in varying degrees of paralysis in almost 200 children and death in 10.[2] Vaccine production was halted until every manufacturing facility was inspected and stricter standards for ensuring full inactivation of the polio virus were employed.

Subsequent litigation regarding purported harms by other vaccines contributed to the decision by many vaccine manufacturers in the United States to get out of the business of developing or producing vaccines. The courts' findings of "liability without fault" meant that vaccine manufacturers were liable for "damage without negligence" even if their product was made using the most current science available and according to industry standards.[3]

National Childhood Vaccine Injury Act

In the mid-1970s and early 1980s, after damages were awarded to groups of patients claiming harm from the diphtheria, pertussis, and tetanus vaccine (DPT)—despite lack of scientific evidence to support those claims—liability insurance costs skyrocketed, several vaccine manufacturers halted production, and vaccine prices soared. The subsequent shortage in the vaccine supply triggered concern by public health officials that we might see a recurrence of epidemic illness as a result. This prompted Congress to pass the National Childhood Vaccine Injury Act (NCVIA) in 1986. Under this act, the National Vaccine Program Office (NVPO) was established to do the following[4]:

1. Coordinate vaccine-related activities between all Department of Health and Human Services (DHHS) agencies, including the FDA, the Centers for Disease Control and Prevention (CDC), the NIH, and the Health Resources and Services Administration (HRSA).
2. Require health care providers who administer vaccines to give a Vaccine Information Statement, which contains a description of the disease and risks and benefits of the vaccine, to each person receiving a vaccine or to their guardian.
3. Require health care providers to report certain possibly vaccine-related adverse events to the VAERS.
4. Establish the National Vaccine Injury Compensation Program (NVICP) to compensate, on a "no-fault" basis, those persons who were potentially injured by vaccines.
5. Establish a committee from the Health and Medicine Division of the National Academies of Science, Engineering, and Medicine (formerly the Institute of Medicine) to review the literature on potential vaccine reactions.

As a result of these actions over the years, there has been significant improvement in the monitoring and testing of vaccines for safety and efficacy, and we can place our faith in the fact that our vaccine supply is one of the best in the world.

THE BIRTH OF A VACCINE

The assertion by the anti-vaccine movement that vaccines are not studied thoroughly enough before being brought to market is unfounded. In fact, vaccines are the most thoroughly studied intervention that we have in modern medicine, so much so that it can actually be a problem to address emergent needs in the setting of illness epidemics and pandemics. (See Appendix C: Vaccine Topics Explained to find videos on how vaccines are made.) The development of a vaccine is an involved and highly regulated process that takes years (typically 10-15) to complete. Following is an outline of the phases of prelicensure vaccine development, as well as the postlicensure monitoring that continues after a vaccine is brought to market, that ensures the safety and efficacy of our vaccine supply[5] (**Figure 5.1**).

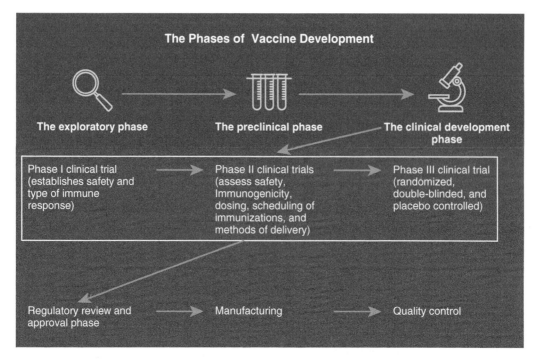

FIGURE 5.1 Phases of vaccine development. (From George Washington University. Producing prevention: The complex development of vaccines. Milken Institute School of Public Health. February 15, 2017. Accessed December 19, 2018. https://publichealthonline.gwu.edu/blog/producing-prevention-the-complex-development-of-vaccines/.)

The Exploratory Phase

The exploratory phase begins with monitoring new, persisting, or mutating infections in the population and then moves to the basic science laboratory where infectious viral and bacterial particles, or antigens, are identified. These laboratories are generally run by academic or government scientists who are funded by the federal government, and this step of the process usually lasts between 2 and 4 years.

The Preclinical Phase

The Preclinical phase tests the safety and immunogenicity (or ability to induce an immune response) of proposed vaccines, using cell and tissue cultures. Animal subjects (mice and monkeys, for example) are commonly used at this stage of vaccine development, allowing researchers to gauge the type of response they may expect to see in humans. In this stage, the researchers may challenge their test subjects by vaccinating them and then exposing them to the targeted illness. Many candidate vaccines fail to achieve the desired immune response and never make it beyond this stage of development. These researchers are most often from private industry, and this phase of testing typically takes between 1 and 2 years.

The Clinical Development Phase

An application for an Investigational New Drug is then placed with the FDA that has 30 days to approve or deny the application. At this phase, those putting forth the application are typically from private companies. They are charged with summarizing the basic science data, describing the manufacturing and testing processes, and putting together a plan for the proposed study which an Institutional Review Board, from the institution where the clinical trials will be conducted, then evaluates for approval. Once this approval takes place, the vaccine candidate is subject to three phases of human testing.

Phase I Clinical Trials

The first stage of testing in humans is conducted on a small number of study participants (typically fewer than 100) and may be nonblinded or open-label, meaning that participants and researchers may know who is getting a vaccine and who is getting placebo. If the proposed vaccine is intended for children, testing will first be done on adults and then, as safety and efficacy are established, testing will occur with younger subjects until the target age population is reached. The goal of this phase is to establish safety and determine the kind of immune response that the vaccine may induce.

Phase II Clinical Trials

If phase I testing is promising, a larger number of study participants (on the order of several hundred) will be enrolled in clinical trials. These participants may be people at risk for acquiring the disease (these vaccines are often tested in other countries where illness may be more prevalent). Typically, these trials are randomized, well controlled, and include a placebo group. The goals in this phase are to assess safety, immunogenicity, dosing, scheduling of immunizations, and method of delivery.

Phase III Clinical Trials

If a vaccine makes it to phase III trials, a much larger group of subjects (thousands to tens of thousands) are enrolled for testing. Phase III trials are randomized, double-blinded, and placebo controlled. The goals here include more of the same. Safety continues to be a primary end point. In these trials, we may expect to find rare side effects that are only detectable in a larger group and may not be seen when fewer subjects are studied. Efficacy is evaluated, looking at whether the vaccine prevents disease, whether it prevents infection with the pathogen, and whether it induces an adequate immune response (measurable antibody response) (**Box 5.1**).

 **Box 5.1   Did You Know?**

You may not have heard of Dr. Maurice Hilleman, but we have all benefitted tremendously from his work. Hilleman was an American microbiologist and vaccinologist. He developed 8 of the 14 routinely recommended US immunizations, including measles, mumps, meningococcus, hepatitis A, hepatitis B, chickenpox, pneumonia, and *Haemophilus influenzae* type b. Although he is not as well known as other vaccine scientists, such as Jonas Salk and Albert Sabin who developed the polio vaccine, he is credited with saving more lives than any other scientist in the 20th century. The documentary, *Hilleman: A Perilous Quest to Save the World's Children*, tells of his contributions to the fields of science, medicine, and public health and his unwavering dedication to ridding the world of deadly diseases.

Regulatory Review and Approval Phase

If phase III clinical development trials are successful, the developer will submit a Biologics License Application to the FDA, which will then inspect the manufacturing facilities and approve labeling of the vaccine. The FDA continues oversight after the licensure to assure safety, purity, and potency of the vaccine.

Manufacturing

This part of the production process is undertaken by major drug manufacturers. They are equipped with the personnel and infrastructure necessary to make and distribute large quantities of vaccines. They also see the benefit of profit from the sale of successful or widely used vaccines.

Quality Control

After a vaccine is brought to market, the monitoring and oversight do not end. The following organizations participate in ongoing safety and efficacy monitoring of our vaccine supply.

The Drug Manufacturer

Phase IV clinical trials are optional trials that the vaccine's manufacturer may choose to conduct after release of the vaccine for general use. These trials monitor effectiveness and safety but also look for other potential uses or applications of the vaccine.

The Vaccine Adverse Events Reporting System

VAERS was established in 1990 as a "national early warning system to detect possible safety problems in US-licensed vaccines."[6] It takes reports of adverse events from any concerned party and investigates the claims to look for any patterns suggesting safety issues with a vaccine. It is managed jointly by the CDC and the FDA.

The Vaccine Safety Datalink

The Vaccine Safety Datalink (VSD) was also established in 1990 as a collaborative venture between the CDC and eight health care organizations from around the country. Its mission is to monitor the "safety of vaccines and conduct studies about rare and serious adverse events following immunizations."[7] Data gathered from these organizations allow researchers to look at adverse events in the context of patients' medical conditions, other vaccines administered at the same time, and other factors.

THE PHARMACEUTICAL INDUSTRY AND ITS INVOLVEMENT IN VACCINE PRODUCTION

As we learned above, drug companies are less often involved in the early research stages of vaccine development. They are more likely to enter the scene at the stage of vaccine production if they view a vaccine to have potential for widespread use. Larger pharmaceutical companies have the necessary funds and infrastructure to produce and market vaccines (and really, we are talking about a select few pharmaceutical companies such as Sanofi-Pasteur, GlaxoSmithKline, Merck, Pfizer, Novartis, etc.). Smaller drug manufacturers simply cannot afford to be involved.

It is difficult, it turns out, to confidently estimate the cost of vaccine production. Estimates exist regarding development of a new drug (depending on the source, it is estimated to cost between 1.2 and 1.4 billion dollars to bring a drug to market in the United States), but it is less clear if this estimate applies equally to vaccine production. In looking at examples of more recent immunizations produced (such as the rotavirus vaccine), we may conclude that these estimates are likely correct. Using publicly available data regarding the phase I through III trials for two different rotavirus vaccines, we know that it costs approximately $200 million to bring each of these vaccines through testing. However, the expense is much greater than just the cost of human trials. There is the laboratory research that happens prior, paying for researcher salaries and equipment, there are costs of registering the vaccine, etc. Moreover, we also have to consider the cost of trials that fail but get us closer to successful vaccine production. In the case of rotavirus, there were four total attempts, each costing an average of $200 million plus the $86 million spent on other costs, which gets us close to that $1.2 billion average.[8] According to Dr. Paul Offit, pediatrician, researcher, vaccinologist, and coinventor of the rotavirus vaccine, "bringing any vaccine from research development through licensure costs approximately one billion dollars."

It is obviously very costly to develop a new vaccine. Although large drug companies hope to make money on their vaccine investments—as we would expect of any company wanting to stay in business—the profit is minimal in comparison to profits made on drugs used to treat disease. The percentage of profit margin for any of these companies involved in vaccine production is usually in the 3% range.[9] As we read about earlier in the chapter, there was a time when drug companies were getting out of the business of making vaccines. Prior to the existence of the NVICP, drug companies themselves were liable if someone suffered a rare but serious adverse reaction to a vaccine. The potential costs to defend themselves against such litigation were astronomical and could have put the companies at real threat of financial collapse. Many companies could no longer run the risk of producing vaccines. In 1990, however, the federal government set up the NVICP to take this risk away from vaccine manufacturers. In order to support an industry that would continue to participate in production of these vital preventive and life-saving interventions, the government opted to take on the risk and deal itself with any claims of harm.

Drug companies are also involved to some degree in legislation. For policymakers who are understaffed or working part time and don't have an employee devoted to health care policy, drug companies can provide education regarding vaccines and the illnesses they prevent that can aid legislators in drafting policies in a more knowledgeable manner. Vaccine manufacturers can also help mobilize organizations in support of pro-vaccine legislation, conduct consumer marketing campaigns, and can help fill gaps in access to vaccines once legislation is enacted. However, transparency in such interactions is extremely important and has not always been present to an ideal degree. Without transparency, there can be a sense, whether correct or not, that these interactions and their outcomes are driven by profit motive rather than what is best for the public servant's constituents. Transparency in drug company interactions with legislators and development of stronger relationships between government officials and the regional health departments that they serve would help ensure that information being presented is unbiased.[10]

A LOOK AT WHO'S INVOLVED IN VACCINE OVERSIGHT AND MONITORING

In looking at the history of regulation of biological products, we have already discussed several of the organizations involved in vaccine oversight. However, to even further counter the argument that immunizations are not monitored well enough, let's look at the primary groups, both federally and privately funded, that are involved in this process.[11] (**Figure 5.2A and B**)

Federally Funded Organizations

The National Vaccine Program Office

Housed under the DHHS, the NVPO "provides strategic leadership and management and encourages collaboration and coordination among federal agencies and other stakeholders whose mandate is to help reduce the burden of preventable infectious disease." It offers "thorough reporting, unbiased advice and expertise to other agencies in identifying and responding to gaps in the vaccine system, making vaccines safer and more effective for all."[12]

The Centers for Disease Control and Prevention

The CDC curates several vaccine safety–related programs and participates in the development of the schedule of vaccines to be used in the pediatric, adolescent, and adult populations.

The Vaccine Adverse Events Reporting System. Established in 1990 as a joint venture between the CDC and the FDA, VAERS takes reports from vaccine manufacturers, health professionals, and the public regarding possible adverse reactions related to vaccines and monitors for any emerging patterns of harm. It investigates those deemed serious (resulting in or prolonging hospitalization, causing life-threatening illness, permanent disability, or death) to determine if they were, indeed, related to the vaccine administered.

The Vaccine Safety Datalink. Established in 1990 to "address gaps in the scientific knowledge of rare and serious adverse events following immunizations," the VSD is a collaboration between the CDC and large health plans, which provide information regarding vaccines, medical encounters, health conditions, birth, and other census data. It allows for planned immunization safety studies and testing of hypotheses that arise from reports to VAERS, review of the medical literature, changes to the immunization schedule, and introduction of new vaccines. The VSD's Rapid Cycle Analysis allows the

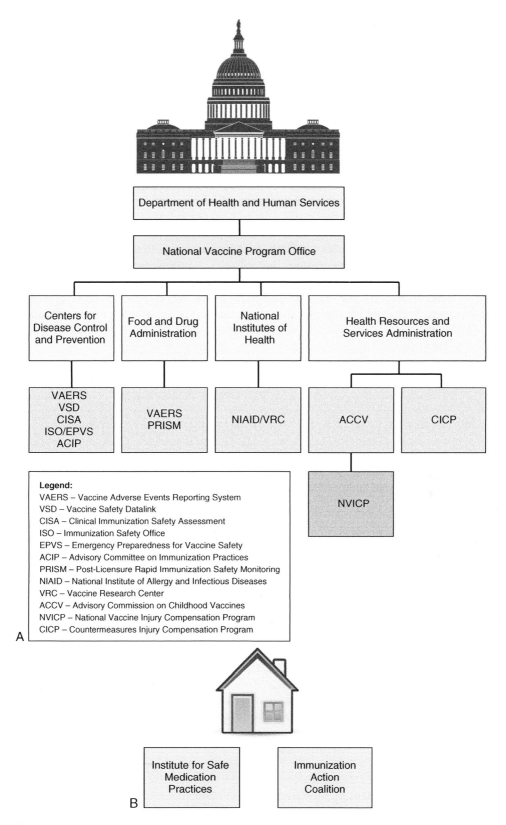

FIGURE 5.2 A, Federally funded government organizations. B, Privately funded organizations.

CDC and coinvestigators, using data taken from its participating health plans that serve more than 9 million people yearly, to monitor in near-real time any adverse events following immunization so that the public can be quickly informed.

The Clinical Immunization Safety Assessment Project. Established to improve understanding of adverse events following immunization (AEFI) at the individual-patient level, this agency serves to assist providers who need consultation regarding clinical and individual vaccine safety issues. (For example, if the refrigerator temperature decreases by 10°, how does this impact the vaccines contained therein?) Clinical Immunization Safety Assessment (CISA) also aids the CDC in developing strategies to identify individuals who may be at increased risk of adverse events following immunization and conducts studies to help identify risk factors for AEFI and prevention in special populations.

Immunization Safety Office and Emergency Preparedness for Vaccine Safety. This program ensures that active systems are in place to rapidly monitor the safety of vaccines in the event of an emergency vaccination program. As large numbers of vaccines may be given in a short timeframe, a greater number of side effects may be reported to VAERS, and, if the vaccines being used are new and less likely to have robust safety data, this would allow for monitoring of unexpected or concerning safety issues.[13]

Advisory Committee on Immunization Practices. This committee includes medical and public health experts who develop recommendations regarding the use of vaccines in the civilian population of the United States. There are 15 voting members (14 with expertise in the areas of immunology, vaccinology, family medicine, pediatrics, infectious disease, virology, public health, and/or preventive medicine, and one member who is a consumer representative, offering perspectives on the community and social aspects of vaccination). There are also eight ex officio members representing other federal agencies that are involved in other US immunization programs and another 30 non-voting representatives of partner organizations that add immunization expertise. The Advisory Committee on Immunization Practices (ACIP) meets at the CDC in Atlanta three times each year, and meetings are open to the public.[14]

The Food and Drug Administration

As learned earlier in the chapter, the FDA is involved in the development and oversight of vaccines, from the Investigational New Drug approval phase to inspection of manufacturing facilities and oversight of labeling, to monitoring of purity and potency in the production phase of vaccine development. They also comanage the VAERS with the CDC and, in 2009, began the Post-Licensure Rapid Immunization Safety Monitoring (PRISM) program. PRISM uses data from national health insurance plans and immunization registries, which represent millions of individuals over geographically diverse areas, to monitor the safety of vaccines.[15]

The National Institutes of Health

The NIH administers the Vaccine Research Center (VRC) as part of the National Institute of Allergy and Infectious Diseases under its Intramural Research Program. It also provides biomedical research funding to non-NIH research facilities through its

Extramural Research Program. The mission of the VRC is to "conduct research that facilitates the development of effective vaccines for human disease."[16] The VRC is currently working on development of vaccines for HIV/AIDS, Ebola, and a more universal influenza vaccine.

The Health Resources and Services Administration

The HRSA administers the NVICP—established under the NCVIA—to compensate individuals who experience certain health events following immunization (see **Box 5.2**, The Vaccine Injury Table, for a list of each vaccine-associated event). Individuals are compensated on a "no-fault" basis, meaning that they are not required to prove fault/negligence on the part of the medical provider or manufacturer to receive compensation. Also housed under the HRSA is the Advisory Commission on Childhood Vaccines (ACCV). The ACCV "advises and makes recommendations to the Secretary of the DHHS on issues relating to the operation of the NVICP," helping to provide oversight and recommend improvements to the program.[17]

 Box 5.2   The Vaccine Injury Table

The Vaccine Injury Table is a comprehensive list of conditions felt to be most likely caused by vaccines—https://www.hrsa.gov/sites/default/files/vaccinecompensation/vaccineinjurytable.pdf.

Privately Funded Organizations

The Immunization Action Coalition

This organization is funded largely by educational grants and donations. Its website lists the following contributors: The National Center for Immunization and Respiratory Diseases (an agency of the CDC), the EJ Wexler and Mark and Muriel Wexler Foundations, the Herbert and Jeanne Mayer Foundation, other anonymous foundation contributors, pharmaceutical companies, the Physician's Alliance of America, Inc., the American Pharmacists Association, as well as other private individuals and organizations. Its mission is to "increase immunization rates and prevent disease by creating and distributing educational materials for healthcare professionals and the public that enhance the delivery of safe and effective immunization services. The Coalition also facilitates communication about the safety, efficacy, and use of vaccines within the broad immunization community of patients, parents, healthcare organizations, and government health agencies."[18]

The Institute for Safe Medication Practices

The Institute for Safe Medication Practices (ISMP) is a 501c[3] nonprofit organization devoted to the prevention of medication errors. As an "independent watchdog organization, ISMP receives no advertising revenue and depends entirely on charitable donations, educational grants, newsletter subscriptions, and volunteer efforts to pursue its life-saving work." The ISMP collects and analyzes "reports of medication-related hazardous conditions, near-misses, errors, and other adverse drug events." Working alongside a variety of patient-safety and educational institutions, as well as government agencies, they conduct research; educate the community about safe medication practices; and support the use of safe medication standards throughout the pharmaceutical, health care, and regulatory industries.[19]

A DEEPER DIVE INTO THE VACCINE ADVERSE EVENTS REPORTING SYSTEM

A misunderstanding of how VAERS works often contributes to the false conclusion that vaccines commonly cause serious adverse events. The following paragraphs take a deeper dive into VAERS to elucidate its role and to help clear up misunderstandings.[20] Although no vaccine or other medical intervention is risk-free, very serious and life-threatening adverse reactions are exceedingly rare. As a passive reporting system, meaning it does not proactively seek out possible untoward vaccine-related events but relies on voluntary reporting (from institutions and health care providers, patients, parents and caregivers, and others) to collect data, VAERS cannot draw conclusions regarding whether a vaccine did or did not cause a particular event or reaction.

There are relatively common reactions to vaccines that are noted in initial testing (such as pain at an injection site or low-grade fever). However, if a reaction is very rare, it may only be discovered by ongoing monitoring after the vaccine is administered to hundreds and thousands or millions of people. Vaccines are also studied in relatively healthy study participants. We may, then, expect to see different or more common reactions after vaccines are administered on a larger scale to those in special populations, with chronic illness or pregnant women for example. VAERS findings do not suggest causality. VAERS primarily serves as an early warning tool. It functions best as a safety signal detection and hypothesis generating system. Understanding this is vital to drawing proper conclusions about VAERS data (**Box 5.3**).

 **Box 5.3   Interpretation of VAERS Data**

Advisory Guide to the Interpretation of VAERS Data—https://wonder.cdc.gov/wonder/help/vaers/VAERS%20Advisory%20Guide.htm.

To help understand the language used in the VAERS reporting data, we must first define some terms.

- A *vaccine adverse event* or an *AEFI* is an adverse health event or health problem that occurs after administration of a vaccine. These events are associated in time with the vaccine administration but may or may not be caused by the vaccine. AEFIs are also related to product quality concerns, anxiety-related events, and vaccine administration errors, as well as those related to inherent properties of the vaccine. An example of an AEFI might be fainting following vaccine administration.

- A *vaccine adverse reaction* or *vaccine adverse effect* are terms that indicate that there is a significant body of evidence to suggest that the adverse health event was indeed caused by vaccination. Examples of vaccine adverse reactions would be things such as redness and swelling at the injection site.

VAERS accepts all reports, whether they be adverse events following immunization or whether they be adverse reactions, without placing judgment on their clinical importance.

There is no time limit on how far past immunization a person can report a suspected adverse event. Of course, reporting is preferred as soon as an event or reaction is suspected so that follow-up data can be gathered more easily. Reports are reviewed and are assigned medical terms for adverse events using the Medical Dictionary for Regulatory Activities to systematically encode information reported to VAERS. Certified coders and software systems are used to facilitate consistency in reporting. These reports are then categorized as serious or nonserious according to the FDA regulatory definitions. Serious events include one or more of the following: death following vaccination, life-threatening health event, hospitalization following vaccination or a prolongation of hospitalization if the vaccine was administered during a hospital stay, or lasting disability.

Serious events are then further investigated by a VAERS contractor who will request health records, hospital discharge summaries, medical and lab results, death certificates, and autopsy reports. If there are serious events where a patient has not recovered, follow-up letters are sent a year later to gather further information. Each report is then placed into a continuously updated database that is then shared with the CDC and FDA that conduct further analysis (**Box 5.4**).

 Box 5.4   VAERS Reporting Data

Data from these reports, cleared of sensitive patient information, are available for viewing by the public at the following:
- VAERS website—www.vaers.hhs.gov/data/index
- CDC's WONDER (Wide-ranging Online Data for Epidemiological Research) site—https://wonder.cdc.gov/VAERS.html

Between 2011 and 2014 there were approximately 30,000 reports submitted annually. Only 7% of these were classified as serious. Health care professionals submitted 38% of the reports, 30% were submitted by vaccine manufacturers and 14% by patients and parents. Although most of the reports to VAERS do not signal a pattern of concern, there have been several cases where vaccine-related adverse reactions were successfully detected. For example, the original rotavirus [RotaShield] was noted to be associated with a higher than expected rate of intussusception in infants. The vaccine was subsequently pulled from the market, issues with the vaccine were addressed, and a safer product was made available to the public.

The strengths of VAERS are as follows:

- It has national reach.
- It is able to rapidly detect possible safety issues because of the size and diversity of the population that can submit reports.
- It includes detailed information about the vaccine in question, the characteristics of the vaccinated individual, and about the event itself.
- Its data are made available to the public, which provides an important transparency.

The weaknesses or limitations of VAERS are several:

- VAERS is subject to reporting bias (for example, common and less worrisome events/reactions are often underreported, whereas clinically serious conditions are reported more often). When the public looks at this information, it can, therefore, erroneously appear that serious conditions are common.
- VAERS can fall victim to "stimulated reporting," a situation where increased media attention and public awareness of an issue may result in increased reporting.
- Since VAERS data do not include an unvaccinated comparison group, it is impossible to compare rates of adverse events in vaccinated versus unvaccinated individuals to determine if vaccination is associated with a higher risk of a particular adverse event.
- Except on rare occasions (for example, when anaphylaxis occurs within an appropriate timeframe following vaccination and no other environmental triggers were encountered), it is generally not possible, using VAERS, to definitively state whether a serious event was caused by vaccination.

CONCLUSIONS YOU CAN SHARE WITH YOUR PATIENTS

- As interventions that are preventative and are given to healthy people, vaccines are rigorously scrutinized and safety standards are set high.
- Vaccines are some of the most highly regulated and monitored interventions that we have in medicine.
- Numerous publicly and privately funded organizations provide oversight of the vaccine production and administration process.
- Oversight does not end with bringing a vaccine to market but continues for decades to follow.
- Drug companies should expect to make a profit on vaccines. If their products didn't make a profit, they wouldn't stay in business. Their returns on investment for vaccines are a minimal part of their profit margin, however.
- VAERS is a passive monitoring system. It cannot prove or disprove causality. It detects signals of possible adverse events that can then be further investigated and studied.

- The NVICP[a] was started, not as an admission of common harm caused by vaccines, but as an attempt to ensure compensation for those suffering from the known, but rare serious harms from vaccines, and to remove the threat of litigation from drug manufacturers, so that they can continue to produce these life-saving interventions. Without the NVICP, we would risk seeing drug companies lose motivation to continue production. This could result in vaccine shortages, greater risk of illness recurrence in the community, and higher cost to patients.

---

[a]Though enacted with the best of intentions, the NVICP is an imperfect program. The intention of Congress in its formation under the National Childhood Vaccine Injury Act (NCVIA) was to compensate the victims of vaccine injury more rapidly and in a more informal and less adversarial manner than lawsuits heard in civil court, to ensure the vaccine supply, and, in not limiting litigation of pharmaceutical companies for vaccine design defects, to contribute to ensuring safety of the vaccine supply. Additionally, under the NCVIA, the Secretary of the DHHS is granted discretionary authority to alter the Vaccine Injury Table (VIT), allowing injuries associated with vaccines developed in the future to be added.

In practice, however, the process of pursuing a claim through the NVICP is lengthy and no less adversarial than civil court. Moreover, despite the addition of multiple new vaccines to the recommended regimen since the Act was instituted, few new compensable events have been added to the VIT (some might argue that very few serious adverse events occur following these vaccinations). The Secretary of the DHHS has even removed some compensable events (seizures following DPT administration, for example) and narrowed the definition of other conditions making it, in effect, more difficult to seek compensation.

It is also important to know that the NVICP does not apply to all vaccines, only those listed in the VIT. The shingles vaccine, for example, is not included on the VIT. Compensation related to harm presumably caused by nonincluded vaccines may be sought in civil court. Additionally, vaccines and other measures utilized during declared public health emergencies are not subject to the NCVIA. In 2005, Congress passed the Public Readiness and Emergency Preparedness (PREP) Act to further protect manufacturers and all medical administrators of covered countermeasures used to respond to biological and chemical threats or illness pandemics. A claim made under the PREP Act cannot be adjudicated under NVICP. The PREP Act sets up its own Countermeasures Injury Compensation Program (CICP) with its own Countermeasures Injury Table. Moreover, as opposed to the NVICP, which requires claims to be made within 3 years of vaccine administration, the CICP offers only a 1 year statute of limitations. "With effective access only to an administrative tribunal, with a one-year statute of limitations, and with no opportunity for appeal or review in any court, consumers have exceptionally limited recourse under the PREP Act."[21]

Although it is important to acknowledge the benefits of the NVICP, it is also important to acknowledge its limitations. We must continue to seek ways to keep the pharmaceutical industry accountable to the ethical and safe production of vaccines and support the processes in place to report and detect adverse reactions so that our vaccine supply grows even safer over time.

References

1. Bren L. The road to the biotech revolution—highlights of 100 years of biologics regulation. *FDA Consum.* 2006;40(1):50-57.

2. Fitzpatrick M. The Cutter incident: how America's first polio vaccine led to a growing vaccine crisis (review). *J R Soc Med.* 2006;99(3):156.

3. Colgrove JK. The Cutter incident: how America's first polio vaccine led to a growing vaccine crisis (review). *Bull Hist Med.* 2007;81(3):677-678.

4. Centers for Disease Control and Prevention. History of Vaccine Safety. https://www.cdc.gov/vaccinesafety/ensuringsafety/history/index.html. Accessed December 19, 2018.

5. George Washington University. *Producing Prevention: The Complex Development of Vaccines.* Milken Institute School of Public Health. February 15, 2017. https://publichealthonline.gwu.edu/blog/producing-prevention-the-complex-development-of-vaccines/. Accessed December 19, 2018.

6. Vaccine Event Reporting System. About VAERS. https://vaers.hhs.gov/about.html. Accessed December 19, 2018.

7. Centers for Disease Control and Prevention. Vaccine Safety Datalink. https://www.cdc.gov/vaccinesafety/ensuringsafety/monitoring/vsd/index.html. Accessed December 19, 2018.

8. Hurford I. *How Much Does It Cost to Research and Develop a Vaccine? Effective Altruism Forum.* February 23, 2018. https://forum.effectivealtruism.org/posts/BjBmcfwg2awqPJLin/how-much-does-it-cost-to-research-and-develop-a-vaccine. Accessed December 19, 2018.

9. Régnier SA, Huels J. Drug versus vaccine investment: a modelled comparison of economic incentives. *Cost Eff Resour Alloc.* 2013;11:23.

10. Mello MM, Abiola S, Colgrove J. Pharmaceutical companies' role in state vaccination policymaking: the case of human papillomavirus vaccination. *Am J Public Health.* 2012;102(5):893-898.

11. Centers for Disease Control and Prevention. Vaccination safety. In: Hamborsky J, Kroger A, Wolfe C, eds. *Epidemiology and Prevention of Vaccine-Preventable Diseases.* 13th ed. Washington, DC: Public Health Foundation; 2015. https://www.cdc.gov/vaccines/pubs/pinkbook/downloads/safety.pdf. Updated September 8, 2015. Accessed December 19, 2018.

12. U.S. Department of Health & Human Services. National Vaccine Program Office (NVPO). https://www.hhs.gov/nvpo/index.html. Accessed December 19, 2018.

13. Centers for Disease Control and Prevention. Emergency Preparedness for Vaccine Safety. Accessed December 19, 2018. https://www.cdc.gov/vaccinesafety/ensuringsafety/monitoring/emergencypreparedness/index.html.

14. Centers for Disease Control and Prevention. *Advisory Committee on Immunization Practices Policies and Procedures.* January 2018. https://www.cdc.gov/vaccines/acip/committee/downloads/Policies-Procedures-508.pdf. Accessed December 19, 2018.

15. Nguyen M, Ball R, Midthun K, et al. The Food and drug Administration's post-licensure Rapid immunization safety monitoring program: strengthening the federal vaccine safety enterprise. *Pharmacoepidemiol Drug Saf.* 2012;21(S1):291-297.

16. National Institute of Allergy and Infectious Diseases. Vaccine Research Center. https://www.niaid.nih.gov/about/vrc. Accessed December 19, 2018.

17. Health Resources & Services Administration. Federal Advisory Committees: Advisory Commission on Childhood Vaccines (ACCV). https://www.hrsa.gov/advisory-committees/vaccines/index.html. Accessed December 19, 2018.

18. Immunization Action Coalition. About Us. www.immunize.org/aboutus/. Updated April 17, 2018. Accessed December 19, 2018.

19. Institute for Safe Medication Practices. ISMP Mission and Vision. https://www.ismp.org/about/mission. Accessed December 19, 2018.

20. Shimabukuro TT, Nguyen M, Martin D, et al. Safety monitoring in the vaccine adverse event reporting system (VAERS). *Vaccine.* 2015;33(36):4398-4405.

21. Holland MS. Liability for vaccine injury: the United States, the European Union, and the developing world. *Emory L J.* 2018;67(3):415-462.

Catching Flies: Approach Matters

A spoonful of honey will catch more flies than a gallon of vinegar.

—Benjamin Franklin

Although the origins and exact meaning of Franklin's phrase are debated, it is generally understood to be a cautionary statement used to convey the notion that approaching someone with words of kindness and understanding is a more successful way to bring them around to your way of thinking than using caustic or acidic statements. If we think about our own interactions when we have disagreed with someone, be it spouse or parent or child, we inherently know this to be true. How do we feel in a discussion when someone comes at us in anger or bitterness? How do we feel when we are cut off mid-sentence? How do we feel when we are speaking and the other person is rolling their eyes or sighing? For most of us, it becomes very difficult to want to understand the other person's point of view. We feel defensive. The listening, understanding, empathetic part of our brains shut down. We tend to become only that much more entrenched in our way of thinking, no longer willing to consider discussion.

This is what can happen if we don't approach our vaccine-hesitant patients with empathy, with a welcoming way, and with words that unite as we try to understand their point of view. They will sense our irritation, they will feel spoken down to, and they will be less likely to hear and accept the vaccine education that we are trying to offer. I know that this is easier said than done. When we find ourselves having a conversation with a vaccine-questioning patient for the fifth time that day, it can be difficult to hide the frustration we feel. But we must. If we want to give ourselves the best chance of success, we must go into each conversation remembering that patients are coming to us as their trusted provider, that they are not trying to make our lives more difficult, and that they are just trying to do what is best for themselves and for their families. They are looking to us to help them make sense of what they are hearing about vaccines on their Facebook feed or from their family and friends.

HOUSTON, WE HAVE A PROBLEM

Science and medicine in the United States currently have a public relations problem. A study by the Robert Wood Johnson foundation and the National Institute of Mental Health, looking at polling data of public trust in physicians between 1966 and 2014, shows a significant decrease in public trust over the decades. In 1966, 73% of Americans expressed great confidence in leaders of the medical profession compared with only 34%

in 2012. A 2014 Gallup poll found only 23% of Americans have great confidence in the medical system as a whole.[1] And although the public generally trusts scientists to understand and communicate the science in their area of expertise more than it trusts others who may comment upon scientific progress (such as the media, business leaders, and elected officials), that level of trust is still not very good. A PEW study looking at public trust of medical, climate, and genetically modified food scientists showed that, for example, only 35% of adults had "soft trust in medical scientists to give full and accurate information about the effects of the MMR vaccine," and medical scientists were the *most* trusted of the three groups. "These findings," the study states, "suggest that the authority of scientists to speak on matters directly relevant to their expertise is often met with some skepticism."[2]

The reasons for this mistrust and skepticism are multifactorial and much of it is out of doctors' and scientists' control. Physicians have less time to spend in each office visit, which often leads to decreasing opportunities to develop a close rapport with patients and families. In addition to the time barriers we encounter, the electronic medical record puts an actual physical barrier between patient and physician. A doctor's time is eaten up with administrative tasks, and our ability to act in the best interests of our patients is sometimes hindered by insurance company roadblocks. Health care costs are rising, but we are not necessarily seeing much improvement in chronic disease or mortality rates. Even though satisfaction with one's individual provider remains relatively high,[1] we are losing public confidence as a profession. For their part, scientists participate in work that, by its very nature, puts forward assertions that are sometimes found to be faulty or, at least, not reproducible. To a public who may not understand the importance of viewing scientific studies on the whole and not individually, and who may not see the benefit of Edison's purported statement, "I have not failed 10,000 times...I have succeeded in proving that those 10,000 ways will not work,"[3] this can erode trust in the scientific process.

LANGUAGE MATTERS

In thinking about the divide between medicine, science, and the public, let's look at something that we *do* have control over—words. The language that we use when talking to patients likely plays a role in our successes or failures in getting our vaccine messaging across. Given the aforementioned uphill battle that we are fighting with respect to the confidence and trust that patients have in physicians as a whole, the words that we use in trying to explain the science and data behind the safety of vaccines take on great importance. I certainly don't lay all of the blame for eroded confidence (or even the majority of the blame) at the feet of scientific language, but I do feel we have to acknowledge the role that our language plays. Communication is key. The Independent Monitoring Board of the Global Polio Eradication Initiative sums up the issue, noting concern over "the Global Programme's weak grip on the communications and social mobilization that could not just neutralize communities' negativity, but generate more genuine demand. Within the Programme, communications is the poor cousin of vaccine delivery, undeservedly receiving far less focus. Communications expertise is sparse throughout and needs to be strengthened."[4]

The words we choose can either make patients feel comfortable with the information we are providing them or put an unintentional distance between us. When we go to medical school or graduate school in the sciences, we essentially learn another language—the language of Science. It is a hybrid of Latin, Greek, German, French, and other languages that takes us 4 or more years to learn and is peppered with acronyms (NSTEMI, EMDR, ARI, COPD, etc.) that are even difficult for those of us in the sciences to keep track of. When explaining scientific information to patients, we must speak in a way that is, of course, respectful but also accessible and understandable to someone who doesn't speak our language. By providing them with easily digestible information, we can help win back their confidence.

In discussing vaccines with our patients, we often entreat them not to rely on what they read on Facebook or Twitter or what the "mommy blogger" they follow is telling them. We encourage them to "do their own research" and not take blog posts or news stories at face value. However, accessing primary source research studies and then understanding that research proves difficult for the average nonmedical, non–science-trained person. Currently, accessing many research articles requires signing up or registering with a research clearing house of sorts, such as PubMed and ScienceDirect. Often, these sites require affiliation with a university or other system that conducts research or payment to access individual papers, the cost of which can be prohibitive (for medical and nonmedical persons alike). A 2016 article in *The New York Times* states that "legally downloading a single journal article when you don't have a subscription costs around $30, which adds up quickly considering a search on even narrow topics can return hundreds if not thousands of articles."[5] In fact, Harvard University, the article reports, with one of the largest academic library budgets in the world, is having a hard time affording the costs of journal subscriptions.[5] And even if the articles are free, the requirement to prove credentials can be off-putting to someone without those credentials.

Although the scientific community is slowly beginning to make primary research articles more readily available through open access journals (like those under the umbrella of the Public Library of Science, or PloS, for example) and other means, the scientific information that is generally available can be very intimidating to the lay reader. In truth, if they are highly specialized articles, they are sometimes even difficult for general medical providers to comprehend. Take the following as an example. It is a segment of an article, titled "Innate Immunity and Toll-like Receptors: Clinical Implications of Basic Science Research," which was published in the April 2004 issue of the *Journal of Pediatrics*: "These receptors bind molecular structures that are expressed by microbes but are not expressed by the human host, eg, lipopolysaccharides (LPS) or double-stranded RNA (dsRNA). Activation of these receptors initiates an inflammatory cascade that attempts to clear the offending pathogen and set in motion a specific adaptive immune response."[6]

Asking a patient to read and understand this statement would be like asking those of us not trained in finance and accounting to understand the following phrase: "Apply to those EPS and/or EBITDA estimates an appropriate P/E ratio or EV to EBITDA ratio based on the following: Industry identification."[7]

For me, and likely for many of you, the finance statement written above is confusing. I have no idea what it means. This is probably how many of our patients feel if asked to read scientific research studies. We need to be available to them to act as interpreters of the scientific information that they are now coming across. And then there's the fact that the words we use in medicine and science often mean something entirely different to patients and the lay public. Take, for example, the word "negative." In medicine, we say this to mean that a test result was normal. However, to most patients, the word "negative" has a negative connotation. It can create significant worry to hear that "Your test results were negative," until results are further explained. Breaking down the data for patients in words and concepts that they can understand and that are meaningful to them will go a long way to helping them feel more comfortable with the information we are trying to present (**Box 6.1**).

Box 6.1   Did You Know?

Other than to serve as a source of confusion when trying to order vaccines, did you know that the capital and lowercase letters in a vaccine (for example, DTaP vs Tdap) have meaning? Uppercase letters mean that the vaccine has a full-strength dose of that component of the vaccine. Lowercase letters mean that the vaccine uses a smaller amount of that particular component in the vaccine. So, for example, in the Tdap immunization, there are full-strength tetanus and lesser-strength diphtheria and pertussis components of that vaccine. This is the "adult" version of the vaccine, given to people aged 10 and older. For younger children, we use the full-strength dose of all three components (DTaP). The "a" in both vaccines means that the pertussis component is "acellular," contrasted with the DTP vaccine (no longer used in the United States), which had a whole-cell pertussis component.[8]

A WAY FORWARD

Those of us currently in practise have not been given specific training on how to translate basic science research and medical concepts into common and easy-to-understand language. We have figured it out through trial and error. But scientists and researchers are beginning to recognize the problems that this communication breakdown is causing. Denial of scientific facts, be it in the area of vaccinations, climate change, or evolution, among others, is real and is becoming increasingly common. In the public health sector, this disconnect is a particular problem as the "change agents who can make the biggest difference in improving health behaviors and social and environmental conditions are generally nonscientists outside of the health professions."[9] Consequently, research is being done and models are being tested to help find ways to successfully educate our future scientists in improved methods of communication and engagement with the public, as well as encouraging the news media to be more responsible to the weight of evidence when writing or talking about one of these "controversial" topics.[10]

Brownell et al. conducted a study on incorporating skills training for communicating science to a layperson audience in undergraduate and graduate students enrolled in the Immunology Program in the School of Medicine at Stanford University. The researchers found a positive impact on the students' self-confidence in communicating science to a lay audience as well as an improved confidence in their basic writing skills.[11,12] Susanne Pelger, in her article titled "Popular Science Writing Bringing New Perspectives into Science Students' Theses," found in similar research that "popular science writing offers a cognitive tool to widen science students' perspectives, and hence, to promote their development of scientific literacy and achievement of scientific writing skills."[13] Still others have proposed the use of science liaisons, a job description currently requiring a PhD, PharmD, or MD. Science liaisons are typically employed in the pharmaceutical, biotechnology, medical device, and other health care industries to maintain peer-peer relationships with key thought leaders (physicians and researchers) at major academic institutions and clinics.[14] Instead of working to develop relationships within the halls of science and industry, however, this newly imagined liaison would serve to communicate and maintain relationships with those who don't have a science background—the lay public, news media, and government officials.

The words we choose and the access granted to patients to try to understand the science behind our vaccine recommendations are extremely important to our endeavors to convince them of the benefit and safety of vaccines. However, there are other factors in the vaccine discussion that are equally as important to keep in mind when working with our questioning or hesitant patients. The remainder of this chapter is devoted to looking at those other factors—proven motivational interviewing approaches that will help you maintain a strong rapport with your patients. These approaches will allow your patients to feel listened to, their concerns heard and respected, and will facilitate getting your message across in a way that the patient or parent will be most likely to accept.

THE PRESUMPTIVE VERSUS PARTICIPATORY APPROACH

The practice of medicine is much different than it used to be. Our technological age has made information more readily available and, despite some of the roadblocks discussed earlier in the chapter, has allowed patients to become increasingly savvy about topics in science and medicine. Patients are significantly more informed than in prior years and the era of "paternalistic medicine," the father-knows-best, do-as-I-say approach to care, is over. Patients now expect to be involved in the decision making about their care. They want to have discussions about the pros and cons of various treatments rather than simply following their provider's recommendation without question. This is a good thing. With patients being participants in their care decisions, they also assume partial responsibility for the outcomes of those decisions. For the majority of our discussions with patients, this shared decision making, termed the *participatory approach*, is very appropriate and is the best course of action.

However, when it comes to the vaccine discussion, it turns out that the participatory approach can introduce doubt into the patient's or parent's mind. In the case of vaccines, what has a much higher rate of success is the *presumptive approach*.[15] This approach goes into the conversation presuming that the patient or parent is going to accept the vaccine recommendation. It leaves no room for doubt that this is what we feel is best for that person's health. Let's look at some examples of these approaches in action.

Participatory approach
   "What would you like to do about vaccines today?"

Presumptive approach
   "Today we need to do your tetanus, HPV, and meningitis vaccines."

You can see how the participatory approach can engender doubts. Parents might be thinking, "Why is the doctor asking me what I want to do about vaccines? Is there some reason we shouldn't be doing the recommended vaccines?" Whereas the presumptive approach helps patients and parents to see that you are firmly committed to your recommendation. Research shows that provider recommendation is the most influential factor in parents' decisions to vaccinate their child, so having a strong message is extremely important.[16]

The glaring difference between these two approaches was demonstrated in a study by Douglas Opel, MD, et al. looking at success rates for acceptance of vaccines when each of these approaches was used during vaccine counseling sessions with parents of 1- to 19-month-old children at their routine health supervision visits. The study looked at both the routinely recommended childhood vaccines and the flu shot (the study was conducted from September 2011 to August 2012), a vaccine that people inherently are less likely to accept without question. The results were virtually identical. When the participatory approach was used, only about 4% of patients were likely to accept vaccines recommended by the provider by the end of the visit, the remainder either refusing (83%) or providing an alternate plan (13%) for vaccines. However, when the presumptive approach was used, a whopping 74% of patients were willing to get the recommended shots, with only 26% continuing to decline. Opel et al. then went on to look at how many parents opted for vaccination after initially declining if the provider continued to pursue their recommendation. Of those parents that were vaccine-resistant at first, 47% went on to accept the vaccines if the provider continued to encourage their initial plan for immunization.[15]

Some may worry that the presumptive approach closes off discussion about vaccines and doesn't allow informed consent. They may feel that they are "bullying" their patient into submitting to vaccines. However, simply stating that the plan is for vaccination doesn't eliminate the possibility of discussion. If you are paying attention to facial expressions and body cues, you will still get a sense of whether the patient or parents are all-in or have persistent doubts. If detecting continued doubts or concerns, you can follow your declaration with further inquiry. "Today we need to do the tetanus, HPV, and meningitis vaccines." Pause. Observe. "I sense that you might have some questions about these vaccines. Tell me what concerns you have." This gives the patient or parent an opening to express any hesitation and lets them know that you are open to a discussion. As for informed consent, if we are reviewing the common risks, such as "Anna might feel a bit under the weather for a day or so or even have a low-grade fever. We consider this a normal reaction when the immune system is kicking into gear after a shot," and ensuring the patient receives a Vaccine Information Statement, then we are providing adequate informed consent. We certainly don't want to bully our patients into a decision that they aren't comfortable with, but we do want to give them the security of knowing that we are fully confident in our recommendations.

THE C.A.S.E, 3-AS, AND A.S.K. APPROACHES TO THE VACCINE DISCUSSION

Health care providers describe a variety of perceived barriers to effective vaccine counseling. For instance, we have a limited amount of time with our patients; we don't have the resources we need to provide vaccines (when the clinic orders too few vaccines, or if the clinic can't afford to offer certain immunizations because of inadequate reimbursement); and we lack confidence in addressing the multitude of patients' very specific concerns about vaccines.[17] Providers also sometimes worry that strong encouragement of vaccines may create an adversarial relationship with our vaccine-hesitant patients. Certainly, there are approaches that may engender hostility; the vaccinate-or-find-another-doctor approach would be unlikely to go over well with most vaccine-hesitant patients. However, there are ways to tackle the vaccine discussion that are effective in leaving both you and your patient feeling like you are on the same team, working together to make the best decisions possible for them or for their child.

TABLE 6.1 C.A.S.E. Approach

Corroborate	Acknowledge the patient's concerns and find some points on which you can agree.
About me	Describe what you have done to build your expertise on the subject.
Science	Review the data and science behind the vaccines.
Explain/Advise	Explain your recommendations, based on the science.

(Adapted from Autism Science Foundation. Making the Case for Vaccines. http://autismsciencefoundation.org/wp-content/uploads/2015/12/Making-the-CASE-for-Vaccines-Guide_final.pdf. Accessed January 1, 2019.)

The C.A.S.E (Corroborate, About me, Science, Explain/Advise) approach to motivational interviewing **(Table 6.1)** was developed by Alison Singer of the Autism Science Foundation,[18] a nonprofit organization whose mission is to "support autism research by providing funding and other assistance to scientists and organizations conducting, facilitating, publicizing and disseminating autism research. The organization also provides information about autism to the general public and serves to increase awareness of autism spectrum disorders and the needs of individuals and families affected by autism."[19] The C.A.S.E. approach has proven to be an effective way to acknowledge the patient's concerns, instill confidence that you are well-versed in the science to be able to address those concerns, and then educate them about the facts and why you feel a particular vaccine is so important.[20] Let's look at a conversation between provider and patient with the C.A.S.E. approach at work:

Provider: *"We are coming up on flu season again. Let's make sure to protect Lily and get her flu shot while you are here today."*

Parent: *"I'm not so sure I want her to have the shot. I heard it can actually make you sick."*

C—Corroborate

Acknowledge the patient's concerns and find some point on which you can agree.

"It sounds like we both want to keep Lily healthy and safe. If the flu shot actually caused the flu, I wouldn't want her to get it either."

A—About me

Describe what you have done to build your expertise on the subject.

"I have been practicing medicine for 18 years and have spent a great deal of time researching the data on vaccinations. Because the flu strains change year to year, I'm particularly interested in the effectiveness of the flu shot."

S—Science

Review the data and science behind the vaccines.

"The flu shot is actually a killed virus vaccine. That means there is no live or active virus in it so it cannot make you sick. Any vaccine can cause a person to feel a little achy or under the weather for a day or two, but that is just your immune system revving up to protect you from the real infection. The body's reaction to the real flu would be much worse."

E—Explain/Advise

Explain your recommendations, based on the science.

"The flu causes hundreds of thousands of hospitalizations and tens of thousands of deaths every year. Of those that died from the flu, 80% to 90% were not vaccinated. I vaccinate my own children to protect them from what can be a very serious illness and this is why I recommend the flu vaccine for your child as well."

TABLE 6.2 The 3-As Approach

Ask	Don't stop with a "No" response. Dig a little deeper.
Acknowledge	Acknowledge the patient's or parent's concerns.
Advise	Advise patients of the facts about vaccines and provide a strong recommendation to vaccinate.

(Data from Hendrikson NB, Opel DJ, Grothaus L, et al. Physician communication training and parental vaccine hesitancy: A randomized trial. Pediatrics. 2015;136:70-79.)

The 3-As (Ask, Acknowledge, Advise) technique **(Table 6.2)** is another approach, studied by Hendrickson, Opel, and partners, in order to test the effectiveness of engaging patients and parents in a respectful, open discussion about vaccines.[21,22] Like the C.A.S.E. approach, it is meant to help us develop a rapport and trusting relationship with our patients while allowing us to educate in a nonjudgmental manner. Let's look at the conversation below.

Provider: *"It's time to do Max's shots. These include some he's had before and, additionally, the MMR, chickenpox, and hepatitis A vaccines."*

Parent: *"I'm fine with the ones he's had before and the hepatitis A and chickenpox shots, but I don't think I want to do the MMR vaccine today."*

A—Ask

Don't just stop with a "No" response. Respectfully dig a little deeper.

"What questions do you have about the vaccines we are recommending today? Tell me what worries you about the MMR vaccine."

A—Acknowledge

Acknowledge the patient's or parent's concerns.

"You are obviously a very caring parent and I know that you want to make the best decision you can for your child. With all the different information that we see on the news and social media, it's not always easy to know what to believe about vaccines."

A—Advise

Advise patients of the facts about vaccines and provide a strong recommendation to vaccinate.

"The original study suggesting a link between MMR and autism included only 12 children. That original study was found to be fraudulent and none of the subsequent studies, looking at hundreds of thousands of children, have found a link between the MMR vaccine and autism. Not vaccinating can leave Max at risk for some very serious infections. I

TABLE 6.3 A.S.K. Approach

Acknowledge concerns	Acknowledge your patient's concerns and ask questions to clarify those concerns.
Steer the conversation	Refute myths and keep the conversation open for future discussion.
Knowledge	Provide tailored information, reinforce your message with discussion of the benefit of vaccination, offer further reading material, and provide a strong recommendation.

(Data from Morgana T, Pringle J. Approaches to families questioning vaccines—the ASK approach for effective immunization communication. Presented at: 48th Annual Meeting of the Infectious Diseases Society of America; October 23, 2010; Vancouver, BC. Abstract 92.)

particularly worry about measles, which is making a comeback and can cause severe illness and death. I care about Max and that is why I strongly advise the MMR vaccine."

A.S.K. (Acknowledge concerns, Steer the conversation, and Know your facts) **(Table 6.3)** is yet another stepwise approach to effective communication with vaccine-hesitant patients that feels relatively intuitive and can be easily incorporated into your vaccine counseling sessions.[23,24] Here is what this approach looks like in action.

Provider: *"Okay, Mrs. Jones. Since you have a brand new grandchild you'll be taking care of, I would highly recommend we update your pertussis, or whooping cough, protection by giving you a Tdap vaccine."*

Patient: *"But I'm not due for a tetanus shot for another couple of years and I had whooping cough as a kid myself."*

A—Acknowledge concerns

Acknowledge your patient's concerns and ask questions to clarify those concerns.

"I'm really glad you've kept up-to-date on your vaccines and these are common questions when we recommend a vaccination earlier than the normal schedule would suggest."

"Tell me what you've heard about whooping cough infections and the Tdap vaccine."

S—Steer the conversation

Refute myths and keep the conversation open for future discussion.

"It's common to think that once you've had whooping cough you can't get it again, but our immunity eventually wears off. We, of course, don't want you to get sick again. But by vaccinating you, we're really protecting your new grandchild."

"Consider talking to your son and daughter-in-law to find out how they feel about protecting their child from whooping cough. If you opt against it today, you can always change your mind and come back for a nurse visit to get it done."

K—Know your facts

Provide tailored information, reinforce your message with discussion of the benefit of vaccination, offer further reading materials, and provide a strong recommendation.

"Whooping cough can be deadly to babies in their first months of life. They are not old enough to get the vaccine themselves, so they rely on a bubble of protection from those around them."

"The Tdap vaccine is safe to get sooner than every 10 years. In fact, we recommend it to pregnant women towards the end of every pregnancy, even if those pregnancies are only a year apart. This vaccine has significantly reduced hospitalizations and deaths from whooping cough."

"Would you like some resources to do further reading about whooping cough and the Tdap vaccine?"

"The best protection for your grandchild is to immunize all of those he'll be spending time with, so let's give you your Tdap vaccine today."

If done properly, the C.A.S.E., 3-As, and A.S.K. approaches will leave both provider and patient satisfied that the other has heard their concerns. Even if your patients ultimately still decide not to vaccinate, they will be more willing to have further discussions because they know that you provide an environment that is open to dialogue and in which their opinions will not be judged.

And you never know. You might just change their mind. It may take persistence and more than a few conversations but they could come around. Let's consider an example from my own practice. I have a patient whom we'll call Sarah who has been in my practice for many years. Every year, we discuss preventive care options. I offer the flu shot, the pneumonia vaccine, the shingles vaccine, her colonoscopy, and so on. And every year, she declines—very respectfully and with voiced appreciation for my concern for her health—but still, she declines. Recently, Sarah came down with a terrible case of shingles. It affected her health for months. This year, when we sat down at her physical to discuss her preventive care options, she had changed her mind. This year she stated, "Shingles was so terrible. I never want to have anything like that happen again. I'm ready to do everything you've been recommending. Give me the shingles vaccine. Give me the flu shot. I'd like a referral for my colonoscopy." Not all changes of heart will be this dramatic, of course, but patients will have events happen in their lives that might bring about a change of mind. A relative may die of throat cancer or a friend may be hospitalized with complications from the flu. There's always the possibility that something will impact your patients' choices. Let them know that you care enough about their well-being to continue to offer vaccines and other preventive care measures.

How we broach the vaccine discussion matters greatly to our chances of success. We want the patient to come away knowing that it is natural to question and to want to know more when it comes to making important decisions about their health and the health of their loved ones. We applaud them for this. This is a good thing. In continuing the discussion, we want our patients to have access to trusted resources for factual information, and we want to use language in our discussion of vaccines that helps them feel like they fully grasp the science behind the safety and efficacy of immunizations. If someone expresses incorrect information and misunderstandings about vaccines, we must remember that it can be really difficult for patients and parents to know which information they read or hear should be believed, and which should not. There is so much bad information out there, and we want patients and parents to know that we don't find them personally misguided but that the information they are working with may be faulty or misleading. We want our patients to feel that we are on their side, that we are on their team, and that we are there to help them understand the research and to sort fact from fiction (see Appendix B: Fast Facts about Vaccines for Patients and Clinic Staff.). In partnering with our patients in this manner, we will be able to facilitate their healthy choices and improve vaccine acceptance.

References

1. Blendon RJ, Benson JM, Hero JO. Public trust in physicians – U.S. Medicine in International perspective. *N Engl J Med.* 2014;371:1570-1572.

2. Funk C. Mixed messages about public trust in science. *Issues Sci Technol.* Fall 2017;34(1). https://issues.org/real-numbers-mixed-messages-about-public-trust-in-science/.

3. Furr N. *How Failure Taught Edison to Repeatedly Innovate.* Forbes. June 9, 2011. Accessed January 15, 2019. https://www.forbes.com/sites/nathanfurr/2011/06/09/how-failure-taught-edison-to-repeatedly-innovate/#5e1e8b8665e9

4. World Health Organization. *Report of the SAGE Working Group on Vaccine Hesitancy.* November 12, 2014. https://www.who.int/immunization/sage/meetings/2014/october/SAGE_working_group_revised_report_vaccine_hesitancy.pdf?ua=1. Accessed January 1, 2019.

5. Murphy K. *Should All Research Papers be Free?* New York Times. March 12, 2016. https://www.nytimes.com/2016/03/13/opinion/sunday/should-all-research-papers-be-free.html. Accessed January 1, 2019.

6. Aubrey MT, Ardith M. Innate immunity and toll-like receptors: clinical implications of basic science research. *J Pediatr.* 2004;144(4):421-429.

7. Whitman MJ. *Value Investing: A Balanced Approach.* Hoboken, NJ: John Wiley & Sons, Inc; 2000.

8. Centers for Disease Control and Prevention. Diphtheria, Tetanus, and Whooping Cough Vaccination: What Everyone Should Know. https://www.cdc.gov/vaccines/vpd/dtap-Tdap-Td/public/index.html. Updated December 17, 2018. Accessed February 7, 2019.

9. Woolf SH, Purnell JQ, Simon SM, et al. Translating evidence into population health improvement: strategies and barriers. *Annu Rev Public Health.* 2015;36:463-482. https://www.annualreviews.org/doi/pdf/10.1146/annurev-publhealth-082214-110901.

10. Seppa N. *Science Denial in the 21st Century.* Science News. April 24, 2012. https://www.sciencenews.org/blog/scene/science-denial-21st-century. Accessed January 1, 2019.

11. Brownell SE, Price JV, Steinman L. A writing-intensive course improves biology undergraduates' perception and confidence of their abilities to read scientific literature and communicate science. *Adv Physiol Educ.* 2013;37:70-79. https://www.physiology.org/doi/full/10.1152/advan.00138.2012?url_ver=Z39.88-2003&rfr_id=ori%3Arid%3Acrossref.org&rfr_dat=cr_pub%3Dpubmed.

12. Brownell SE, Price JV, Steinman L. Science communication to the general public: why we need to teach undergraduate and graduate students this skill as part of their formal scientific training. *J Undergrad Neurosci Educ.* 2013;12(1):E6-E10.

13. Pelger S. Popular science writing bringing new perspective into science students' theses. *Int J Sci Educ B Commun Public Engagem.* 2018;8(1):e1-e13.

14. Medical Science Liaison Society. What is a Medical Science Liaison? https://www.themsls.org/what-is-an-msl/. Accessed January 1, 2019.

15. Opel DJ, Heritage J, Taylor JA, et al. The architecture of provider-parent vaccine discussions at health supervision visits. *Pediatrics.* 2013;132(6):1037-1046.

16. Paterson P, Maurice F, Stanberry LR, et al. Vaccine hesitancy and healthcare providers. *Vaccine.* 2016;34:6700-6706.

17. Esposito S, Principi N, Cornaglia G. Barriers to the vaccination of children and adolescents and possible solutions. *Clin Microbiol Infect.* 2014;20(5):25-32.

18. Autism Science Foundation. Making the Case for Vaccines. http://autismsciencefoundation.org/wp-content/uploads/2015/12/Making-the-CASE-for-Vaccines-Guide_final.pdf. Accessed January 1, 2019.

19. Autism Science Foundation. Mission Statement. https://autismsciencefoundation.org/about-asf/our-mission/. Accessed January 6, 2019.

20. Jacobson RM, Van Etta L, Bahia L. The C.A.S.E. approach: guidance for talking to vaccine hesitant patients. *Minn Med.* 2013;96:49-50.

21. Henrikson NB, Opel DJ, Grothaus L, et al. Physician communication training and parental vaccine hesitancy: a randomized trial. *Pediatrics.* 2015;136:70-79.

22. Loehr J, Savoy M. Strategies for addressing and Overcoming vaccine hesitancy. *Am Fam Physician.* 2016;94(2):94-96.

23. Morgana T, Pringle J. *Approaches to families questioning vaccines—the ASK approach for effective immunization communication.* Presented at: 48th Annual Meeting of the Infectious Diseases Society of America; October 23, 2010; Vancouver, BC. Abstract 92.

24. Domachowske JB, Suryadevara M. Practical approaches to vaccine hesitancy issues in the United States: 2013. *Hum Vaccin Immunother.* 2013;9(12):2654-2657.

7

A Risk Worth Taking

Nothing in life is to be feared, it is only to be understood. Now is the time to understand more, so that we may fear less.

—Marie Curie

In prior chapters, we touched on some of the unfounded claims that the anti-vaccine community makes about vaccines, medical providers who encourage immunization, pharmaceutical companies, and more. In the coming chapters, we will dispel the many myths about vaccines, but this chapter seeks to recognize and acknowledge the risks that *do* come with vaccinating. Contrary to what anti-vaccination supporters would assert, these risks are not being kept secret from patients to knowingly put them in harm's way. Instead, they are readily available for people to read about, and they are typically much less common or worrisome than people opposed to vaccination would have us believe.

Most of you know this, but if there are any nonmedical people reading this book (and I hope that there are), I want to make it clear that no doctor or scientist has ever claimed that vaccines are 100% safe. As we read in chapter 5, vaccines undergo rigorous testing and retesting, both before and after licensure, to discover any safety issues present. Many vaccines never make it to market because they either didn't achieve their goals or their risks were too great. But when a vaccine proves to be effective and safe enough for widespread use, like any other medical intervention, it still has possible risks. The staunch anti-vaccine folks are likely to take those last two sentences and twist them to make it sound as if doctors are knowingly harming people. So, let's put it into context (**Figure 7.1**).

The risk of major adverse reactions (anaphylaxis, Guillain-Barré syndrome [GBS], etc) happening as a result of vaccination is exceedingly small—1 to 2 persons in a million. This pales in comparison to the risks of the diseases themselves. Measles, for instance, results in hospitalization for 1 in 4; encephalitis with the possibility of permanent brain damage for 1 in 1000; and death for 1 to 2 in 1000 patients infected. Meningitis infection results in death for 10 to 15 out of 100 patients infected, even with proper treatment. And what about some of the other things we do every day without thinking about *their* potential risks? Seat belts, if improperly fitted, have the potential to injure or kill people, but we don't stop wearing seat belts.[4] We know that the benefit of wearing a seat belt in the event of a car crash far outweighs the risks of the seat belt itself. Physicians recommend exercise to everyone to maintain overall health and to reduce the incidence of heart disease, stroke, diabetes, and other serious diseases; yet, every year people are seriously injured or die while exercising.[5] Do we stop exercising because of what happens to those unfortunate few? No. We continue on because we know that the chance of serious injury is small compared with the greater benefit from getting regular exercise.

The Odds an American Will...

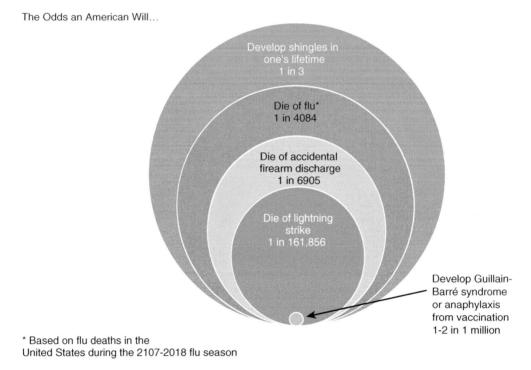

* Based on flu deaths in the
United States during the 2107-2018 flu season

FIGURE 7.1 These risks of common and uncommon events give perspective on the risks of vaccines.[3,10,11]

Now, should we do our best to make sure that these potential risks are minimized? For instance, should we ensure that our children's seat belts are fitted properly? Yes. Should we check with our physicians to make sure we are healthy enough to engage in a vigorous exercise program? Absolutely! Should we choose the proper people to receive live-attenuated vaccines so that we don't give an illness to someone whose immune system is compromised? Of course! Should we avoid giving a vaccine to someone during a serious illness or high fever? Most certainly! The point is, everything we do—in life and in medicine—has risks, and we *do* take measures to reduce those risks. The potential upside to pursuing preventative health measures is so great that we still do them despite the very minimal potential downside. We should think of vaccination in much the same way—the benefits far outweigh the risks.

That being said, we don't want to downplay the possible adverse effects of vaccination just like we wouldn't want to minimize the possible risks of any other intervention we do in medicine. We would never think of skipping a risk/benefit discussion with our patients who are headed into surgery, for example. We need to have a similar informed consent discussion when it comes to immunizations. However, I would argue that just handing someone a Vaccine Information Statement (VIS) prior to immunizing may not be adequate. How often do we thoroughly read the paperwork that we are given at the doctor's office? Providing the VIS is required and important, but providing verbal informed consent will likely be more meaningful. This doesn't mean that you have to have a long and detailed discussion of every possible risk and side effect of vaccines. Even a short discussion of the most common side effects following vaccination can set expectations so that patients and parents aren't surprised or unnecessarily frightened if they experience an adverse reaction.

I suspect two reasons for why many people believe that the flu shot can make them sick. The first is our failure to adequately express the limitations of the vaccine in the first 2 weeks after administration (that it takes 2 weeks for the vaccine to become fully effective). The second is our failure to caution our patient's about the common and normal symptoms of a person's immune system kicking into gear after vaccination (aches, fatigue, headache, low-grade fever, etc), an omission that leads people to attribute these symptoms to the flu shot making them "sick." Setting up appropriate expectations is key, and patients will have greater confidence that we are not trying to "pull one over on them" if we are up front about possible risks. So, what *are* some common and not-so-common side effects or risks of vaccines? This chapter seeks to answer this question while giving a bit of perspective so that we can see these risks for what they are—mild or highly uncommon.

RISKS THAT ARE COMMON TO ALL VACCINES

There are some generalities that we can make regarding possible side effects of all vaccines. Some are obvious, and one would think barely need mention, but others may be less intuitive and require some explanation so that patients know what to expect.

1. Vaccines hurt. Everyone's pain threshold is different, but we can generally say that receiving a vaccine will likely cause some mild discomfort, both at the time of injection and possibly for a few days following. However, we should help our patients and parents understand that they don't have to be afraid of this discomfort. The pain from vaccination is minimal and temporary and, in the case of infants and toddlers, almost immediately forgotten, but the benefit of vaccination can last a lifetime.

2. Redness and swelling at the injection site are common. Some reactions are more robust than others, but any penetration of the skin and muscle by a needle with injection of a "foreign" substance will bring about an inflammatory reaction (an expected part of the immune response). Sometimes this results in modest soreness, and other times we get more notable redness, warmth, swelling, and pain at the injection site. These are temporary reactions that aren't considered worrisome, although they can certainly be bothersome to patients. We can counsel use of ice and anti-inflammatory medications, if tolerated, to reduce symptoms.

3. Allergic reactions can happen. People can have allergic reactions to almost anything. We can use a new lotion and develop an allergic contact rash. Babies can eat a strawberry or a nut for the first time and develop hives. The same is true for vaccines. However, these events are relatively uncommon and typically mild. More serious allergic reactions (anaphylaxis, angioedema, recurrent vomiting, etc) are exceedingly uncommon. But if they do happen, the doctor's office is the perfect place to be. For all vaccines, a life-threatening reaction to a dose of the vaccine or to any of its components is a contraindication to future immunization with that same vaccine.

4. We might feel "under the weather" after vaccination. When we give a vaccine, we are essentially triggering the immune system in a much milder and more controlled way than it would be triggered by exposure to the live virus or bacteria. How do we feel when we develop an infection? We likely have many days of fever, aches, and fatigue. When our immune system encounters a killed or weakened virus or bacterium in the form of a vaccine, it kicks into gear to start making antibodies, and this can give us a very mild and short-lived version of those same symptoms. This is not "sickness." This is proof that our immune system is working! It is important that patients know that this is common, expected, and not worrisome.

Risks of Live-Attenuated or Weakened Vaccines

1. Live-attenuated vaccines can rarely trigger the illness against which they are meant to protect. As stated previously, live-attenuated or weakened virus vaccines should not be given to people who have a suppressed immune system (for example, patients with leukemia, patients on chemotherapy, patients without a spleen, or pregnant women). A healthy immune system is strong enough to handle the weakened form of a virus and will either keep us from getting sick at all or will help us to have only minimal symptoms. However, people without a fully functioning immune system could become ill from the viruses or bacteria present in live-attenuated vaccines. We screen patients prior to administering these immunizations to prevent this from happening, but rarely, mistakes are made or patients have an underlying immune dysfunction that has yet to be recognized.

Vaccine-Specific Risks

In this section, we will delve into individual vaccines and discuss the adverse reactions of which physicians and other medical professionals providing immunizations should be aware (**Table 7.1**). I will include both the routinely administered, US-recommended vaccinations,[1] and less commonly given travel vaccines,[6] as some of us provide or recommend these in our clinics for patients traveling internationally.

1. Diphtheria:
Diphtheria vaccine only comes in combination with tetanus (Td) or tetanus and pertussis (DTaP or Tdap).

- Specific incidence is not established, but pain, redness, and swelling (termed a local reaction) is noted to be common after injection with diphtheria toxoid. These are short-lived and typically do not require treatment. Development of a nodule or abscess at the injection site has also been reported but is not common.

TABLE 7.1 Rates of Adverse Reactions Occurring with Vaccination

RATE OF RISK	ADVERSE REACTION
Common (>1/100)	Redness, swelling, and pain at the injection site occur relatively commonly with all injectable vaccines.
Occasional (up to 1/10,000)	Fever, malaise, muscle aches, headache, nausea, abdominal pain, syncope, and dizziness occur less commonly with certain vaccines.
Uncommon (up to 1/100,000)	Intussusception, brachial neuritis, febrile seizures, idiopathic thrombocytopenic purpura, Arthus-type reactions, and allergic reactions (hives) are uncommon responses to certain vaccines.
Rare (1-2/1 million)	Life-threatening reactions, such as anaphylaxis, angioedema, and Guillain-Barré syndrome (GBS), are exceedingly rare occurrences.

No medical intervention is without risk, but, when it comes to vaccines, most are very mild. Other more serious risks do occur but are extremely rare. Risks vary depending on the vaccine. Rates shown here represent overall risk.

- Fever and other systemic symptoms are uncommon.
- Arthus-type reactions (local exaggerated responses, such as painful swelling from shoulder to elbow) are reported and can occur 2 to 8 hours after injection. Frequency is listed as "occasional" and is thought to be more common in those that have had frequent doses of diphtheria or tetanus toxoid.

2. *Haemophilus influenzae* type b (Hib):
   - Local reactions at the injection site occur in approximately 5% to 30% of recipients and typically resolve within hours.
   - Fever and irritability are uncommon.
   - More serious reactions are very rare.

3. Hepatitis A:
   - Local reactions occur in 20% to 50% of vaccine recipients.
   - Fewer than 10% of patients will develop fever, fatigue, or malaise.
   - No serious adverse events have been reported.

4. Hepatitis B:
   - Frequency of local reactions is not described.
   - Anaphylaxis related to the hepatitis B vaccine is described in one case per 1.1 million doses.

5. Human papillomavirus (HPV):
   - Local reactions occur in 20% to 90% of patients.
   - Fever (defined as minimum temperature of 100°F) happens in 10% to 13% of recipients.
   - Syncope (fainting) is reported uncommonly in teens receiving this vaccine. The percentage affected is not described, but an increase in fainting with any vaccine is more common in teens. For this reason, we recommend administering the vaccine while the recipient is seated and monitoring the recipient for 15 minutes after each dose.
   - As with any immunization, allergic reactions, including very rare anaphylactic events, have been reported. People with a severe yeast allergy are cautioned about taking the HPV vaccine. However, the only current contraindication to getting the vaccine is a life-threatening allergic reaction to a prior dose or to a component of the vaccine. No serious adverse events at rates above those in the general population have been noted.

6. Influenza:
   There are two types of influenza vaccine—inactivated influenza vaccine (IIV—the shot) and live-attenuated influenza vaccine (LAIV—the nasal spray). We will discuss their potential adverse reactions separately.
   - IIV:
     - Local reactions occur in 15% to 20% of recipients.
     - Fewer than 1% of people will develop fever, malaise, or fatigue.
     - Allergic reactions, such as hives, angioedema, or anaphylaxis happen rarely.
     - Following use of the 2009 H1N1 pandemic influenza vaccine in Finland, Iceland, and Sweden, a higher rate of narcolepsy was reported in children vaccinated with the Pandemrix flu vaccine (4-9 times the rates seen in unvaccinated individuals). Narcolepsy is strongly genetically linked, and the proposal is that there was some interplay between the suspected genotype, the vaccine, and other environmental factors that increased the risk in this population.

However, this finding has not been noted in other countries that utilized the Pandemrix vaccine.[7] Moreover, the more recent SOMNIA Global Collaborative Study, looking at the incidence of narcolepsy diagnoses before, during, and after vaccination at the time of the H1N1 pandemic (evaluating both the AS03- and MF59-adjuvanted vaccines), does *not* support an association between the pandemic H1N1 vaccine and narcolepsy.[8]

) GBS occurs in 1 to 2 in 1 million persons vaccinated. People who have previously suffered from GBS may be at higher risk for recurrence, regardless of vaccination status. However, it is prudent to avoid repeat influenza vaccination if a person developed GBS within 6 weeks of prior influenza vaccination. For others who have a history of GBS and who are at high risk for severe complications of influenza, the proven benefits of influenza vaccination would suggest the need for continued yearly immunization.

- LAIV:
) In children, there is *no* reported increased risk of upper respiratory infection symptoms (cough, sore throat, fever, etc); however, in children aged 6 to 23 months, there is an increased risk of wheezing reported.
) In adults, there is a significantly higher rate (10%-40% of LAIV recipients) of cough, runny nose, sore throat, nasal congestion, and chills, whereas there is no significant increase in the occurrence of fever following vaccination.
) No serious adverse events have been reported in either children or adults.
) As a live-attenuated virus vaccine, the risk exists for people with suppressed immune systems to develop influenza if given this version of the flu vaccine. People with a suppressed immune system should be offered IIV.

7. Japanese encephalitis:
   - Local reactions occur in 4% to 33% with injection site discomfort being the most common.
   - Systemic adverse events (including headache, muscle pain, nausea, fatigue, flulike illness) occur in 5% to 19%.
   - Hypersensitivity reactions are rare and there are no reports of anaphylaxis or death.

8. Measles:
   In the United States, the measles vaccine is only available in combination with mumps and rubella vaccines (MMR).
   - Local reaction percentage is not described, but reactions can occur as with any immunization.
   - Fever of 103°F or higher can occur in 5% to 15% of recipients, typically occurring 7 to 12 days after immunization and lasting 1 to 2 days. Rarely, febrile seizures can occur with high fever. An increased rate of febrile seizures was primarily noted only with the MMRV (MMR and varicella combined) vaccine, showing one extra case of febrile seizure per 2300 to 2600 children vaccinated. For this reason, it is recommended to give the MMR and varicella injections separately (separate needle sticks; not separated in time).

- Rash can occur in 5% of vaccine recipients 7 to 10 days after immunization.
- Immune thrombocytopenic purpura can occur in 1 in 30,000 to 40,000 recipients (based on estimates from Europe) immunized with the MMR vaccine. This typically occurs within 2 months following vaccination, and the clinical course is usually mild and temporary.
- Allergic reactions are uncommon and most typically involve a hivelike (wheel and flair) reaction at the injection site.
- Anaphylaxis is exceedingly rare.

9. Meningococcal vaccines:

Routine vaccination with meningococcal polysaccharide vaccine (MPSV4) is not recommended and should only be used in people older than 55 years of age or when neither of the meningococcal conjugate vaccines (MenACWY-D and MenACWY-CRM) is available. Serogroup B meningococcal vaccination (MenB) is currently optional in 16- to 18-year olds but is recommended for certain high-risk groups (researchers working with *Neisseria meningitidis* in the lab, patients without a spleen, people exposed during a meningitis outbreak, patients with persistent complement component deficiency, or patients using the drug eculizumab).[9]

- Local reactions occur in 13.7% to 19.7% of recipients, depending on the vaccine brand used.
- Fever can occur in up to 16.8% of people vaccinated with the meningococcal conjugate vaccines and in up to 3% of people vaccinated with MPSV4. This typically occurs within 7 days of immunization.
- Headache occurs in 16% and dizziness in 13.4% of people vaccinated.
- Syncope occurs in 8.8% to 10%, depending on the product used.
- Serious adverse events occur exceedingly rarely. Keep in mind that the reporting of serious events does not necessarily mean that causality was established (**Box 7.1**).

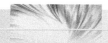 Box 7.1 Adverse Events Versus Adverse Reactions[10]

Adverse Event:

Any health problem that occurs following immunization. It may be truly caused by the vaccine or it may not.

- For example, fainting after an injection could be a side effect of the vaccine or it could be a vasovagal reaction due to fear of needles.

Adverse Reaction:

An adverse health problem that occurs following immunization that is *known* to be caused by the vaccine.

- For example, redness and swelling at the injection site; or, in the absence of any other triggering exposures, an anaphylactic reaction following immunization.

10. Mumps:

    Mumps vaccine is available in the United States only as a part of the MMR vaccine.

    - Local reaction percentage is not described, but reactions can occur as with any immunization.
    - Most adverse reactions reported after administration of the MMR vaccine (joint pain, fever, rash, etc) are likely attributable to the measles or rubella components of the vaccine.
    - Parotitis (inflammation/swelling of the parotid glands) and orchitis (inflammation of the testes) have been reported but have not been proven related.
    - Rare incidences of central nervous system symptoms, such as deafness, aseptic meningitis, and encephalitis have also been reported, but the Health and Medicine Division (HMD) of the National Academies of Sciences, Engineering, and Medicine (formerly the Institute of Medicine) has not found adequate evidence to confirm or deny a causal relationship with vaccination.

11. Pertussis:

    Pertussis is not offered as an individual vaccine. It is only given in combination with tetanus and diphtheria in the form of the DTaP vaccine (given to children younger than 10 years of age) and Tdap vaccine (approved for people at the age of 10 years and older). Adverse reactions are, therefore, reported as part of those seen with these immunizations in combination.

    - Local reactions occur in 20% to 40% of children after the first three doses. Incidence seems to increase after the fourth and fifth doses. Of the adults receiving Tdap, injection site pain is the most common adverse reaction to the vaccine, occurring in up to 66% of people.
    - A temperature of 101°F or higher occurs in 3% to 5% of DTaP recipients. A fever of 100.4°F or higher occurs in 1.1% to 1.4% of Td and Tdap recipients.
    - Systemic reactions, such as drowsiness, fretfulness, headache, and GI symptoms, are reported infrequently.
    - More severe reactions, such as high fever (to 105°F), febrile seizures, uncontrolled crying lasting longer than 3 hours, and hypotonic-hyporesponsive episodes, are reported but are less common. Since the pertussis component of the vaccine became acellular, these reactions now occur in fewer than 1 in 10,000 people vaccinated.

12. Pneumococcal vaccines:

    - Pneumococcal conjugate vaccine (PCV13):
        - Local reactions occur in 5% to 49% of patients receiving the vaccine; 8% are considered severe (such as pain that interferes with arm movement). Reactions are more common after the fourth dose than with the first three.
        - Fever (100.4°F or higher) and muscle pain occur in 24% to 35% of recipients. High fever occurs in fewer than 1% of patients.
        - Febrile seizures occur in 1.2 to 13.7 patients per 100,000 (0.0012%-0.013%) vaccinated and occur slightly more often if administered at the same time as the trivalent influenza vaccine. However, after evaluating risks and benefits of vaccination, the Advisory Committee on Immunization Practices made no recommendations for changes to the schedule based on this information.

- Pneumococcal polysaccharide vaccine (PPSV23):
  - Local reactions are common, occurring in 30% to 50% of people receiving the PPSV23 vaccine. These typically resolve within 48 hours.
  - Fever and muscle pain are described in fewer than 1% of vaccine recipients.
  - Severe adverse reactions are rare.

13. Polio:

    The use of inactivated polio vaccine (IPV) has been recommended exclusively since 2000 and oral polio vaccine (OPV), which is a live-attenuated virus vaccine, is no longer available in the United States.

    - IPV:
      - Minor local reactions are noted, but frequency has not been established.
      - Allergic reactions can occur as trace amounts of streptomycin, neomycin, and polymyxin B are contained in this vaccine. People allergic to these antibiotics may have an allergic response to IPV (however, allergic reactions that are not anaphylactic in nature are not a contraindication to this vaccine).
    - OPV:
      - This vaccine is still used in other parts of the world. Rare reports of vaccine-associated paralytic polio have occurred following use of the oral vaccine.

14. Rabies:

    There are two rabies vaccines—RAB-HDC (rabies-human diploid cell) and RAB-PCEC (rabies-purified chick embryo cell). Both are killed virus vaccines.

    - RAB-HDC:
      - Local reactions occur in 60% to 90% with local injection site pain being the most common at 21% to 77%.
      - Systemic reactions, such as fever, GI complaints, headache, and dizziness, occur in 7% to 56%.
      - Systemic hypersensitivity reactions, such as hives and angioedema, can occur in 6% of people receiving booster doses.
    - RAB-PCEC:
      - Local reactions happen 11% to 57% of the time with injection site pain noted in 2% to 23% of recipients.
      - Mild systemic symptoms are noted in up to 31% of recipients.

15. Rotavirus:

    - RV5 (RotaTeq):
      - Diarrhea occurs in 18.1% of vaccine recipients and vomiting in 11.6%.
      - There are increased rates of otitis media, bronchospasm, and nasopharyngitis.
      - Postlicensure risk of intussusception is unconfirmed because of the small number of cases.
    - RV1 (Rotarix):
      - More common with RV1 are irritability in 11.4% of recipients, cough or runny nose in 3.6%, and flatulence in 2.2%.
      - Postlicensure assessment of intussusception showed an extra 1 to 3 per 100,000 cases (0.001%-0.003%), following the first dose.

16. Rubella:

    The rubella vaccine is only available in the United States as part of the MMR vaccine.

    - As with any vaccine, local injection site reactions are possible.
    - Most common reactions are fever, lymphadenopathy (swollen lymph glands), and arthralgia (joint pain). Joint symptoms occur more commonly in adults than in children (yet another reason to vaccinate on schedule) and typically affects more women than men. Up to 25% of postpubertal females will develop sudden joint pain following vaccination. This typically begins 1 to 3 weeks after vaccination and can last up to 3 weeks, recurring rarely.

17. Tetanus:

    Administered as part of the Td or DTaP and Tdap vaccines.

    - Local reactions (redness, swelling, pain) are common but short lived. Development of a nodule or abscess at the injection site has been reported but is infrequent.
    - Fever and other systemic symptoms are uncommon.
    - Arthus-type reactions, as described under diphtheria, have occurred.
    - Brachial neuritis (a form of peripheral nerve pain affecting the chest, shoulder, arm, and hand)[11] can occur up to 1 month after immunization and affects up to 0.5 to 1 patient per 100,000 vaccinated.
    - The HMD rejects a causal relationship between tetanus toxoid and type 1 diabetes. It reports inadequate evidence to accept or reject association with peripheral neuropathy or GBS but does find causal relationship with anaphylaxis, which occurs rarely.

18. Typhoid:

    There are two forms of typhoid vaccine. The injectable form (Typhim Vi) gives 2 years of immunity and is a killed virus vaccine. The oral form (Vivotif) provides 5 years of immunity and is a live-attenuated (weakened) vaccine.

    - Injectable:
        - Injection site tenderness is the most common local reaction, occurring in up to 98% of recipients. Swelling occurs in 5% to 15% and redness in 4% to 5%.
        - Systemic symptoms are less common: malaise (4%-34%), headache (16%-20%), muscle pain (3%-7%), and nausea (2%-8%).
        - Fever occurs in <2% of vaccine recipients.
    - Oral:
        - Intestinal symptoms (nausea, vomiting, abdominal pain, diarrhea) occur in 2% to 6% of patients, but only nausea occurs more frequently than in placebo groups.
        - Fever occurs in 3%, headache in 5%, and rash in 1% of patients.
        - In postmarketing surveillance of 60 million doses, only one serious allergic reaction occurred.

19. Varicella (chickenpox):

    - Local reactions occur in 19% of children receiving the vaccine and in 24% of adolescents and adults.
    - Injection site varicella-like rash occurs in 3% of children and 1% of adolescents and adults with a median of two lesions. These typically occur within 2 weeks of injection and are usually maculopapular, not vesicular.
    - Generalized varicella-like rash occurs in 4% to 6% of recipients, with an average of five lesions. These occur generally within 3 weeks of injection and are commonly maculopapular, not vesicular.

- Fever can occur within 42 days of immunization in 15% of children and 10% of adolescents and adults. These are attributed to concurrent illness rather than to vaccination. Other systemic reactions are rare.

20. Yellow fever:
    - Reactions are generally mild. Fewer than 5% of recipients will have local reactions, headache, or fever within 5 to 7 days following immunization.
    - Two serious adverse events have been described:
      - Vaccine-associated viscerotropic disease—this occurs in approximately 1 in 250,000 doses. Symptoms include fever, nausea, vomiting, myalgia, diarrhea, shortness of breath, and can result in end-organ damage (liver, kidneys, heart, etc), which rarely progresses to cardiorespiratory failure and death. Men older than 56 years of age, young women, people with autoimmune disease, and people who have had their thymus gland removed for treatment of thymoma seem to be at greatest risk.
      - Vaccine-associated neurotrophic disease—this occurs in approximately 1 in 125,000 doses. Symptoms include fever, headache, and localized or generalized neurologic dysfunction. It may be more common in people older than 60 years of age.

21. Zoster (shingles):
    - The live-attenuated herpes zoster virus vaccine (Zostavax) is no longer recommended for routine use now that we have a much more effective and killed herpes zoster virus vaccine option in Shingrix. However, it is still given on occasion as Shingrix is currently in short supply. Local reactions are not uncommon and occur in 34% of people vaccinated. There is no significantly increased risk of fever or other systemic or serious reactions. Zostavax should not be given to anyone with a suppressed immune system.
    - Shingrix is much more effective than Zostavax (>90% vs around 50% effective) and is now recommended even for those who have already had the Zostavax vaccine. Injection site redness, pain, and swelling are relatively common, and about one in six people will have a more vigorous reaction (such as, fatigue, muscle pain, fever, chills, stomach pain, or nausea) that prevents them from doing normal daily activities. These effects typically resolve on their own within 2 to 3 days (**Box 7.2**).

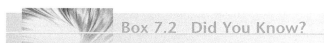

Box 7.2   Did You Know?

In rare instances, in people who received the chickenpox vaccine, the vaccine strain of the varicella zoster virus can cause a latent infection in the dorsal root ganglia and reactivate as herpes zoster (shingles). This occurs much less commonly than shingles resulting from an infection with the wild-type chickenpox virus. About one in three people who had a wild-type chickenpox infection will develop shingles in their lifetime. It is also possible that people who received the vaccine for chickenpox, given waning immunity and the ongoing potential to come into contact with the wild-type virus, can contract chickenpox, which can later reactivate and cause shingles. Both of these situations happen uncommonly, but, for now, it is recommended that those who were vaccinated against chickenpox still get the shingles vaccine at the age of 50 years.[12]

We know that vaccines have risks, but these risks are mild or extremely rare compared with the much more serious risks of vaccine-preventable illness. Some in the anti-vaccine community claim that they are "not against vaccines, per se." They just want vaccines to be "safer." Vaccines are already extremely safe, with extensive preproduction and postproduction monitoring and oversight. If they weren't safe, their use would not be permitted. No government agency, or private entity for that matter, would knowingly put themselves at risk for thousands of lawsuits by releasing unsafe vaccines to be used on healthy children and adults. Nothing we do in life is free from risk. There is risk in walking, eating, and even breathing. If we are waiting for vaccines to be risk-free, we will die waiting…and maybe from a vaccine-preventable disease.

References

1. Centers for Disease Control and Prevention; Hamborsky J, Kroger A, Wolfe C, eds. *Epidemiology and Prevention of Vaccine-Preventable Diseases.* 13th ed. Washington, DC: Public Health Foundation; 2015. Updated December 2016. Accessed December 13, 2018. https://www.cdc.gov/vaccines/pubs/pinkbook/downloads/table-of-contents.pdf.

2. National Safety Council. What are the Odds of Dying From. Accessed December 13, 2018. https://www.nsc.org/work-safety/tools-resources/injury-facts/chart.

3. Miller ER, Moro PL, Cano M, et al. Deaths following vaccination: what does the evidence show? *Vaccine.* 2015;33(29):3288-3292.

4. National Highway Traffic Safety Administration. Seat Belts. Accessed December 13, 2018. https://www.nhtsa.gov/risky-driving/seat-belts.

5. O'Brien C, Rutherford G, Marcy N; Consumer Product Safety Commission. *Hazard Screening Report -- Sports Activities and Equipment (Excluding Major Team Sports).* May 2005. Accessed December 13, 2018. https://www.cpsc.gov/s3fs-public/pdfs/hazard_sports.pdf.

6. Marshall G. *The Vaccine Handbook: A Practical Guide for Clinicians.* 7th ed. West Islip, NY: Professional Communications Inc; 2018.

7. World Health Organization. *Statement on Narcolepsy and Vaccination.* April 21, 2011. Accessed December 13, 2018. https://www.who.int/vaccine_safety/committee/topics/influenza/pandemic/h1n1_safety_assessing/narcolepsy_statement/en.

8. Weibel D, Sturkenboom M, Black S, et al. Narcolepsy and adjuvanted pandemic influenza A (H1N1) 2009 vaccines -- multi-country assessment. *Vaccine.* 2018;36(41):6202-6211.

9. Centers for Disease Control and Prevention. *Serogroup B Meningococcal (MenB) VIS: What You Need to Know.* August 9, 2016. Accessed December 13, 2018. https://www.cdc.gov/vaccines/hcp/vis/vis-statements/mening-serogroup.html.

10. Centers for Disease Control and Prevention. Understanding Side Effects and Adverse Events. Accessed January 15, 2019. https://www.cdc.gov/vaccinesafety/ensuringsafety/sideeffects/index.html.

11. Johns Hopkins Medicine. Brachial Neuritis. Accessed December 13, 2018. https://www.hopkinsmedicine.org/healthlibrary/conditions/nervous_system_disorders/brachial_neuritis_134,33.

12. Vaxopedia. Can the Shingles Vaccine Cause Shingles? Accessed February 6, 2019 https://vaxopedia.org/2017/07/12/can-the-shingles-vaccine-cause-shingles/.

8

The Lie That Started It All

If we've been bamboozled long enough, we tend to reject any evidence of the bamboozle. We're no longer interested in finding out the truth. The bamboozle has captured us. It's simply too painful to acknowledge, even to ourselves, that we've been taken. Once you give a charlatan power over you, you almost never get it back.

—Carl Sagan, The Demon-Haunted World: Science as a Candle in the Dark

As stated in chapter 2, anti-vaccine sentiment has been alive and well since the advent of immunizations and immunization programs. However, our modern-day movement is built primarily upon the work of a single man, Andrew Wakefield. With the aid of rapid dissemination of faulty information via the Internet and social media platforms, Wakefield has transformed a once small and localized group into an increasingly organized and vocal fringe with worldwide reach. Some see him as a hero, a martyr of sorts, sacrificing his professional practice and reputation for the good of the poor unsuspecting families who are being duped by pharmaceutical companies, government, and the medical profession. He would have people believe that these institutions are in cahoots to bilk everyday citizens out of their money and their health. It is hard to comprehend how anyone could imagine this to be true. It sounds utterly paranoid and delusional. Yet, every day, people make ill-informed vaccine decisions based upon his lies that affect their health, the health of their loved ones, and the health of their communities. Moreover, even though his assertions have been proven wrong time and again, and his "research" shown to be factually inaccurate and unethically conducted, people are still buying what he's selling. It is remarkable that we, as a society, are not more incensed at the chaos that Wakefield has created in the medical and public health sector. Indeed, we should be outraged at the illnesses he has caused our children to suffer and the deaths that are on his hands as a result of the self-serving seed of doubt he planted with the publication of his study suggesting a link between the measles, mumps, and rubella (MMR) vaccine and the development of an intestinal illness and autism.

This chapter will dig deeper into Wakefield's 1998 *Lancet* article. It will examine Wakefield's methods, his misrepresentation of facts, his unethical scientific practices, and his ultimate aims to profit financially from his claims. As medical practitioners, most of us are aware that his research was debunked and that he was stripped of his medical license for falsifying data, but I suspect we are not as familiar with the incredible depths and degrees of his deception. Using the comprehensive investigative journalism of award-winning reporter Brian Deer on behalf of London's *The Sunday Times*, and the insightful and scientifically grounded evaluation of Wakefield's research by retired researcher Joel A. Harrison, PhD, MPH, as a foundation, this chapter will hopefully revive our sense of outrage at the costly and dangerous hoax that Wakefield perpetrated upon an unsuspecting public.

WHO IS ANDREW WAKEFIELD?

Andrew Jeremy Wakefield was born in 1957 in Eton, Berkshire, England. He graduated medical school in 1981 at what is now the Imperial College School of Medicine. Before being discredited and having his name stricken from the UK medical register for unethical behavior, misconduct, and fraud, he was a gastroenterologist and researcher at the Royal Free Hospital School of Medicine. In 1998, Wakefield, along with 12 other coauthors on the study, published an article in *Lancet* titled "Ileal-Lymphoid-Nodular Hyperplasia, Non-specific Colitis, and Pervasive Developmental Disorder in Children." The study suggested a link between the combined MMR vaccine and a syndrome that the researchers termed "autistic enterocolitis," a combination of inflammatory bowel disease and regressive autism. In an unusual move for a researcher, Wakefield didn't just submit his paper for publication in an academic medical journal, where it may have raised questions and concerns in the academic sphere and would have encouraged further study, as is common in the process of scientific research. Instead, he launched a public relations campaign with a video news release and press conference, calling for a boycott of the combined MMR vaccine in favor of individual MMR vaccines spaced apart by a year, thus spreading news of his unconfirmed data to the world and giving us a sense of the media spectacle that Wakefield seems to thrive in.

As concerns began surfacing about the truthfulness of his data, he refused requests to attempt validation of his *Lancet* paper with a controlled study. After reportedly being asked to leave his post at the Royal Free Hospital, he moved to the United States in 2001 with his family where he lives to this day. He established and served as executive director of the Thoughtful House Center for Children, an organization that "studies" autism, continuing to put forth his theory of a link between autism and the MMR vaccine. He resigned from Thoughtful House in 2010 when, after a record-setting 2 1/2 years of deliberation, the British General Medical Council Fitness to Practice Panel stripped him of his medical license for "dishonest and irresponsible" research practices. Despite all of this, he continues to be held up by anti-vaccine activists, such as J. B. Handley of the group Generation Rescue, as "Nelson Mandela and Jesus Christ rolled up into one."[1]

His recent activities include speaking out against legislation that would make it more difficult to seek exemption from vaccination, holding counsel with President Trump—a meeting that resulted in Trump's proposal to create a committee to look into the safety of vaccines (not a bad idea, but these committees already exist and the proposal only served to alarm and further confuse the populace), and producing a film shot in documentary style titled *Vaxxed: From Cover-Up to Catastrophe*. Of the film, the *Washington Post's* Michael O'Sullivan gave the following review: "It's hard to know which of the film's many flaws to cite first, so here's one thing it does fairly well: scare the bejesus out of you. That's assuming you have read nothing about the subject of vaccines and autism, and are of a generally lax and incurious mind when it comes to the rigors of scientific inquiry."[2] (See Appendix E: Journal Articles Addressing Specific Vaccine Concerns for a list of reliable research papers on vaccines.)

THE LANCET STUDY—A SUMMARY OF DECEPTIONS

Wakefield's *Lancet* study was published on February 28, 1998. It described 12 children with a "history of a pervasive developmental disorder with loss of acquired skills and intestinal symptoms" and asserted that the "onset of behavioral symptoms was associated, by the parents, with measles, mumps, and rubella vaccination in eight of the 12 children."[3] The article also reported that the onset of these behavioral and intestinal symptoms generally began within 14 days after administration of the MMR immunization. Following release of the article, the United Kingdom saw a significant drop in vaccination rates below those required to maintain herd immunity, from 92% in 1996-1997 to 80% in 2003-2004, with a subsequent increase in outbreaks of vaccine-preventable disease.[4] (**Box 8.1**) Although the study itself did not claim to *prove* an association, the inclusion of the parents' observations certainly suggested one, and the public bought into the claim with disastrous consequences in communities across the world.

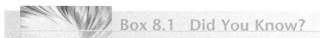 Box 8.1   Did You Know?

Scientists believe that having a measles infection "resets" or "disables" immune memory, such that prior immunity built to other infections is lost and people become increasingly susceptible to infectious disease for at least 2 to 3 years following the measles illness. It's not just that people getting the measles vaccine are more likely to receive other vaccines and better health care in general. Research looking at epidemiological data from the United States, Wales, England, and Denmark dating back to the 1940s shows that the number of measles cases noted in these countries predicted the number of deaths from other infectious diseases 2 to 3 years later. Conversely, when a population is vaccinated against measles, the rates of other infectious diseases drop, and we see a decrease in rates of child mortality overall. So, not only does vaccination against measles provide herd immunity to measles, but it also provides herd immunity against other infectious pathogens as well.[5]

In the years of confusion and fear that followed, an investigative journalist named Brian Deer was engaged by *The Sunday Times* to look into the veracity of Wakefield's claims. In 2004, Deer wrote his first in a series of articles for the *Times*, highlighting numerous incidences of dishonesty and unethical practices associated with the article, triggering 10 of Wakefield's 12 coauthors to retract their part of the study. In 2010, following the longest professional misconduct hearings by the UK General Medical Council ever held, Wakefield was found guilty of "serious professional misconduct"[6] and his name was stricken from the medical register. Shortly thereafter, the *Lancet* retracted his paper (**Figure 8.1**).

Despite retraction of the misrepresented and unsubstantiated data, a spark had been lit. Wakefield's claims spread rapidly across developed nations, serving as fodder for existing anti-vaccine organizations and triggering numerous other concerns about vaccines. If it wasn't the MMR vaccine itself that caused autism, then perhaps it was the thimerosal preservative used in vaccines, or the aluminum adjuvant, or the sheer number of vaccines that contributed to neurologic regression and to rising rates of cancers and autoimmune diseases. The anti-vaccine movement had found itself a spokesperson and a hero, and we medical professionals have been fighting his deceptions ever since.

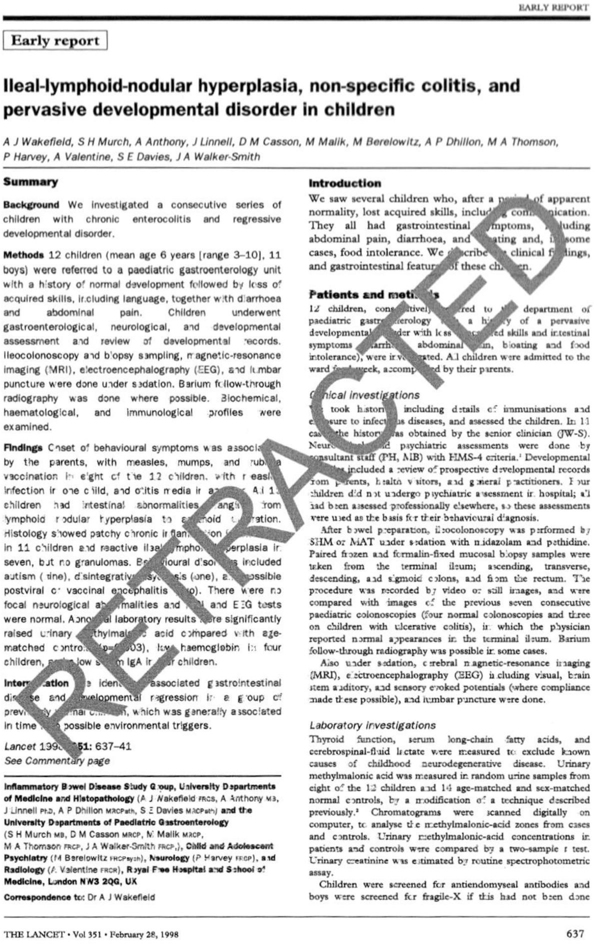

FIGURE 8.1 Image of Andrew Wakefield's retracted paper. (Reprinted from Wakefield AJ, Murch SH, Anthony A, et al. RETRACTED: Ileal-lymphoid-nodular hyperplasia, non-specific colitis, and pervasive developmental disorder in children. *Lancet.* 351(9103):637–641, Copyright 1998, with permission from Elsevier.)

Deer's work was subsequently published in a 2011 article in the *British Medical Journal* titled "How the Case against the MMR Vaccine Was Fixed." The following are highlights from Deer's findings.[7]

A FINANCIAL CONFLICT OF INTEREST

One of the most shocking findings from Deer's investigations was that Wakefield held very significant, and undisclosed, conflicts of interest regarding his study's claims; conflicts which, if disclosed to *Lancet* on submission of his paper, would have disqualified the work from publication. First, 2 years prior to enrollment of any of his 12 test subjects, Wakefield was hired by attorney Richard Barr to find evidence of what the two dubbed a "new syndrome," which was to be the focal point of a class action lawsuit against companies manufacturing the MMR vaccine. He was paid by Barr with money from the UK legal defense fund, a governmental fund used to help poor people have access to justice. The money, totaling approximately US $750,000, plus expenses, was billed through his wife's company (the two have now split). He was also granted further startup funds for the purpose of conducting his MMR-related research but, again, never disclosed this to the *Lancet* on submission of his paper. Finally, demonstrating an even more gross abuse of procedures for the ethical performance of research, 9 months before the public release of Wakefield's study, he applied for a patent for a supposedly "safer" single measles vaccine, which would have potentially seen great commercial success if the reputation of the combined MMR vaccine was damaged by his research.[8] His plans to financially profit from the reported findings of the study are undeniable.

A BIASED SELECTION OF STUDY PARTICIPANTS

Wakefield's selection of patients for his study was also highly suspect. These patients were not put forward for participation by concerned medical providers as is common in research studies. They were, Deer discovered, largely clients or contacts of the attorney, Richard Barr. They were not merely a run-of-the-mill group of children seeking care from the London Hospital for digestive symptoms or developmental disorder, as was asserted. In all cases, none of the children lived in London (one was even brought over from the United States), and in most cases, they had been preselected by "MMR campaign groups" for participation in the study.[8] Wakefield also submitted as evidence the parents' claims that neurologic regression had occurred days after the MMR vaccination, when recollections were vague and unverified. When they got to the hospital for study, parents were more likely to draw a link between their child's symptoms and the MMR vaccine because that is why they had been brought to the hospital in the first place.

MANIPULATION AND FABRICATION OF DATA

Using the General Medical Council hearings to his advantage, Deer was able to gain access to the test subjects and their families, as well as patient data and laboratory and pathology results, which allowed him to attempt substantiation of Wakefield's claims. However, what he found, after numerous interviews with the families involved, was that "Wakefield had repeatedly changed, misreported and misrepresented diagnoses, histories and descriptions of the children, which made it appear that the syndrome had been discovered."[8] Upon review of the study data, Deer found that unreported data from standard blood tests for inflammation in the children were normal. He also noted that what was found in the guts of most of the test subjects was constipation and that biopsies of intestinal tissue had been benign, though this was not what was reported in the *Lancet* article. In addition, in speaking with the parents of the test children, Deer found that some of the subjects who had reportedly developed a regressive autism following MMR immunization had suspicions by their primary physicians of developmental delay and issues with bowel concerns *prior* to administration of their first MMR vaccine. One was noted to have had repair of a coarctation of the aorta at age 14 months, which her physicians felt coincided closely with her delay. One child's medical report noted a "very small deletion within the fragile X gene."[7] Three children were not admitted to the study with a diagnosis of autism, nor discharged from the study with this diagnosis. Moreover, the one child in the study who truly did have suspicion of regressive autism following vaccination did not have onset of symptoms within 2 weeks, as Wakefield claimed. On discussion with the child's mother, Deer noted that the mother recollected the onset of regression to be between 2 and 6 months following vaccination.[7] "When taken together with developmental histories and diagnoses," Deer writes, "…not one case was free of critical mismatches between the paper which launched the vaccine crisis and the kids' contemporaneous records."[8]

UNETHICAL RESEARCH PRACTICES

In light of the findings above, the fact that Wakefield subjected the children in his study to invasive procedures (lumbar punctures, colonoscopies, barium follow-through studies, and others), often requiring anesthesia, which is not without risk, puts him in obvious violation of the Helsinki Declaration, a "formal statement of ethical principles published by the World Medical Association (WMA) to guide the protection of human participants in medical research."[9] Knowing that no institutional review board (IRB) or respected medical or academic journal would approve his methods or publish a blatantly biased and ethically questionable study, Wakefield falsely reported to the *Lancet*, when submitting his paper for publication, that his study had been approved by his institution, the Royal Free Hospital's, ethics committee. When faced with Deer's discoveries to the contrary, Wakefield initially denied the claims. However, when confronted with proof of his lies during the General Medical Council hearings, he backpedaled to state that he hadn't actually needed the ethics committee's blessing (a claim that is in direct violation of clear laws regarding the process of IRB approval).

BENEFITTING FROM CONTROVERSY

Wakefield very obviously hoped to benefit financially and by reputation from the results of his study. Although perhaps not in the original way that he envisioned, he has certainly done so. Records from the General Medical Council proceedings note that "On behalf of Dr. Wakefield, no evidence has been adduced and no arguments or pleas in mitigation have been addressed to the Panel. In fact Mr. Coonan [Dr. Wakefield's lawyer] specifically submitted: 'we call no evidence and we make no substantive submissions on behalf of Dr. Wakefield at this stage.…I am instructed to make no further observations in this case.'"[10] Instead of arguing on his behalf, however, Wakefield soon after self-published his book *Callous Disregard: Autism and Vaccines—The Truth behind a Tragedy*, which "contains much of what one would assume would have been used in an appeal."[4] Wakefield's behavior around the time of the hearings was aptly criticized by one of the High Court judges, stating that Wakefield "wished to extract whatever advantage he could from the existence of the proceedings while not wishing to progress them."[8]

Since his discrediting, Wakefield has been both reviled and lauded as a savior. He keeps company with anti-vaccine celebrities, such as Jenny McCarthy, attended Trump's inaugural ball, has directed a "documentary" film, and is, at the time of this writing, dating supermodel Elle Macpherson. Following his very public announcement proposing a link between the MMR vaccine and autism, Wakefield's scientific career has ended, but his fame and sphere of influence seem only to have skyrocketed at the expense of the health of our children and the health of our communities (**Box 8.2**).

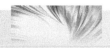 Box 8.2   Impact of Wakefield's Work on
Resurgence of Disease

Even though Andrew Wakefield's inflammatory article was ultimately retracted, damage had already been done. This list represents only a fraction of the outbreaks and deaths that occurred as a result of his actions:

- 2006: A 13-year-old British boy died from measles, making him the first person to die from the disease in Britain in over a decade.[11]
- 2010: The worst whooping cough outbreak in 50 years hit California, affecting 9,120 and killing 10. Nonmedical exemptions to required school vaccinations likely contributed to the spread of the illness.[12]
- 2013: Eagle Mountain International Church in Texas had 21 members of its congregation contract measles. The head of the ministry was known to be skeptical of vaccinations.[12]
- 2015: A measles outbreak in Disneyland California affected 147 people. Subsequently, several other states, Canada, and Mexico reported measles cases related to the Disneyland outbreak.[13]
- 2016-2017: More than 800 people became infected with mumps in the state of Washington. As a result, 5,000 more people opted for the MMR vaccination than in previous years.[14]
- 2017: Between April and May, 65 cases of measles were reported in a Somali community in Minnesota. Of those, 62 patients were unvaccinated due to the fear of a link between the MMR vaccine and autism.[15]
- 2018: New York saw clusters of measles outbreaks across several counties. In Brooklyn, NY, the outbreak likely began with under-vaccinated travelers.[16]
- 2018: Measles outbreak across Europe sickened nearly 80,000 and killed 72. In some areas of Europe, vaccination rates were below 70%.[17,18]

References

1. Dominus S. The crash and burn of an autism guru. *New York Times Magazine*; April 20, 2011. https://www.nytimes.com/2011/04/24/magazine/mag-24Autism-t.html. Accessed January 8, 2019.

2. O'Sullivan M. *'Vaxxed: From Cover-Up to Catastrophe": Closer to Horror Film Than Documentary.* Washington Post; May 19, 2016. https://www.washingtonpost.com/goingoutguide/movies/vaxxed-from-cover-up-to-catastrophe-closer-to-horror-film-than-documentary/2016/05/19/7129aaf4-1c5d-11e6-8c7b-6931e66333e7_story.html?noredirect=on&utm_term=.58b4dcdff7e6. Accessed January 15, 2019.

3. Wakefield AJ, Murch SH, Anthony A, et al. Ileal-lymphoid-nodular hyperplasia, non-specific, colitis, and pervasive developmental disorder in children [retracted in: *Lancet.* 2010;375(9713):445]. *Lancet.* 1998;351(9103):637-641.

4. Harrison JA. Wrong about vaccine safety: a review of Andrew Wakefield's callous disregard. *Open Vaccine J.* 2013;6:9-25.

5. Mina MJ, Metcalf JE, de Swart RL, et al. Long-term measles-induce immunomodulation increases overall childhood infectious disease mortality. *Science.* 2015;348(6235):694-699.

6. Deer B. *MMR Scare Doctor Faces List of Charges.* September 11, 2005. https://briandeer.com/wakefield/gmc-alleges.htm. Accessed January 8, 2019.

7. Deer B. How the case against the MMR vaccine was fixed. *BMJ.* 2011;342:c5347.

8. Deer B. *Andrew Wakefield – the Fraud Investigation*. 2018. https://briandeer.com/mmr/lancet-summary. htm. Accessed January 8, 2019.

9. Dik BJ, Doenges TJ. *Declaration of Helsinki*. In: *Enyclopædia Britannica*. October 28, 2014. https://www. britannica.com/topic/Declaration-of-Helsinki. Accessed January 8, 2019.

10. General Medical Council. *Determination on Serious Professional Misconduct (SPM) and Sanction: Dr Andrew Jeremy WAKEFIELD*. May 24, 2010. https://briandeer.com/solved/gmc-wakefield-sentence.pdf.

11. Hannaford A. Andrew Wakefield: Autism Inc. *The Guardian*. April 6, 2013. https://www.theguardian. com/society/2013/apr/06/what-happened-man-mmr-panic. Accessed January 8, 2019.

12. Krans B. Anti-vaccination Movement Causes a Deadly Year in the U.S. https://www.healthline.com/health-news/children-anti-vaccination-movement-leads-to-disease-outbreaks-120312#3. Accessed January 8, 2019.

13. Centers for Disease Control and Prevention. *Year in Review: Measles Linked to Disneyland*. December 2, 2015. https://blogs.cdc.gov/publichealthmatters/2015/12/year-in-review-measles-linked-to-disneyland/. Accessed January 8, 2019.

14. Centers for Disease Control and Prevention. Controlling a Mumps Outbreak in Washington. https://www. cdc.gov/cpr/readiness/stories/wa.htm. Updated March 19, 2018. Accessed January 9, 2019.

15. Centers for Disease Control and Prevention. Measles Outbreak — Minnesota April–may 2017. *MMWR Morb Mortal Wkly Rep*. 2017;66(27):713-717. https://www.cdc.gov/mmwr/volumes/66/wr/mm6627a1. htm.

16. Hackett DW. *Visitors to NYC's Rockefeller Center Should be Wary of Measles*. December 14, 2018. https:// www.precisionvaccinations.com/new-york-state-measles-outbreaks-are-related-under-vaccinated-international-travelers. Accessed January 9. 2019.

17. Thornton J. Measles cases in Europe tripled from 2017 to 2018. *BMJ*. 2019;364:l634.

18. Dunn L, Carroll L. Measles outbreak raging in Europe could be brought to U.S., Doctors Warn. *NBC News*. October 20, 2018. https://www.nbcnews.com/health/kids-health/measles-outbreak-raging-europe-could-be-brought-u-s-doctors-n922146. Accessed January 15, 2019.

9

Addressing Your Patients' Vaccine Doubts: Point-Counterpoint, Part 1

Doubt can only be removed by action.

—Johann Wolfgang von Goethe

Health care providers encounter a myriad of anti-vaccine claims, some of which we are readily equipped to discuss ("The flu shot causes the flu," for example). Yet, others seem so far out in left field (such as, the "formaldehyde and aluminum in vaccines cause cancer" assertion) that we are sometimes caught off guard and may be unprepared to discuss the research and data that support the effectiveness and safety of our immunizations. Sometimes our patients' anti-vaccine claims represent a fundamental misunderstanding of how vaccines work. Sometimes they are based on erroneous interpretation of science and statistics. And sometimes they play into the fears of parents or of laypeople trying to make sense of complicated and often confusing research. It is our job to educate our patients with the facts that justify our recommendations and to set our patients' minds at ease. (See Appendix B: Fast Facts about Vaccines for Patients and Clinic Staff.)

But when does the average clinician have time to do all the investigation necessary to provide counterarguments to their patients' many assertions? We spend long hours taking care of patients, sometimes barely having time for family, friends, and self-care. The task of researching the science and data to counter arguments to anti-vaccine claims can seem daunting. Below you will find the most commonly heard anti-vaccine assertions (and some not so commonly heard) and the information you will need to counter them. Chapter 10 will continue the discussion and address those concerns that are specific to certain groups (religious groups, children, pregnant women, and immune-suppressed patients). Finally, chapter 11 will look at the two most "controversial" vaccines—influenza and HPV. These chapters are laid out in a question and answer or point-counterpoint format that you can use to provide quick and easy education to your patients.

1. How do vaccines even work?
    - Our bodies attempt to protect us from harm by mounting an immune response when exposed to foreign proteins (such as viruses and bacteria). Through vaccination, we harness the benefit of this response by

exposing the body to killed or weakened viral or bacterial proteins in a safe and controlled manner. Our body then develops memory cells (antibodies), which live on for years and are quickly mobilized to protect us in the event of future exposure to that same virus or bacterium. To draw an analogy to war, instead of a surprise attack where all of our "troops" are ill-prepared for the onslaught and we suffer large losses in the battle; through vaccination, we are now equipped with weapons to defend ourselves, and our bodies are prepared to successfully fight off an attack.[1] (See Appendix C: Vaccine Topics Explained for a video explaining how our immune systems respond to vaccines).

2. If vaccines are so beneficial, why don't we have vaccines against the common cold? Colds make more people sick each year than tetanus and whooping cough do.

- The common cold is, well, common, and it certainly can make us feel miserable, but there are several reasons why we don't have vaccines against cold viruses. First, it is extremely costly to produce a vaccine—costing billions of dollars (see chapter 5 for more discussion of this topic). Second, it is not an easy process. It takes 10 to 15 years on average to develop and produce a vaccine. Third, and perhaps most importantly, cold viruses don't typically land people in the hospital and cause serious health consequences or death. We immunize against viruses and bacteria that have the potential to be severely damaging and deadly.

3. What are the different types of vaccines? What is the difference between a "killed virus vaccine" and a "live-attenuated virus vaccine" (**Table 9.1**)?

- There are generally considered to be four different types of vaccines. We can subdivide these into those vaccines that are safe for all (inactivated/killed, subunit, and toxoid vaccines) and those that are not safe for people with a weakened immune system (live-attenuated vaccines).

  - Live-attenuated vaccines—These vaccines contain live viruses or bacteria that have been weakened. These are most similar to a natural infection and provide the longest immunity. Because they contain the live germ, they cannot be used in people who have a compromised immune system (pregnant women, newborns, AIDS patients, or patients on chemotherapy or other types of immuno-suppression, for example). Another challenge with this type of vaccine is that it also has to be kept cool. This renders them difficult to transport and use in parts of the world where access to refrigeration is scarce.

  - Inactivated/killed virus vaccines—These vaccines contain viruses or bacteria that have been inactivated or killed. There is no live germ present in these vaccines, therefore they cannot induce the infection against which they are meant to protect. Their immunogenicity (ability to induce an immune response) is less than a live-attenuated vaccine, so they may require boosters to provide life-long immunity.

  - Subunit, recombinant, polysaccharide, and conjugate vaccines—These use pieces of the virus or bacterium (such as sugars, proteins, or the casing around the germ, called a capsid) to induce an immune response. These also are safe for all but may need boosters to maintain immunity.

> Toxoid vaccines—These vaccines don't use the virus or bacterium itself, but instead use the toxin that is produced by the virus or bacterium to induce an immune response. Toxoid vaccines are also safe for everyone and need boosters to provide lasting immune protection.

TABLE 9.1 Types of Vaccines

LIVE-ATTENUATED[a]	INACTIVATED	SUBUNIT	TOXOID
MMR	Hep A	Pneumococcal (PPSV23, PCV13)	Dtap
LAIV (nasal flu)	IIV (flu shot)	Hep B	Tdap
Varicella	IPV	Hib	Td
Zoster (Zostavax)	Rabies	Meningococcal (MenACWY/B)	
Oral typhoid	Japanese encephalitis	Zoster (Shingrix)	
Oral polio		Pertussis	
Rotavirus		HPV	
Yellow fever		Injectable typhoid	
Tuberculosis			

[a]*Live-attenuated vaccines are contraindicated in immune-compromised people.*

4. What about the aluminum in vaccines. Isn't that toxic?
   - Aluminum is used as an adjuvant to boost the immune response to vaccines. Aluminum is used only in inactivated, subunit, and toxoid vaccines, not in live-attenuated vaccines. The Agency for Toxic Substances and Disease Registry (ATSDR) monitors minimum risk levels (MRLs)—levels below which we will not see any harm—of aluminum and other compounds in vaccines. The amount of aluminum in vaccines is definitively below MRLs (1.0 mg/kg/d).[2]
   - Aluminum is the most abundant element in the earth's crust. In nature, it is found most commonly in combination with other elements in the form of potassium aluminum sulfate and aluminum oxide.[3] Aluminum is extracted from these compounds and placed into products we use every day (pots, pans, aluminum foil, seasonings, cereals, baby formula, paints, fuels, antiperspirants, etc.). It also leaches in small amounts from the earth's surface into our food and water supply. We are exposed to and consume more aluminum (the average adult consumes 7-9 mg of aluminum per day)[4] than we are ever administered in any series of vaccines. Babies, for example, consume more aluminum from breast milk or formula in the first 6 months of life than they receive from all the immunizations given in that same time period (**Box 9.1**).

 Box 9.1   Facts About Aluminum in Vaccines

1. Infants get about 4.4 mg of aluminum in the vaccines given in the first 6 months of life.
2. Infants get *more* than that in their diets during the first 6 months of life.
    - Breast milk—~ 7 mg/6 mo
    - Formula—~ 38 mg/6 mo
    - Soy formula—~117 mg/6 mo[5]

If we take the weight of an average 6 month old (around 16.5 pounds—a little less for girls and a little more for boys), the amount of aluminum that they could safely receive (calculated using the MRL) would be approximately 7.5 mg/d. If we were to give every vaccine recommended at the 6-month well-child check (Hep B, rotavirus, DTaP, Hib, PCV13, IPV, and influenza),[6] we would only be giving 1.4 mg of aluminum, much below the allowable MRL.[5] Note that some children may receive fewer vaccines at 6 months as there is some flexibility in dosing per the Centers for Disease Control and Prevention (CDC) vaccine schedule. Also note that vaccines given in combination form often have even less aluminum per dose than if given separately—yet another reason *not* to space out immunizations (**Box 9.2**).

 Box 9.2   Did You Know?

Children ages 6 months through 8 years, who have never had an influenza immunization, need to begin with the two-dose series. This is also true for children who only ever received the first of the two-dose series. These first two influenza vaccines should be administered at least 28 days apart. Any person who has already received their first two-dose series, or is at the age of 9 years or older, only needs one dose per flu season going forward. The reason for the two-dose series is that the first dose, given to those ages 6 months through 8 years, is not likely to cause a full immune response by itself. It "primes" the immune system. The second dose is where we get a more robust immune response. By the age of 9 years, however, we are likely to have already come in contact with an influenza infection naturally and have developed some aspect of immune memory. After the age of 9 years, one dose of influenza vaccine is, therefore, all that is needed to mount a full response to the vaccine.[7,8]

5. I heard there is formaldehyde in vaccines. Doesn't formaldehyde cause cancer?
    - Formaldehyde is used in the vaccine production process to inactivate viruses and to render bacterial toxins no longer toxic. It is diluted during manufacturing to the degree that there is only a minuscule amount remaining in some vaccines.
    - Formaldehyde is listed by the ATSDR as a possible human carcinogen but this requires much higher levels of exposure than what is present in vaccines, and toxicity is typically greatest through inhalation. The ATSDR lists MRLs (levels below which are considered to be nontoxic) for

formaldehyde as 0.3 mg/kg/d on an intermittent basis.[2] Considering our same 6-month-old baby, weighing an average of 16.5 pounds, he or she could safely be exposed to 2.25 mg of formaldehyde per day. In all of the shots recommended at the 6-month checkup (if we include influenza), there is only approximately 0.2 mg given. Again, much below the MRL.

- What is not commonly understood by the general public is that our bodies *require* formaldehyde for cellular function. Our bodies actually make their own formaldehyde to aid in the production of amino acids, the building blocks of proteins, and in the metabolism of some fats. Our bodies contain approximately 2.6 mg of formaldehyde per liter of blood. Given that humans have around 5 liters of blood, we have about 13 mg of formaldehyde circulating in our systems at any given time.[9] Even the average newborn, weighing only 6 to 8 pounds, has approximately 50 to 70 times more formaldehyde in his or her system[10] than the newborn would be exposed to in any one vaccine or series of vaccines.

- In addition to the formaldehyde made by our own bodies, we are exposed to formaldehyde through our environment as well. It is in products that we use every day, such as household cleaners and building materials, and in the foods that we eat.

- Whether it is with aluminum or formaldehyde or any other ingredient in vaccines, what we need to remember is that *anything* in too great a quantity can be toxic. Even water can be harmful to our health, diluting the salts in our body and causing heart arrhythmias, weakness, and confusion if we drink too much of it. As the saying goes, "The dose makes the poison," and the doses of these components of vaccines are *significantly* below levels that should worry us (see chapter 12 for a more detailed discussion regarding vaccine ingredients).

6. There's squalene in vaccines. Wasn't that given to soldiers in the anthrax vaccine and is the cause of Gulf War Syndrome?

- We have Joseph Mercola to thank for espousing this bit of misleading information. In his article titled "Squalene: The Swine Flu's Dirty Little Secret," he lays out these claims and others that are completely unfounded.

- First, squalene is a naturally occurring molecule found in plants, animals, and humans. In humans, it is produced in the liver and circulates in the bloodstream. It is felt to have antioxidant properties when consumed in foods, such as olive oil and fish oils.

- Second, there is no squalene in most US-licensed vaccines. Only the influenza vaccine, Fluad, licensed for use in patients older than 65 years of age, contains squalene. When combined with surfactants (which help particles in a liquid remain in suspension), it works as an adjuvant to boost the immune response in this vaccine.

- Third, according to the World Health Organization (WHO), squalene was neither added to nor used in the manufacturing process of the anthrax vaccine that was given to Gulf War military.[11,12]

- Lastly, studies looking at the levels of antisqualene antibodies in Gulf War veterans showed no elevation of antibody levels beyond those in the baseline population. They also showed no increase in antibody levels generally in patients vaccinated with squalene-containing vaccines versus nonimmunized people.[13,14]

7. Exposure to these chemicals through our food is one thing. But aren't these chemicals way more toxic if we *inject* them into our bodies?
   - Remember, whether ingested or injected, these substances are present in such tiny amounts that they do not cause any harm.
   - Injected substances don't just sit there. The body has ways of processing these "foreign particles" that penetrate the skin, just as it would the "toxins" that are injected when you are stung by a bee.
   - Whether through the digestive tract or via the skin, these substances eventually make their way to the bloodstream. Once in the bloodstream, the body processes the substances in the same way.
   - The substances are either broken down into their harmless component parts (for example, monosodium glutamate will break down into sodium and glutamate) or are metabolized rapidly (like formaldehyde, which is metabolized in around 10 minutes).[15]

8. Don't vaccines make you sick?
   - In triggering our immune system, vaccines do sometimes cause us to feel a little under the weather for a day or two (fatigue, low-grade fever, mild body aches, etc.). This is just our immune system kicking into gear. It doesn't happen every time we get a vaccine, but it does happen commonly enough that we want patients to know about it. We should consider this a sign that the vaccine is doing its job.
   - Some people claim that they got sick with the flu after getting the flu shot. See chapter 11 for a more detailed discussion of this specific concern.

9. I'm healthy. Why do I need vaccinations?
   - Saying you don't need to vaccinate because you never get sick is like saying you don't need to wear a seat belt because you have never been in a car accident. Prevention saves lives.
   - Even healthy people can suffer serious consequences from infection. Most children who are unvaccinated and contract measles naturally are "healthy." But healthy children can develop encephalitis and permanent brain damage or die from the illness. Even healthy children who survive their illness can go on to develop subacute sclerosing panencephalitis (SSPE) 7 to 10 years later. SSPE is a universally fatal measles-related neurodegenerative condition. Ongoing observation of pediatric deaths from influenza show that, of all children who die from the flu, approximately 50% were entirely healthy to start.[16] These illnesses do have the potential to cause greater devastation in those who have chronic illness, the elderly, infants, and the immune compromised, but none of us are immune from risk.
   - We seek to vaccinate all members of a community, not just those who are sick or at high risk, to protect each individual, but also to provide something called *herd immunity* or *community immunity* as it is also known. Herd immunity is resistance to the spread of a contagious disease that results if a sufficiently high number of people (depending on the illness, typically 80%-95%) are immune to the disease, especially through vaccination.[17,18] See chapter 11, **Figure 11.2** for an excellent graphical representation of herd immunity in action.
     - Herd immunity provides protection to all of us but is most notably aimed at protecting those in our community who cannot take vaccines themselves. People who are immune suppressed cannot receive

live-attenuated virus vaccines. Others may have allergic reactions to certain components of vaccines. Newborns, for example, cannot take the pertussis vaccine until they are 2 months old, but the newborn period is the most risky time were they to acquire this infection. These people are at much higher risk if we don't surround them with a bubble of protection by vaccinating those with whom they come in contact.

› Vaccinations are not perfect. For example, the flu shot at its best is about 60% effective. As a result, it's all hands on deck for individual and population-level protection from this potentially serious infection. Even the ones that are generally highly effective (for example, complete measles vaccination is 97% effective at protecting against infection) require the assistance of vaccinating as many as possible to limit spread. Measles is highly contagious. It can linger in the air for 2 hours, which means that no direct contact is required for transmission. One person has the ability to infect up to 18 others. It is easy to see how the infection can spread rapidly in unvaccinated or under-vaccinated communities. Only by vaccinating the greatest number possible do we hope to limit spread throughout the population. (See Appendix C: Vaccine Topics Explained for a video depicting herd immunity in action.)

› Most vaccine-preventable illnesses are contagious before the person carrying it has even one symptom. Many of us like to think of ourselves as taking steps to protect others when we are sick (covering coughs, washing hands, avoiding contact with babies or immune-suppressed persons), but how many of us are this vigilant when we are feeling perfectly healthy?

› If vaccination levels fall below levels required to provide herd immunity, we see an increase in the cases of vaccine-preventable illness (as was seen during the 2017 measles outbreak in the Somali community of Minnesota,[19] the 2018 measles outbreak in New York, pertussis outbreaks across the country, etc.).

• We have an ethical obligation, as members of society, to protect each other for the common good. We do not live in isolation. We are part of a wider world. When I vaccinate myself and my children, I am protecting you and your children. For the public's health, we hope that each member of the community will return the favor.

10. Isn't it true that we don't see as many serious illnesses because of the introduction of better hygiene and sanitation, not because of vaccines?

• Our current US sanitation standards were established under the Safe Drinking Water Act of 1974.[20] Improvements in sanitation, hygiene, nutrition, and other public health measures have certainly helped decrease the spread of disease and have improved survival rates. However, there is no denying the significant drop in the incidence of disease that happens after the introduction of a vaccine for that particular illness or the increase in cases of disease when vaccine rates fall.

› In the early 1990s, our sanitation standards were already well established. Yet we didn't see a significant drop in the incidence of Hib (dropping from around 20,000 cases per year to 1419 cases by 1993) until *after* the conjugate Hib vaccines were introduced in the late 1980s to early 1990s.[21]

> In Britain, a drop in the rates of pertussis (whooping cough) vaccination in 1974 resulted in an epidemic of more than 100,000 cases with 36 deaths by 1978. No lessening of hygiene or sanitation standards had occurred to explain this rise[21] **(Figure 9.1)**.

11. We eat all organic foods, avoid exposure to chemicals, and take supplements such as vitamin A, which I've read can prevent measles. Won't keeping our immune systems strong naturally protect us from getting sick?

- Living a healthy lifestyle is extremely important, and there is no denying that death rates from vaccine-preventable disease in some other countries are higher in part because of a general lack of nutrition. Undernourished people do not have the reserves to fight off disease such as those with good nutrition. But in this country, where we have fortified foods and where most people are afforded the luxury of regular meals, we still see significant death rates from vaccine-preventable disease (for example, 80,000 people died from the flu in the 2017-2018 flu season). Illnesses, such as influenza, pertussis, and measles, do not discriminate based on race, gender, socioeconomic background, or nutritional status, be it organic or otherwise.

- The discussion of vitamin A is an interesting one. First, we must make it known that chronic excessive vitamin A intake can be harmful, causing vision changes, bone pain, increased intracranial pressure, and liver toxicity, and that use of any supplements in children should be discussed with the child's primary care provider.

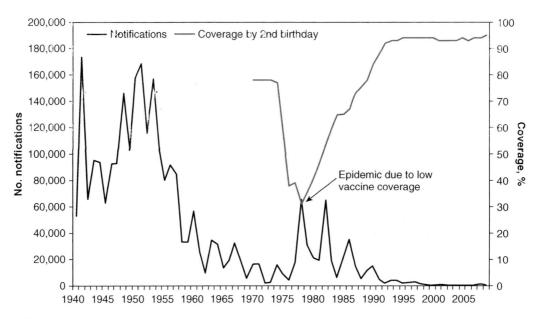

FIGURE 9.1 Graph showing the drop in cases of whooping cough in England and Wales after introduction of the pertussis vaccine in the 1950s. It also shows a subsequent rise in cases of whooping cough after vaccination rates temporarily decreased in the 1970s. (Modified from Campbell H, Amirthalingam G, Andrews N, et al. Accelerating control of pertussis in England and Wales. *Emerg Infect Dis.* 2012;18(1):38-47. doi:10.3201/eid1801.110784.)

- The WHO recognizes vitamin A deficiency as a contributing risk factor for severe measles. Not only are those with poor nutritional status and relative vitamin A deficiency at increased risk, but an acute measles infection also "precipitates vitamin A deficiency by depleting vitamin A stores and increasing its utilization."[22] There is evidence to suggest that children in generally undernourished communities see less morbidity and mortality from measles infection if administered a vitamin A supplement on a daily preventative basis.[23] There is also evidence that administration of a prescribed dose of vitamin A over 2 days to children hospitalized with measles decreases overall and pneumonia-specific mortality in those younger than 5 years of age.[23]
- That is *not* to say that vitamin A supplementation prevents measles infection, only that vitamin A administration may help decrease the severity of the illness once acquired.

12. Aren't vaccines just another way for Big Pharma and doctors to make money?
    - In the earlier days of vaccines, drug companies actually moved away from production because vaccines were very expensive to make, liability was high, and they did not bring in large profits. These days, with worldwide distribution, drug companies are back in the swing of making vaccines and, like we would expect from any other company, are in business to make money. Even though they are now a more profitable endeavor, money made on vaccines typically represents no more than 3% of a pharmaceutical company's total profits.[24] Drug (medication) manufacturing is a much more lucrative business.
    - Some smaller health care clinics are not able to offer a full complement of vaccinations because the reimbursement they receive isn't enough to cover the growing costs of immunizations. A 2010 study in the *Annals of Family Medicine* showed that approximately 44% of family physicians surveyed referred patients to other locations for some of the routinely recommended childhood and adolescent vaccines. Nearly 53% referred patients out for adult vaccines. Half of those who referred patients to other vaccine providers cited lack of adequate payment as the reason.[25]
    - Health care providers receive no payments from drug companies for offering vaccines or for offering one vaccine over another. With the move toward medical provider reimbursement based on outcomes and prevention of disease, physicians *are* seeing an increasing percentage of their compensation coming from "bonuses" based on achievement of certain quality measures. The emphasis on this type of compensation makes intuitive sense, at least in the primary care world. If providers can help prevent illness and disease from happening, decreasing the devastating effects on patients' lives and the cost to the health care system, then we all benefit.
    - We recommend vaccinations and other preventive measures because they have been *proven* to reduce disease, suffering, hospitalizations, loss of life, medical costs, and costs to society.

13. We don't see illnesses such as polio in our country anymore, so why would I need to vaccinate against it?
    - One of the factors contributing to the rise in anti-vaccine sentiment is that we rarely see vaccine-preventable illnesses anymore (such as polio, measles, and mumps), thanks to prior years' vaccination efforts. These illnesses no longer feel like an ever-present danger, and the small risks of vaccinating can falsely seem greater than the risk of contracting a vaccine-preventable disease. However, our world is much smaller than it used to be. International travel is common and illnesses can be reintroduced into a community with relative ease. There are a few countries in the world where polio still occurs (Pakistan, Afghanistan, and Nigeria). If we are to keep polio from returning to the United States, we need to stay vigilant!
    - This concern is not only for polio but also for other illnesses that have been declared no longer endemic (originating) in the United States. In the state of Washington in 2017, we saw an outbreak of mumps brought to the state by travelers from the Marshallese community. In 2018, US travelers to Israel brought measles back to New York City, which is now experiencing its largest measles outbreak seen in recent history. In both cases, outbreaks occurred in largely unvaccinated or under-vaccinated groups.
    - Some historic perspective—smallpox, a deadly and disfiguring disease that killed millions of people and contributed to the downfall of the Roman, Aztec, and Incan empires, was eradicated from the face of the planet in 1979, thanks to focused vaccination efforts by WHO. Today's children no longer need to receive vaccination against smallpox. Vaccination works, but we have to keep at it!

14. Shouldn't this be my decision? How does my health or illness impact the community?
    - In addition to the importance of maintaining herd immunity, as discussed previously, we also have to consider the social and economic impact of these illnesses.
        - There is the personal cost to the patient or family members of being out of school or work for extended periods.
        - There is the potential for incredible personal expense if a complication arises that requires hospitalization.
        - The cost to the community is also significant. A study looking at the cost of four major adult vaccine-preventable illnesses (influenza, pneumococcal disease, shingles, and whooping cough) in the United States in 2013 estimated the annual cost for these illnesses in adults older than 50 years of age to be $26.5 billion.[26] Imagine the costs if we looked at *all* vaccine-preventable diseases for both adults *and* children!

15. I heard that people can die, be paralyzed, or stop breathing after getting a vaccination. Why would I want to take that risk?
    - One of the most feared reactions to a vaccination is called Guillain-Barré syndrome (GBS), a neurologic condition that can cause paralysis. When this happens, it is certainly terrible and frightening. Fortunately, the majority of people will recover. The CDC estimates

the risk of GBS following influenza immunization to be only one to two cases out of 1 million people vaccinated,[27] whereas the risk of developing GBS after an influenza infection is 17 cases per 1 million people infected. In preventing influenza, the vaccine actually *lessens* your chances of developing GBS.

- Severe allergic reactions (such as anaphylaxis or angioedema) occur very rarely. There are components of select vaccines to which people may be allergic (neomycin and other antibiotics, yeast, latex, etc.). We are pretty good about screening for these allergies and the Vaccine Information Statement (VIS) that is required to be given to patients prior to vaccine administration reviews these possible allergic concerns with the patient as well. A 2016 study in the *Journal of Allergy and Clinical Immunology* reported that the rate of anaphylaxis in all vaccines combined was only 1.31 in 1 million people vaccinated.[28] This type of an allergic reaction generally happens very quickly, and the doctor's office is the right place to be to care for someone in case of such an event.

- The risk of developing severe complications from a vaccine-preventable disease is much greater than the rare risk of developing severe or life-threatening reactions to a vaccine (see chapter 7, A Risk Worth Taking, for a more detailed discussion). Let's use GBS as an example. In 2018, the CDC recorded 80,000 deaths from influenza in the United States, 185 of whom were children. The US population in 2018 was around 326.7 million people. If we divide 80,000 by 326.7 million, then the risk of dying from influenza in the 2017 to 2018 flu season was approximately 1 in 4084 people. The risk of developing GBS, as stated above, is about 1 in 1 million people. If I were a betting person, I'd put my bets on the flu vaccine!

16. I've heard that there's a concern about being vaccinated if you have a *MTHFR* gene mutation. If either I or my children have that mutation, couldn't we be harmed by getting vaccines?

- *MTHFR* stands for methylenetetrahydrofolate reductase. It is an enzyme that plays a role in the conversion of 5, 10-methylenetetrahydrofolate to 5-methylenetetrahydrofolate. 5-MTHF is a molecule that is required in the multistep process (the methionine cycle) that converts homocysteine to methionine, an amino acid used to make proteins and other important compounds in the body. The *MTHFR* gene encodes the instructions for making the enzyme. *MTHFR* is also part of the folate cycle, which produces the essential nutrient, folate (or folic acid), required for RNA and DNA synthesis.[29]

- There are multiple *MTHFR* gene mutations that have been identified. Some sources suggest that up to 50% of us have one of these mutations.[30] However, in all but a very few cases, residual enzyme activity remains. There is a range of affectedness, from almost no activity to nearly normal enzyme activity. One source suggests that we think of these mutations as normal variants, such as those that we have with eye color, and not as anything more pathologic.[31] What matters in this discussion is not the degree to which the enzyme is affected, but how much homocysteine and folate are present. Without adequate *MTHFR*, a buildup of homocysteine and a reduction in folate levels occur. High homocysteine levels are felt to contribute to DNA damage and both conditions are suspected of playing a role in various conditions, such as peripheral vascular disease, stroke, heart disease, dementia, psychiatric disorders, and possible cancers, though more investigation is necessary before we can draw correlation.

- The presence of the *MTHFR* gene mutations can be easily surmised without expensive genetic testing, though anti-vaccine websites will often try to sell patients expensive tests. There are simple blood tests that can detect the presence of high levels of homocysteine and low levels of folate in the blood.

- One of the anti-vaccine assertions on this topic is that vaccines may induce a genetic mutation in the *MTHFR* gene that then renders a person susceptible to outcomes related to high homocysteine and low folate levels. However, mutations of these genes are generally handed down from parent to child. Even if a mutation could be "triggered," it is highly unlikely that the mutation would occur in every cell of the body, putting that person at risk for systemic disease.[32]

- Another assertion of vaccine skeptics is that lack of folate and high levels of homocysteine as a result of *MTHFR* gene mutation lead to a decreased ability for the body to produce glutathione, an antioxidant, which in turn allows "toxins" to build up in the body, leading to anything from autism to fibromyalgia to addiction. Interestingly, a meta-analysis looking at this question did find a slightly higher risk of autism associated with the C677T polymorphism of the *MTHFR* gene. However, this risk was only seen in countries *without* folate fortification of the food supply (which we do have in the United States).[33] Most importantly, if it is true that a large percentage of us have some form of *MTHFR* gene mutation, which vaccine skeptics assert impacts our ability to tolerate vaccines and increases our exposure to "toxins,"[34] shouldn't we be seeing significantly higher rates of vaccine adverse reactions than we do?

- In the end, all of these concerns are a relative nonissue. Assuming we are eating a reasonably healthy diet (containing dark green vegetables and folate-fortified foods or taking a daily multivitamin), our diets provide enough natural folate for proper methylation.

17. Why are we seeing such an increase in autoimmune diseases and cancer? I've heard vaccinations have led to this increase.

- Although it is enticing to try to lay the blame for all of the world's ills at the feet of a single agent, in this case vaccines, the reality is much less tidy. It is undoubtedly a complicated interplay between genetics, chemical exposures, infectious agents, situational stresses, hormones, weight, aging, and other factors.[35] As we are increasingly exposed to hormones and chemicals through our foods, environment, and the use of plastics and as the population is becoming heavier, and living longer, we are seeing more autoimmune diseases and cancers occurring. In addition, as science continues to advance, we have gotten better at defining and diagnosing many of these conditions. Though much is still uncertain, we strongly suspect that infections are one trigger that can cause the body to attack itself, resulting in autoimmune diseases such as type 1 diabetes and thyroid disease. We *know* that certain viruses (HPV and hepatitis B) can cause cancer. The best advice we can offer at this time is to let your kids get dirty, avoid chemicals and preservatives, eat lots of vegetables and other healthy foods, drink lots of water, get regular exercise, don't smoke or drink heavy amounts of alcohol, get adequate sleep, and vaccinate to help prevent those infectious triggers from happening. (See Appendix E: Journal Articles Addressing Specific Vaccine Concerns for a list of articles showing no link between vaccines and autoimmune disease.)

18. What about the National Vaccine Injury Compensation Program? Doesn't it prove that vaccines are risky if we are paying out millions of dollars in claims?

   - The National Vaccine Injury Compensation Program (NVICP) was established in the 1980s under the National Childhood Vaccination Injury Act after lawsuits against vaccine manufacturers threatened to cause vaccine shortages, which could have reduced vaccination rates and caused a resurgence in vaccine-preventable disease.[36] In recognizing that there are known, but rare, serious side effects from vaccination and that the people who suffer those consequences deserve to be compensated, the federal government set up the NVICP to reduce the burden on vaccine manufacturers and to provide restitution to those seriously affected by vaccine adverse reactions (see **Box 5.2**: The Vaccine Injury Table).

   - Individuals are compensated on a "no-fault" basis, meaning that they are not required to show fault or negligence on the part of the medical provider or manufacturer to receive compensation. According to the CDC, between the years 2006 and 2012, more than 3.1 billion doses of covered vaccines were distributed in the United States. During this time period, 5576 petitions were adjudicated by the Court and only 3785 received compensation. This means that, for every 1 million doses of vaccine, only one person was found to have reaction severe enough to warrant compensation.[37] This is in line with what we know about the risk of serious or life-threatening events following vaccination (they occur in about 1-2/million cases). The NVICP is not "proof" that adverse events following vaccination are common or that there is some conspiracy on the part of the medical establishment or government to put people at risk. It is simply a safety net that the government provides in the very unlikely event that a patient does suffer a serious vaccine-related outcome.

19. What about all the adverse reactions listed on vaccine package inserts? Isn't that proof that vaccines are harmful?

   - The first thing to know is that package inserts (PIs) are developed by the vaccine manufacturer. That's right, Big Pharma is putting out this informational sheet. Anti-vaccine proponents claim that Big Pharma lies to cover up the truth about vaccines. But in the same breath, they will swear that the PIs produced by the pharmaceutical companies are the gospel truth and should be believed. A slight contradiction, yes?

   - Second, the "Adverse Reactions" that are listed in the PI are required by the Federal Food and Drug Administration (FDA) to be included. They represent every event that was reported during vaccine testing or in postmarketing analysis, whether caused by the vaccine or not. This section of the PI must, by mandate, include any effect reported during the Biologics Licensing Application process. This is history. It doesn't change with the growing knowledge and understanding that we gain from future research. For example, years after multiple studies have shown *no* link between vaccines and autism; autism still exists as a listed "Adverse Reaction" in PIs.

- The "Warnings" section of the PI, however, is a listing of events that *do* have evidence supporting a causal relationship with the vaccine. The FDA can mandate a change to this section of the PI as new scientific evidence arises. It is important to note that none of the PIs list autism under the "Warnings" section.
- If you'd like proof of the fact that there is not necessarily a correlation between those observed adverse reactions listed in the PI and vaccines, look no further than the reaction of "teething" listed in the Varivax PI.[38] How many of us would actually believe that a vaccine induced teething in a child? We call this "true, true, and unrelated"—a coincidence. Just because the two occurred together in time, does not mean that one caused the other (see chapter 3—Psychology of the Anti-vaccine Movement—for discussion of the *post hoc, ergo propter hoc* fallacy of logic).
- The PIs themselves provide the following disclaimer:

These adverse events were reported voluntarily from a population of uncertain size; therefore, it is not always possible to reliably estimate their frequency or establish a causal relationship to vaccination.[39]

20. Do doctors even get training on vaccines, or are they just regurgitating recommendations from government agencies and Big Pharma that they don't really understand?
    - This is a relatively common refrain heard from the staunch anti-vaccine community. They feel that their hours of "research" equates to, or is greater than, the years of learning about vaccines that we get in medical school, residency, advanced training, and practice.
    - It is true that there is no one class or curriculum in medical school called "Vaccines." It is also true that we can do better at teaching our students and residents how to deal with the questions surrounding vaccines that they will encounter in the "real world" of day-to-day clinical practice (hence, the need for this book!) However, it is patently *untrue* that physicians receive inadequate training on the topic of immunizations.
    - For years, we study the building blocks of illness and disease. Our knowledge builds upon the foundation laid by those who have come before us—Jenner, Salk, Hilleman, and other giants in the field.
    - Medical school and residency curriculum addressing vaccines involves *longitudinal* study over time and crosses numerous disciplines. It includes the studies of immunology (how the immune system works), infectious disease (the pathogens that invade the body), pathophysiology (how our body responds to those pathogens), pharmacology (the mechanism of action of medications and other interventions to treat disease), toxicology (study of adverse effects of substances on living organisms), and preventive medicine and public health (preventing widespread disease in communities), among others.
    - We also benefit from our subspecialty rotations, each of which deals with vaccine-preventable disease in their own way.
      - In pediatrics, family medicine, obstetrics, and internal medicine/geriatrics, we learn the importance of vaccines as we see the immediate and long-term complications of diseases that could have been prevented by immunization (for example, recurrent otitis media

from Hib in toddlers; precancerous changes of the cervix and genital warts in our young adults, and invasive cervical, vaginal, and vulvar cancers from HPV in women as they age; preterm labor in our pregnant patients from influenza; and postpolio syndrome and shingles in our elderly).

) In our emergency department rotations, we see the crises that can happen as a result of vaccine-preventable illness (seizures from meningitis, respiratory failure from pneumonia and whooping cough, heart attacks and strokes triggered by influenza, and more).

) In our ENT and oncology rotations, we see the devastation caused by head and neck cancers related to preventable HPV infection.

) In urology and reproductive health, we see penile cancers from HPV and male sterility caused by mumps infections.

) In psychiatry, we treat the emotional scars that these devastating diseases leave on individuals and families. The list goes on and I can think of no specialty that is spared.

Our training is not minimal. In fact, it is prolonged and extensive. What we are missing, I would argue, is a "putting it all into practice" curriculum at the end of training—a curriculum that synthesizes what we have learned into an approach (much as this book tries to do) that better allows us to communicate the importance and safety of vaccines to our patients and our communities.

References

1. LaSalle G. When the answer to vaccines is "no.". *J Fam Pract*. 2018;67(6):348-364.

2. Agency for Toxic Substances and Disease Registry. Minimal Risk Levels (MRLs) for Hazardous Substances. https://www.atsdr.cdc.gov/mrls/mrllist.asp. Updated August 2, 2018. Accessed January 10, 2019.

3. Jefferson Lab. The Element Aluminum. https://education.jlab.org/itselemental/ele013.html. Accessed January 10, 2019.

4. Agency for Toxic Substances and Disease Registry. Toxic Substances Portal – Aluminum. https://www.atsdr.cdc.gov/phs/phs.asp?id=1076&tid=34. Updated January 21, 2015. Accessed January 10, 2019.

5. Children's Hospital of Philadelphia. Vaccine Ingredients – Aluminum. https://www.chop.edu/centers-programs/vaccine-education-center/vaccine-ingredients/aluminum. Accessed January 10, 2019.

6. Centers for Disease Control and Prevention. Recommended Immunization Schedule for Children and Adolescents Aged 18 Years or Younger, United States, 2018. https://www.cdc.gov/vaccines/schedules/hcp/imz/child-adolescent.html. Updated February 6, 2018. Accessed January 10, 2019.

7. Centers for Disease Control and Prevention. Children & Influenza (Flu). https://www.cdc.gov/flu/protect/children.htm. Updated February 5, 2019. Accessed February 7, 2019.

8. Zibners L. *Why Some Kids Need a Second Dose of Flu Vaccine*. December 5, 2012. https://shotofprevention.com/2012/12/05/why-some-kids-need-a-second-dose-of-flu-vaccine/. Accessed February 7, 2019.

9. Staropoli N. *Apple Pie, Mashed Potatoes and Natural Formaldehyde*. American Council of Science and Health. November 23, 2015. https://www.acsh.org/news/2015/11/23/apple-pie-mashed-potatoes-and-natural-formaldehyde. Accessed January 10, 2019.

10. U.S. Food and Drug Administration. Common Ingredients in U.S. Licensed Vaccines. https://www.fda.gov/biologicsbloodvaccines/safetyavailability/vaccinesafety/ucm187810.htm. Updated April 30, 2018. Accessed January 10, 2019.

11. World Health Organization. *Weekly Epidemiological Record*. July 4, 2006; 28:273-284.

12. Spanggord RJ, Wu B, Sun M, et al. Development and application of an analytical method for the determination of squalene in formulations of anthrax vaccine absorbed. *J Pharm Biomed Anal*. 2002;29(1-2):183-193.

13. Phillips CJ, Matyas GR, Hansen CJ, et al. Antibodies to squalene in US Navy Persian Gulf War veterans with chronic multisystem illness. *Vaccine*. 2009;27(29):3921-3926.

14. Del Giudice G, Fragapane E, Bugarini R, et al. Vaccines with the MF59 adjuvant do not stimulate antibody responses against squalene. *Clin Vaccine Immunol.* 2006;13(9):1010-1013.

15. *Injection vs Ingestion. Myths and Facts. Vaxplanations.* February 25, 2015. https://vaxplanations.wordpress.com/2015/02/25/239/. Accessed January 14, 2019.

16. Shang M, Blanton L, Brammer L, et al. Influenza-associated pediatric deaths in the United States, 2010–2016. *Pediatrics.* 2018;141(4):e20172918.

17. Orenstein W, Seib K. Mounting a good offense against measles. *N Engl J Med.* 2014;371:1661-1663.

18. Plans-Rubió P. The vaccination coverage required to establish heard immunity against influenza viruses. *Prev Med.* 2012;55(1):72-77.

19. Hall V, Banerjee E, Kenyon C, et al. Measles outbreak – Minnesota April-May 2017. *MMWR Morb Mortal Wkly Rep.* 2017;66(27):713-717.

20. *History of U.S. water and wastewater systems.* In: *Privatization of Water Services in the United States: An Assessment of Issues and Experience.* Washington, DC: The National Academies Press; 2002:35:chap 4. https://www.nap.edu/read/10135/chapter/4#35. Accessed January 16, 2019.

21. World Health Organization. Global Vaccine Safety: Six Common Misconceptions About Immunization. http://www.who.int/vaccine_safety/initiative/detection/immunization_misconceptions/en/index1.html. Accessed January 10, 2019.

22. Melenotte C, Brouqui P, Botelho-Nevers E. Severe measles, vitamin A deficiency, and the Roma community in Europe. *Emerg Infect Dis.* 2012,18(9):1537-1538.

23. Imdad A, Mayo-Wilson E, Herzer K, et al. Vitamin A supplementation for preventing morbidity and mortality in children from 6 months to 5 years of age. *Cochrane Database Syst Rev.* 2017;3. https://www.cochranelibrary.com/cdsr/doi/10.1002/14651858.CD001479.pub3/full. Accessed February 20, 2019.

24. Kaddar M. Global Vaccine Market Features and Trends. World Health Organization Web site. https://www.who.int/influenza_vaccines_plan/resources/session_10_kaddar.pdf?ua=1. Accessed January 10, 2019.

25. Campos-Outcalt D, Jeffcot-Pera M, Carter-Smith P, et al. Vaccines provided by family physicians. *Ann Fam Med.* 2010;8(6):507-510.

26. McLaughlin JM, McGinnis JJ, Tan L, et al. Estimated human and economic burden of four major adult vaccine-preventable diseases in the United States, 2013. *J Prim Prev.* 2015;36(4):259-273.

27. Mistry RD, Fischer JB, Prasad PA, et al. Severe complications in influenza-like illnesses. *Pediatrics.* 2014;134(3):e684-e690.

28. McNeil MM, Weintraub ES, Duffy J, et al. Risk of anaphylaxis after vaccination in children and adults. *J Allergy Clin Immunol.* 2016;137(3):868-878.

29. U.S. National Library of Medicine. *MTHFR Gene.* January 15, 2019. https://ghr.nlm.nih.gov/gene/MTHFR. Accessed January 10, 2019.

30. 23andMe. *Our Take on the MTHFR Gene.* January 5, 2017. https://blog.23andme.com/health-traits/our-take-on-the-mthfr-gene. Accessed January 10, 2019.

31. Smith J. *A Pediatrician Goes In-Depth into MTHFR.* Cook Children's. July 7, 2017. https://www.check-upnewsroom.com/a-pediatricians-goes-in-depth-into-mthfr/. Accessed January 10, 2019.

32. Skeptical Raptor. *MTHFR Gene and Vaccines – What are the Facts and Myths.* November 18, 2018. https://www.skepticalraptor.com/skepticalraptorblog.php/mthfr-gene-vaccines-facts-myths/. Accessed January 10, 2019.

33. Pu D, Shen Y, Wu J. Association between MTHFR gene polymorphisms and the risk of autism spectrum disorders: a meta-analysis. *Autism Res.* 2013;6(5):384-392.

34. Marino S. *MTHFR Mutations.* National Vaccine Information Center. May 18, 2017. https://thevaccinereaction.org/2017/05/mthfr-mutations/. Accessed January 10, 2019.

35. Schmidt CW. Questions persist: environmental factors in autoimmune disease. *Environ Health Perspect.* 2011;119(6):A249-A253.

36. Health Resources and Services Administration. National vaccine injury compensation program. https://www.hrsa.gov/vaccine-compensation/index.html. Accessed January 10, 2019.

37. Health Resources and Services Administration. Vaccine Injury Compensation Data. https://www.hrsa.gov/vaccine-compensation/data/index.html. Updated January 2019. Accessed January 10, 2019.

38. *Varivax* [package insert]. Whitehouse Station, NJ: Merck Sharp & Dohme; 2018.

39. *Infanrix* [package insert]. Triangle Park, NC: GlaxoSmithKline; 2018.

10

Vaccine Concerns in Specific Populations: Point-Counterpoint, Part 2

Don't believe every worried thought you have. Worried thoughts are notoriously inaccurate.

—RENEE JAIN

In the last chapter, we discussed general questions and concerns that you may hear about vaccines and how to reply to or counter them. In this chapter, we will continue the discussion but look at questions that specifically relate to certain groups of patients or segments of the population. First, we will delve into the common childhood-specific vaccine claims you may encounter as well as those that relate to immunization during pregnancy. Next, we will look at the religious objections that we hear regarding vaccines and why most of them, based on the tenets of the world's leading religions, are unfounded. Finally, the chapter will speak to some of the specific issues surrounding vaccination of immune-compromised patients.

As parents, or prospective parents, we worry. We are really good at it. It is a skill that grows and gestates right along with the growing fetus. Worry isn't all bad though. It does serve some purpose. It keeps us vigilant and cautious so that we may protect the new and delicate life whose care has been entrusted to us. But, for some, worry and fear can become paralyzing and keep us from making decisions that are best for our littlest loved ones. The anti-vaccine movement does a brilliant job of playing on our parental worries. If we allow ourselves to fall prey to anti-vaccine fearmongering, we can inadvertently increase, not decrease, the risk to our children. The following are some of the most common concerns that you will hear during your vaccine counseling discussions and the information you need to help reassure parents that vaccines are safe, effective, and are truly one of the best things we can do to protect our children (also see Appendix B: Fast Facts about Vaccines for Patients and Clinic Staff for a helpful patient handout addressing many common vaccine-related concerns).

SPECIFIC CONCERNS RELATED TO CHILDHOOD VACCINATIONS

1. I've heard that vaccines cause autism.

   Autism is a developmental disorder that negatively affects a child's ability to communicate and interact with others. Features of autism often include repetitive behaviors and obsessive interests. Referred to as Autism Spectrum Disorder (ASD), it has a broad range and severity of symptoms that often begin to be recognized by parents and clinicians when the child is around the age of 2 to 3 years, but sometimes not until the child is of school-age.

   - Although physicians and scientists have yet to discover the exact causes of autism, we can say with confidence that there is no *one* event or *one* cause, such as vaccines. There are likely multiple factors at play, such as older maternal age, the in utero environment, nutrition, and genetics.
     - In review of home movies from infancy in children who were later diagnosed with ASD, we know that symptoms of autism often developed many months *before* administration of the measles, mumps, and rubella (MMR) vaccine (typically given at 12-15 months).[1,2]
     - As we learned in the last chapter, in discussion of *MTHFR* gene mutations, nutritional status and lack of adequate folate levels may play a role.
     - We know that there are higher rates of ASD in identical twins (77% concordance in identical twin boys and 50% in identical twin girls) than in fraternal twins (31% in male fraternal twins, 36% in female fraternal twins, 5.3% for female twin of affected male twin, and 50% for male twin of affected female twin).[3,4]
     - We know that there are higher rates of autism in siblings, regardless of vaccination status.[5] A Kaiser Family Foundation study showed that children with an older sibling carrying the diagnosis of ASD were approximately 14 times more likely to be diagnosed with ASD themselves.[6]
     - We also know that autism affects boys four times more often than girls.[7]
     - All of these findings suggest a strong genetic link.
   - As discussed in chapter 8, the largest setback to vaccination efforts in recent history was the 1998 study by Andrew Wakefield suggesting that vaccination with the MMR vaccine was linked to the development of autism. Wakefield's study involved only 12 children. Subsequent studies involving *hundreds of thousands* of children have found no such relationship. There is even some data to suggest that MMR vaccination may provide a protective benefit against ASD.[8,9] Wakefield's claims have been debunked numerous times over. His paper was found to be fraudulent, and he was stripped of his medical license for falsifying data. However, the damage to vaccination efforts was done, and this claim persists today, despite much evidence to the contrary (See Appendix E: Journal Articles Addressing Specific Vaccine Concerns for a list of studies you can recommend to your patients that *disprove* any link between vaccines and autism).
   - Regarding the specific concern that exposure to mercury increases the risk of autism, it is interesting to note that rates of autism have actually

increased since thimerosal was removed from all US-licensed vaccines in 2001. As of writing this book, the CDC's Autism and Developmental Disabilities Monitoring Network now estimates that 1 in 59 children has been identified as having ASD.[10] If there were a true association between the two, we would have expected the opposite to occur. The rates of autism should have declined as children were no longer exposed to ethyl mercury in vaccines, but they didn't.[11-13]

- Much to pediatricians' and family physicians' dismay, the MMR-autism claim is not the only vaccine-autism assertion that exists. The anti-vaccine community casts their net wide and also asserts the following: The mercury in vaccines causes autism, the aluminum and formaldehyde in vaccines cause autism, and the sheer number of vaccines that we give children causes autism. Yet, in study after study looking to investigate these concerns, none of this has proven to be true.[8,14]

2. Aren't all the vaccines they recommend for kids going to overwhelm or weaken their immune systems?

- Studies looking for a link between vaccination, or the number of viral and bacterial proteins in a series of vaccines and the development of autism and other health concerns, show *no* increased risk of autism[15]; no increased risk of autoimmune disease[16]; no increased risk of other non-vaccine targeted infections[17]; no increased risk of childhood cancer, and in fact, show a possible protective effect on rates of childhood leukemia.[18]

- Kids are exposed to more proteins on a daily basis (crawling around on the floor, constantly sticking their hands in their mouths, sharing germs with kids at school or day care) than they are ever exposed to in a series of vaccines. Moreover, the infant immune system has a remarkably large capacity to respond to antigenic challenges. Modeling would suggest that an infant's immune system could actually handle up to 10,000 vaccines given at once. It also indicates that if 11 vaccines were given to an infant all at one time, only 0.1% of their immune system would be "used up."[19] An infant's immune system is not overwhelmed or weakened by the current immunizations recommended.

- Exposure to environmental proteins (antigens), and to those in vaccines, serves to boost an infant's immune system and to keep the infant safer in the long run. For example, studies show that children who are exposed to animal dander in their younger years have lower rates of asthma, eczema, and allergies.[20,21] Moreover, kids who have been vaccinated with a measles-containing vaccine show a lower rate of all-cause mortality than those who have not been vaccinated.[22]

- Thanks to advances in vaccine production, the immunologic load in today's vaccines is even less than it used to be. The 14 vaccines given today contain fewer than 200 bacterial and viral proteins or polysaccharides, compared with greater than 3000 of these immunologic components in the 7 vaccines administered in 1980.[23]

- Vaccines continue to be perfected. With scientific advancement and better understanding of how to "train the immune system" to defend against disease, vaccines are becoming more precise. When the pertussis (whooping cough) vaccine was first developed in the 1930s, for example, it contained approximately 3000 bacterial proteins. Now, it contains two to five.[23,24]

3. That's so many pokes at one time. Can't we just space out the shots? What about the Dr. Sears schedule for vaccines?

- There are multiple ways in which *The Vaccine Book: Making the Right Decision for Your Child*, written by Dr. Robert Sears and published in 2007, misrepresents vaccine science and leads patients astray in making their vaccination decisions.[25,26]
- Most important to note is that Dr. Sears' Alternative Vaccine Schedule, in seeking to make it so that children receive no more than two shots at one visit, would require doctor's visits at 2, 3, 4, 5, 6, 7, 9, 12, 15, 18, 21, and 24 months and at 2.5, 3, 3.5, 4, 5, and 6 years old.
  - This significantly increases the number of office visits, the number of injections kids receive, and raises the age at which vaccines are given. The result is an increase in the risk of illness outbreaks and a decrease in the likelihood that parents will get their kids back to the office to complete the full series.
- If parents are concerned about the exposure to adjuvants or formaldehyde in vaccines (not that they should be, as discussed in the last chapter), spacing out the vaccines into individual shots has the potential to *increase* the exposure to those substances (for example, aluminum in Dtap is <0.33-0.625 mg/dose and in Hib is 0.225 mg/dose for a maximum cumulative dose of 0.85 mg). Whereas, using the combination vaccine of Dtap/IPV/Hib (given all at one time, in one injection) exposes a child to only 0.33 mg/dose.[27]

4. Kids produce a better immune response to the real thing. I prefer for my child to get chickenpox (or any other vaccine-preventable illness) naturally.

- Although the antibody response may be more vigorous following a "natural" infection than that induced by a vaccine, the "natural" infection carries with it significantly greater risk to life and health. As stated previously, we don't make vaccines against benign diseases. We vaccinate against viral and bacterial infections that have the potential to kill or seriously harm.
- Although most children will recover from chickenpox without incident, some children will develop pneumonia or encephalitis (inflammation of the brain that can cause permanent brain damage). Some will die from the illness. A natural infection from chickenpox also puts people at much higher risk of a devastatingly painful condition in later years called shingles.
- For measles, the statistics regarding "natural" infection are even worse. Of those infected, 1 in 4 will be hospitalized; 1 in 1000 will develop encephalitis; and 1 to 2 in 1000 will die from the infection. Even if a child recovers without incident, they can still develop subacute sclerosing panencephalitis years later. Acquiring an infection naturally can put children at significant risk. (See Appendix C: Vaccine Topics Explained for a video about the devastating effects of subacute sclerosing panencephalitis.)
- Natural infection from tetanus often means death. Natural infection from meningococcal meningitis results in high rates of seizures, loss of limbs, and death. Natural infection from human papillomavirus (HPV) can result in cancer. Natural is not always better.

5. Why do kids need to be vaccinated against hepatitis B at such a young age if it is a sexually transmitted or blood transmitted infection?

    ◦ The hepatitis B virus (HBV) is an infection that can be transmitted via blood or body fluids (including saliva, tears, seminal fluid, and vaginal secretions).[28] Although certain factors (such as intravenous drug use, unprotected sex with multiple partners, and working in a medical field where accidental blood exposure can occur) may certainly put one at greater risk for contracting HBV, it can still be acquired without risky activity. In fact, initial efforts at identifying "at risk" groups and targeting vaccination to those individuals were unsuccessful at limiting rates of HBV infection.[29] It wasn't until we started vaccinating the general pediatric population that we began to see a decrease in rates of HBV infection (**Figure 10.1**).

    ◦ A baby can acquire HBV by being born to a mother who is carrying the virus. A child could be bitten by another child who is carrying the virus. A teen could decide to use her friend's razor to shave her legs at a sleep over and contract the virus. None of these things seem inherently risky, but any activity where the skin is broken and permits exposure to infected blood or body fluids could result in virus transmission.

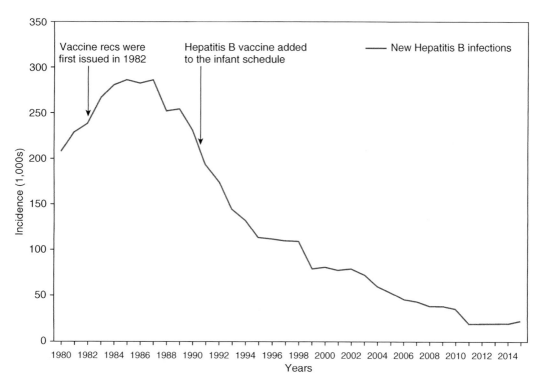

FIGURE 10.1 Graph showing impact when hepatitis B vaccine became available but was used only in "at risk" populations versus dramatic improvement seen when the vaccine was added to the infant schedule recommended for all children. (Adapted from Schillie S, Vellozzi C, Reingold A, et al. Prevention of hepatitis B virus infection in the United States: Recommendations of the Advisory Committee on Immunization Practices. *MMWR Recomm Rep.* 2018;67(No. RR-1):1-31. doi:10.15585/mmwr.rr6701a1.)

- HBV increases the risk of cirrhosis and liver cancer. This is one of only two cancer-prevention vaccines that we have, the other being the HPV vaccine. None of us like to think that our children will engage in risky behavior, but we know that many kids will make choices in their teen years that they might not make as wiser adults. Moreover, these decisions may have unintended consequences. HBV vaccination is one very important way that we can protect our kids from one such potentially lifelong and deadly consequence.

- Finally, and perhaps most importantly, we know that kids who contract HBV at a young age are much more susceptible to the lasting effects of HBV infection. Babies don't fight off the virus as well as older individuals. 9 out of 10 babies who become infected in their first year will develop chronic HBV, staying infected for life. Up to 25% of children who become infected during the first 5 years of life will die an earlier death from HBV-related liver disease, including liver failure or liver cancer.[28,30]

6. Can't vaccines cause sudden infant death syndrome (SIDS)?

- SIDS is a condition of unexplained death, typically during sleep, in a previously healthy infant younger than 12 months old. It is also known as "crib death." In most cases, the exact cause of death is unknown and research is ongoing to try to determine contributing factors. It is suspected that SIDS may be associated with defects in the part of the infant brain that controls breathing and arousal from sleep.

- People who speak out against vaccines will claim that vaccines are known to cause SIDS. However, studies looking at the relationship of this phenomenon to vaccines have shown *no* increased risk of SIDS following immunization,[31,32] with some studies showing that vaccination may *reduce* the risk of SIDS.[33,34]

- What has made the biggest difference in decreasing rates of SIDS has been the American Academy of Pediatrics recommendation originating in 1992 and the Back to Sleep campaign, now called the Safe to Sleep campaign, beginning in 1994, which encouraged parents to put infants to sleep on their backs. Since this campaign was introduced, we have seen a 40% to 50% reduction in cases of SIDS in the United States **(Figure 10.2)**.

7. Vaccines aren't well studied, and when a new one comes out, they just combine it with other vaccines without testing them together to make sure that the combination is safe for our kids.

- We have spent an entire chapter (chapter 5—Who's Minding the Shop?) talking about how rigorously vaccines are tested and monitored, both before and after marketing to the general public.

- Vaccines *are*, in fact, tested together to ensure that the combination of vaccines in our pediatric dosing schedule is safe and effective. Skepticalraptor.com,[35] offers a list of some of the many studies of vaccines in combination, proving this anti-vaccine argument to be false.

8. Vaccines aren't tested using double-blinded, placebo-controlled trials.

- To address this concern, we have to get into a discussion of ethics in research. Use of a placebo-controlled trial is acceptable when there is no safe or efficacious vaccine against a particular disease already in existence. Novel vaccines (for example, Shingrix) are, indeed, tested this way.

- If we do have a vaccine in use that has been shown to safely decrease illness, however, then it would be unethical to place children into an arm of a trial that purposefully put them at risk (by denying access to the effective vaccine) of acquiring a vaccine-preventable illness.

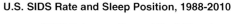

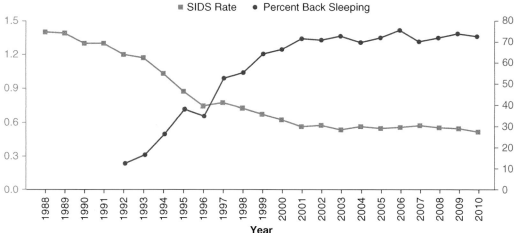

FIGURE 10.2 Graph showing visual reduction of sudden infant death syndrome (SIDS) after the American Academy of Pediatrics (AAP) recommendation and introduction of the Back to Sleep campaign. (Reprinted from National Institute of Child Health and Human Development, Progress in Reducing SIDS. Safe to Sleep. https://safetosleep.nichd.nih.gov/activities/SIDS/progress.)

      The double-blinded aspect of a trial also merits discussion. This means that neither the researcher nor the subject know in which arm (test or placebo) the child is enrolled. This is necessary to prevent bias from impacting study results. In response to concerns over the ethics of a placebo-controlled trial, anti-vaccine parents will offer to enroll their children in the placebo arm of research trials. However, this renders the blinding of the study null and void and has the potential to introduce bias, which would then call the study results into question.

9. You may be an expert in your field but I am an expert when it comes to my children. I know what my children need and what is best for their health.

      This is a difficult declaration to argue against. It basically takes away all ability to reference science and research and data to support your point of view.

      The only thing that may work in this situation is to bring to light the fact that parents of children who died of vaccine-preventable diseases likely felt that they, too, were experts in what their children needed. But disease doesn't discriminate based on whether you have a caring or attentive parent or not. It is an equal-opportunity killer.

10. I can't afford vaccines for my child.

      The Vaccines for Children (VFC) program is a federally funded program that covers all vaccines for children younger than 19 years of age who are Medicaid-eligible, Alaskan Native, American Indian, uninsured, or underinsured.[36] Depending on the clinic, the patient or family may incur a small administration fee, but the vaccine itself is free under this plan. See chapter 14 (Making Your Clinic a Lean, Mean, Vaccinating Machine) for a discussion of how to become a VFC provider.

SPECIFIC CONCERNS RELATED TO VACCINES IN PREGNANCY

There are three vaccines that we need to concern ourselves with in and around the time of pregnancy: MMR, pertussis, and influenza. The following are the common questions you will likely encounter regarding these vaccines.

1. I'm not sure if I got the MMR vaccine as a kid. But why does that matter now? That's a vaccine to prevent childhood illness.
   - Rubella infection is of particular concern in the prenatal period (though contracting measles or mumps in pregnancy could also be significantly problematic). Documenting rubella immunity (by measuring antibody titers) prior to pregnancy, and vaccinating if that immunity is lacking, is extremely important. Rubella infection during pregnancy can result in pregnancy loss or congenital rubella syndrome in the infant (see Appendix A: Vaccine-Preventable Diseases Information to learn more about this condition). The MMR vaccine is a live-attenuated virus vaccine and, as such, should not be given during pregnancy. If vaccination is needed, the vaccine should be administered at least 1 month prior to becoming pregnant.

2. Why do I need a pertussis vaccine in pregnancy? Can't we just wait and give it to the baby during their normal vaccinations?
   - Pertussis causes whooping cough, a respiratory condition that causes prolonged and terrifying spasms of coughing that can stop breathing and decrease a child's ability to feed. Before the vaccine became available in the 1940s, up to 200,000 children were infected yearly in the United States and up to 9000 children died of the illness. Still today, 50% of the babies younger than 1 year of age who contract it will have to be hospitalized for treatment and 20 children per year will die from this terrible infection.[37]
   - Infants cannot receive their first pertussis vaccine until 2 months old. Prior to this, they are completely vulnerable unless we vaccinate the mother during *every* pregnancy (recommended between 27 and 36 weeks' gestational age). This allows her to pass important antibodies to the baby before birth so that he or she is protected in those first months of life.
   - It is also important for those individuals who will be spending time around the newborn to get updated on their pertussis vaccines since immunity wanes over time. The Centers for Disease Control and Prevention (CDC) estimates that 7 out of 10 people will be protected against pertussis 1 year after immunization. By 4 years after immunization, only 3 to 4 out of 10 are protected. In my practice, I recommend repeat vaccination to anyone who is going to be around a newborn if their most recent vaccine was given more than 5 years prior.

3. I'm worried about getting the flu shot during pregnancy. Won't the mercury in the flu vaccine harm the baby?
   - Influenza immunizations given to pregnant mothers are of the single-dose variety. Since 2001, these are "preservative-free," no longer containing ethyl mercury.

- The physical and hormonal changes that occur during pregnancy result in increased heart rate, increased consumption of oxygen, and decreased lung capacity, all of which combine to make a pregnant woman much more susceptible to the potentially serious effects of an influenza infection. Studies of pandemic and seasonal flu show that pregnant patients are at significantly greater risk of severe cardiorespiratory illness (such as pneumonia and asthma exacerbation) and death due to influenza than their nonpregnant counterparts.[38]

- Fetuses also suffer. Though placental transmission of the virus is rare, the fever and maternal inflammation that accompany influenza infection contribute to higher rates of miscarriage, fetal death, and preterm delivery. Some studies also suggest an association between maternal influenza infection and higher rates of birth defects, such as cleft lip and palate, congenital heart defects, and neural tube defects.[38]

- When the pregnant mother gets the influenza vaccine, some of those protective antibodies are also passed on to the baby. This helps protect infants during those first 6 months of life until they are able to receive a flu vaccine themselves.[39]

RELIGIOUS CONCERNS REGARDING VACCINATION

As discussed in chapter 2, religious concerns over vaccination have been around for centuries. However, based on the fundamental teachings of the world's major religions, much of what is expressed as a religious concern actually turns out to be more of a philosophical leaning. As states begin to limit philosophical exemptions, we can expect to see a rise in reported "religious" reasons for not vaccinating. It is important to be able to speak to the religious concerns of our patients so that we can pay respect to their faith and set their consciences at ease. The following are some of the more commonly voiced concerns that you will hear. These tend to fall into three categories. The first is "violation of prohibitions against taking life," the second, "violations of dietary laws," and the third is "interference with natural order by not letting events take their course."[40]

1. Vaccines are made from aborted fetal tissue. I don't support abortion and can't take any vaccine that uses tissue from an aborted fetus.
   - You will hear patients speak about the WI-38 and MRC-5 cell lines, which are the cell lines currently in use that are derived from fetal tissue.[41]
   - There are six vaccines that were originally made using aborted fetal tissue (varicella, rubella, hepatitis A, the original shingles vaccine, adenovirus, and rabies vaccines). Only the first three are now routinely used in the United States. In 1960, tissue was taken from two fetuses aborted by maternal choice (not performed for the purpose of vaccine production) in order to propagate cell lines that are still used in vaccine development today.
   - Human cells can provide advantages for vaccine production that other cells do not.
     - Some viruses don't grow as well in animal cells.

> Animal cells can introduce contamination by viruses or bacteria that are not carried in human cell lines.

> Vaccine production can be hindered or halted, resulting in a shortage of vaccine, if animal products used in development are threatened (if illness were to strike egg-producing chickens, for example, which are used to make much of the influenza vaccine supply).[41]

- Some patients, particularly our Catholic patients, may have concerns about these vaccines. Some years ago, the National Catholic Bioethics Center (NCBC) prepared a statement regarding the use of these vaccines that may help put our patients' minds at ease.

  > "The cell lines under consideration were begun using cells taken from one or more fetuses aborted almost 40 years ago. Since that time the cell lines have grown independently. It is important to note that descendant cells are not the cells of the aborted child. They never, themselves, formed a part of the victim's body."[42]

  > "There would seem to be no proper grounds for refusing immunization against dangerous contagious disease, for example, rubella, especially in light of the concern that we should all have for the health of our children, public health, and the common good."[42]

  > The NCBC *does* encourage use of any available alternative vaccines that are not developed using fetal tissue (there are currently no alternative vaccines available in the United States) and urges families to voice their concerns to government agencies and vaccine manufacturers and to call for development of future vaccines in ways that do not support abortion.

2. Vaccines are made using cow and pig tissues. My faith teaches me to respect all life and doesn't allow me to eat these meats, so I can't take vaccines that are produced this way.

   - The majority of gelatin used in vaccines is porcine derived. Gelatin is a protein used in the production of vaccines to preserve their effectiveness after manufacture and to protect them from freezing or heat.[43]

   - Cow-derived components are used in vaccines in a variety of ways. Cow milk can be used as a source of amino acids and sugar to facilitate growth of viruses or bacteria. Cow tallow can be used to provide glycerol. Gelatin can be made from cow bones. Cow skeletal muscle can be used to prepare broths for growth media, and cow blood may be used to help propagate difficult-to-grow organisms.[44]

   - Our Jewish and Muslim patients are among those whose faiths may express concern over the use of pork in vaccine manufacture. Our Hindu and Buddhist patients and followers of Jainism may express concern over the use of animals based on teachings of vegetarianism in certain texts (though Buddhist attitudes toward vegetarianism vary) or based on teachings of nonviolence (*ahimsa*) and respect for all life, even that of microorganisms.

     > In Judaism, acting to protect one's own or another's life is a *mitzvah* or positive commandment. Remember Maimonides' quote: "Anyone who is able to save a life, but fails to do so, violates 'You shall not stand idly by the blood of your neighbor." He also taught that "One must avoid those things which have a deleterious effect on the body, and accustom oneself to things which heal and fortify it."[40]

> Jewish dietary laws prohibit consumption of impure animals (for example, pork and shellfish) or products of improperly slaughtered animals. However, multiple Jewish authorities agree that these limitations relate only to products used orally and not those given by injection. Even orally administered porcine products are deemed acceptable if doing so is necessary to preserve life and if the amount present is diluted beyond a 1:60 ratio and to the point of loss of taste.[40,45]

> The teachings of the Qur'an forbid our Muslim patients to consume pork flesh while consumption of other animals is forbidden (*haram*) or permitted (*halal*) based on the conditions of slaughter. However, the Qur'an also teaches that a person is not guilty of sin if a lack of a halal alternative creates a necessity to consume that which is otherwise haram (Qur'an 2:173). This is the basis of the Islamic jurisprudence "law of necessity."[40]

> The Qur'an also speaks to protecting life, preventing harm, and the principle of public interest. The concept of *wiqaya* (meaning to safeguard) is used in multiple situations to refer to taking preventive measures. Prevention is deemed to be one of the laws of Allah. This has very obvious applications to medicine.[40]

> Hindu, Buddhist, and Jain teachings promote a respect for all life. However, they also acknowledge that the preservation of human life sometimes requires the unfortunate destruction of other life-forms. Mahatma Gandhi observed that "The very fact of [humanity's] living—eating, drinking and moving about—necessarily involves some himsa, destruction of life, be it ever so minute."[46] Jains recognize a hierarchy of life-forms and may benefit from discussion of the severity of diseases for which we vaccinate. The loss of lives of microorganisms in the production of vaccines may be acceptable in that it prevents the loss of human lives, a higher life-form.

> Hindu, Buddhist, and Jain teachings also accept "violence" in self-defense. In this case, the violence is against microorganisms and other animals used in vaccine production and the self-defense is for the protection of human health and life.[40]

3. Vaccination interferes with God's will. If God desires for me to remain well, I will remain well. If I become sick, I will pray for God to heal me.

○ The Church of Christ, Scientist and Jehovah's Witnesses, along with other smaller denominations that rely on faith healing, are groups whose members may express resistance to vaccination.

> The Church of Christ, Scientist was founded by Mary Baker Eddy in 1879. According to Grabenstein in his study of the world's religions as they relate to vaccination, Eddy called believers to "unmask the devil's lies, one manifestation of which is disease." Christian Scientists deny the reality of disease and believe it to be something that can be dispelled or "prevented by prayer that affirms human perfection as God's child."[40] However, in later discussion of the issue of contagious disease and vaccination, Eddy is quoted as saying, "Where vaccination is compulsory, let your children be vaccinated,

and see that your mind is in such a state that by your prayers vaccination will do the children no harm. So long as Christian Scientists obey the laws, I do not suppose their mental reservations will be thought to matter much."[47]

> The Jehovah's Witnesses trace their roots to 1870, organized under the Watch Tower Bible and Tract Society. Their teachings regarding the use of blood and blood products express their beliefs that only the blood of Jesus can bring redemption and save lives. Teachings on the matter of vaccinations (which sometimes are manufactured using blood products) have varied over time with *The Watchtower*, in 1961, taking a neutral stand, neither prohibiting nor promoting vaccination. In 1990, *Awake!* magazine began to acknowledge the value of vaccination, and the current Watchtower webpage acknowledges the effectiveness of vaccination for the prevention of hepatitis A and B.[48] Today's Jehovah's Witnesses are taught that acceptance of various blood fractions (such as albumin, immune globulins, and coagulation factors) is not absolutely prohibited and is a matter of personal choice.[49]

SPECIFIC CONCERNS RELATED TO IMMUNE-COMPROMISED PATIENTS

1. I have a suppressed immune system. That means I can't get vaccines, right?
   - Wrong! People with suppressed immune systems should not get live-attenuated vaccines, but they absolutely *should* get killed virus vaccines. Immune suppression increases the risks associated with contracting a vaccine-preventable illness. If someone with a suppressed immune system gets the flu, pneumonia, or pertussis, for example, they are more likely than people with healthy immune systems to progress to serious disease or death.
   - When it comes to illnesses that are protected against with live-attenuated or weakened vaccines, we need to vaccinate those around the immune-suppressed person to create a bubble or layer of protection for that person until their immune system recovers. This is herd immunity in action!

2. I am on medications that suppress my immune system, so vaccines won't work on me.
   - Although medications that suppress the immune system may make it less likely to produce a robust response to a vaccine, the body will still develop antibodies in response to vaccination.
   - For people on immune-suppressant medications, the question is when to give the vaccine so that it will be most effective. We don't yet have clear recommendations in this regard. We may try to vaccinate them toward the end of their immune-suppressant dosing interval. For example, if a patient is on once-monthly injections of secukinumab to treat psoriatic arthritis, we might want to aim their pneumococcal

pneumonia immunization in the week or two prior to their next injection, when the effects of the immune suppressant are waning and the individual can, presumably, mount a better immune response (**Box 10.1**).

 Box 10.1   Did You Know?

The timing of the PCV13 and PPSV23 vaccines can be confusing. Vaccines are recommended at certain ages and certain intervals determined by studies looking at immune response based on age, the order of vaccines given, the intervals between vaccines, and more. All of this information is considered by the Advisory Committee on Immunization Practices when setting guidelines for immunization administration. The same is true for the available vaccines against strains of pneumococcus, which can cause upper respiratory infections and more severe disease, such as pneumonia, bacteremia, and meningitis. PCV13 is most effective against the strains that produce pneumococcal disease in children, whereas PPSV23 does not produce a reliable immune response in children younger than 2 years of age.[50] The strains in the PPSV23 vaccine affect older adults to a greater degree, and this vaccine has been recommended to all adults of age 65 years and older for some time. The 2014 recommendation to offer the PCV13 vaccine to all adults of age 65 years and older was based on a study of 85,000 people in the Netherlands, showing a reduction in community-acquired pneumonia by 45%, and a reduction in invasive pneumococcal disease by 75%, compared with that of controls.[51] In adults over 65, PCV13 is recommended to be given before PPSV23 based on studies showing a better response to the serotypes that are common to both vaccines if PCV13 is administered first.[52] Certain extenuating circumstances may indicate that a PPSV23 vaccine be given before age 65 years (people without a spleen, people with immune suppression, and others). In this case, the PPSV23 would be boosted no sooner than 5 years later (after age 65 years) and at least 1 year from the PCV13 vaccine.

- Based on a recent study out of Seoul, Korea, looking at response rates to influenza immunization in patients being treated with methotrexate for rheumatoid arthritis, there *are* now guidelines recommending holding methotrexate for 2 weeks after influenza vaccination to improve immune response. According to the American College of Rheumatology, this approach could be applied to other vaccines as well.[53]

3. I am immune suppressed. Do I need any additional vaccines?
   - Certain people with chronic illness and immune-suppressed states are recommended to receive some vaccines at an earlier age or at a different interval than they would otherwise be recommended. See **Figure 10.3** and **Box 10.2** for discussion of use of pneumococcal vaccines outside the routine guidelines and for vaccination recommendations specific to those with asplenia.

Medical indication	Underlying medical condition	PCV13 for ≥19 y Recommended	PPSV23* for 19 through 64 y Recommended	PPSV23* for 19 through 64 y Revaccination	PCV13 at ≥65 y Recommended	PPSV23 at ≥65 y Recommended
None	None of the below				✓	✓ ≥1 y after PCV13
Immunocompetent persons	Alcoholism					
	Chronic heart disease†					
	Chronic liver disease		✓		✓	✓ ≥1 y after PCV13 ≥5 y after any PPSV23 at <65 y
	Chronic lung disease§					
	Cigarette smoking					
	Diabetes mellitus					
	Cochlear implants	✓	✓ ≥8 wk after PCV13		✓ If no previous PCV13 vaccination	✓ ≥8 wk after PCV13 ≥5 y after any PPSV23 at <65 y
	CSF leaks					
Persons with functional or anatomic asplenia	Congenital or acquired asplenia	✓	✓ ≥8 wk after PCV13	✓ ≥5 y after first dose PPSV23	✓ If no previous PCV13 vaccination	✓ ≥8 wk after PCV13 ≥5 y after any PPSV23 at <65 y
	Sickle cell disease/other hemoglobinopathies					
Immunocompromised persons	Chronic renal failure	✓	✓ ≥8 wk after PCV13	✓ ≥5 y after first dose PPSV23	✓ If no previous PCV13 vaccination	✓ ≥8 wk after PCV13 ≥5 y after any PPSV23 at <65 y
	Congenital or acquired immunodeficiencies¶					
	Generalized malignancy					
	HIV infection					
	Hodgkin disease					
	Iatrogenic immunosuppression‡					
	Leukemia					
	Lymphoma					
	Multiple myeloma					
	Nephrotic syndrome					
	Solid organ transplant					

*This PPSV23 column only refers to adults 19 through 64 y of age. All adults 65 y of age or older should receive one dose of PPSV23 5 or more years after any prior dose of PPSV23, regardless of previous history of vaccination with pneumococcal vaccine. No additional doses of PPSV23 should be administered following the dose administered at 65 y of age or older.
†Including congestive heart failure and cardiomyopathies
§Including chronic obstructive pulmonary disease, emphysema, and asthma
¶Includes B- (humoral) or T-lymphocyte deficiency, complement deficiencies (particularly C1, C2, C3, and C4 deficiencies), and phagocytic disorders (excluding chronic granulomatous disease)
‡Diseases requiring treatment with immunosuppressive drugs, including long-term systemic corticosteroids and radiation therapy

FIGURE 10.3 Currently recommended pneumococcal vaccination schedule for adults. (From CDC. Pneumococcal Vaccine Timing for Adults. https://www.cdc.gov/vaccines/vpd/pneumo/downloads/pneumo-vaccine-timing.pdf.)

 Box 10.2   Vaccination for Asplenic Patients

Vaccination for patients without a spleen has some notable differences, particularly the need to vaccinate every 5 years for PPSV23 and MenACWY. Refer to the resource below for vaccine recommendations for this special population:
    https://www.ncbi.nlm.nih.gov/pmc/articles/PMC5328222/pdf/khvi-13-02-1264797.pdf.

References

1. Zakian A, Malvy J, Desombre H, et al. Early signs of autism and family films: a new study by informed evaluators and those unaware of the diagnosis. *Encephale*. 2000;26(2):38-44. https://www.ncbi.nlm.nih.gov/pubmed/10858914.

2. Webb SJ, Jones EJ. Early identification of autism. Early characteristics, onset of symptoms, and diagnostic stability. *Infants Young Child*. 2009;22(2):100-118. https://www.ncbi.nlm.nih.gov/pmc/articles/PMC5232420/

3. Tick B, Bolton P, Happé F, et al. Heritability of autism spectrum disorders: a meta-analysis of twin studies. *J Child Psychol Psychiatry*. 2016;57(5):585-595. https://www.ncbi.nlm.nih.gov/pmc/articles/PMC4996332/.

4. Hallmayer J, Cleveland S, Torres A, et al. Genetic heritability and shared environmental factors among twin pairs with autism. *Arch Gen Psychiatry*. 2011;68(11):1095-1102. https://www.ncbi.nlm.nih.gov/pmc/articles/PMC4440679/.

5. Jain A, Marshall J, Buikema A, et al. Autism occurrence by MMR vaccine status among US children with older siblings with and without autism. *JAMA*. 2015;313(15):1534-1540.

6. Kaiser Permanente. *Kaiser Permanente Study Finds Risk for Autism in Younger Children Increases Significantly if They Have Older Sibling With Disorder*. August 5, 2016. https://share.kaiserpermanente.org/article/kaiser-permanente-study-finds-risk-autism-younger-children-increases-significantly-older-sibling-disorder/. Accessed January 10, 2019.

7. Baio J, Wiggins L, Christensen DL, et al. Prevalence of autism spectrum disorder among children aged 8 years – autism and developmental disabilities monitoring network, 11 Sites, United States, 2014. *MMWR Surveill Summ*. April 27, 2018;67(6):1-23. https://www.cdc.gov/mmwr/volumes/67/ss/ss6706a1.htm

8. American Academy of Pediatrics. Vaccine Safety: Examine the Evidence. HealthyChildren.org. https://www.healthychildren.org/English/safety-prevention/immunizations/Pages/Vaccine-Studies-Examine-the-Evidence.aspx. Updated July 24, 2008. Accessed January 10, 2019.

9. Taylor LE, Swerdfeger AL, Eslick GD. Vaccines are not associated with autism: an evidence-based meta-analysis of case-control and cohort studies. *Vaccine*. 2004;32(29):3623-3629. https://vaccinepapers.org/wp-content/uploads/Vaccines-are-not-associated-with-autism-An-evidence-based-meta-analysis-of-case-control-and-cohort-studies.pdf.

10. Centers for Disease Control and Prevention. Autism and Developmental Disabilities Monitoring (ADDM) Network. https://www.cdc.gov/ncbddd/autism/addm.html. Updated November 15, 2018. Accessed January 15, 2019.

11. Fombonne E, Zakarian R, Bennett A, et al. Pervasive developmental disorders in Montreal, Quebec, Canada: prevalence and links with immunizations. *Pediatrics*. 2006;118(1):e139-e150. http://pediatrics.aappublications.org/content/118/1/e139.

12. Hviid A, Stellfeld M, Wohlfahrt J, et al. Association between thimerosal-containing vaccine and autism. *JAMA*. 2003;290(13):1763-1766.

13. Stehr-Green P, Tull P, Stellfeld M, et al. Autism and thimerosal-containing vaccines: lack of consistent evidence for an association. *Am J Prev Med*. 2003;25(2):101-106. https://www.ncbi.nlm.nih.gov/pubmed/12880876.

14. Immunization Action Coalition. MMR Vaccine Does not Cause Autism. Examine the evidence! http://www.immunize.org/catg.d/p4026.pdf. Accessed January 10, 2019.

15. DeStefano F, Price CS, Weintraub ES. Increasing exposure to antibody-stimulating proteins and polysaccharides in vaccines is not associated with risk of autism. *J Pediatr*. 2013;163:561-567. https://www.jpeds.com/article/S0022-3476%2813%2900144-3/pdf.

16. Miranda S, Chaignot C, Collin C, et al. Human papillomavirus vaccination and risk of autoimmune diseases: a large cohort study of over 2 million young girls in France. *Vaccine*. 2017;35(36):4761-4768. https://www.sciencedirect.com/science/article/pii/S0264410X17308071.

17. Glanz JM, Newcomer SR, Daley MF, et al. Association between estimated cumulative vaccine antigen exposure through the first 23 months of life and non-vaccine-targeted infections from 24 through 47 months of age. *JAMA*. 2018;319(9):906-913. https://jamanetwork.com/journals/jama/fullarticle/2673970.

18. MacArthur AC, McBride ML, Spinelli J, et al. Risk of childhood leukemia associated with vaccination, infection, and medication use in childhood: the Cross-Canada Childhood Leukemia Society. *Am J Epidemiol*. 2008(5):598-606. https://academic.oup.com/aje/article/167/5/598/211885.

19. Offit PA, Quarles J, Gerber MA, et al. Addressing parents' concerns: do multiple vaccines overwhelm or weaken the infant's immune system? *Pediatrics*. 2002;109(1):124-129. http://pediatrics.aappublications.org/content/109/1/124.long.

20. Langan SM, Flohr C, Williams HC. The role of furry pets in eczema: a systematic review. *Arch Dermatol*. 2007;143(12):1570-1577. https://www.ncbi.nlm.nih.gov/pubmed/18087010.

21. Remes ST, Iivanainen K, Koskela H, et al. Which factors explain the lower prevalence of atopy amongst farmer's children? *Clin Exp Allergy*. 2003;33(4):427-434. https://www.ncbi.nlm.nih.gov/pubmed/12680856.

22. Higgins JP, Soares-Weiser K, Reingold AL, et al. Association of BCG, DTP, and measles containing vaccines with childhood mortality: systematic review. *BMJ*. 2016;355:i5170. https://www.ncbi.nlm.nih.gov/pmc/articles/PMC5063034/?report=reader.

23. Fact or Fiction. Too Many too Soon. Immunize For Good. Accessed January 10, 2019. http://www.immunizeforgood.com/fact-or-fiction/too-many-too-soon.

24. Sun L. *Why It's a Bad Idea to Space Out Your Child's Vaccination Shots*. Washington Post; April 17, 2017. https://www.washingtonpost.com/news/to-your-health/wp/2017/04/17/why-its-a-bad-idea-to-space-out-your-childs-vaccination-shots/?utm_term=.d5b9f5768c5f.

25. Offit PA, Moser CA. The problem with Dr. Bob's alternative vaccine schedule. *Pediatrics*. 2009;123(1):e164-e169.

26. Sears R. *The Vaccine Book: Making the Right Decision for Your Child*. 2nd ed. NY: Little, Brown, and Company; 2011.

27. Children's Hospital of Philadelphia. Vaccine Ingredients – Aluminum. https://www.chop.edu/centers-programs/vaccine-education-center/vaccine-ingredients/aluminum. Accessed January 10, 2019.

28. Franco E, Bagnato B, Marino MG, et al. Hepatitis B: epidemiology and prevention in developing countries. *World J Hepatol*. 2012;4(3):74-80. https://www.ncbi.nlm.nih.gov/pmc/articles/PMC3321493/.

29. Van Herck K, Van Damme P. Benefits of early hepatitis B immunization programs for newborns and infants. *Pediatr Infect Dis J*. 2008;27(10):861-869. https://journals.lww.com/pidj/Abstract/2008/10000/Benefits_of_Early_Hepatitis_B_Immunization.2.aspx.

30. Immunization Action Coalition. Hepatitis B shots are Recommended for All New Babies. Hepatitis B Vaccine Helps Protect Your Baby's Future! www.immunize.org/catg.d/p4110.pdf. Accessed January 10, 2019.

31. Griffin MR, Ray WA, Livengood JR, et al. Risk of sudden infant death syndrome after immunization with the diphtheria-tetanus-pertussis vaccine. *N Engl J Med*. 1988;319(10):618-623. https://www.ncbi.nlm.nih.gov/pubmed/3261837.

32. Institute of Medicine (US) Immunization Safety Review Committee; Stratton K, Almario DA, Wizemann TM, et al. *Immunization Safety Review: Vaccination and Sudden Unexpected Death in Infancy*. Washington, DC. National Academies Press; 2003. https://www.ncbi.nlm.nih.gov/pubmed/25057654.

33. Vennemann MM, Höffgen M, Bajanowski T, et al. Do immunisations reduce the risk for SIDS? A meta-analysis. *Vaccine*. 2007;25(26):4875-4879. https://www.sciencedirect.com/science/article/pii/S0264410X07002800?via%3Dihub.

34. Vennemann MM, Butterfaß-Bahloul T, Jorch G, et al. Sudden infant death syndrome: no increased risk after immunisation. *Vaccine*. 2007;25(2):336-340. https://www.sciencedirect.com/science/article/pii/S0264410X06008978?via%3Dihub.

35. Skeptikal Raptor. *Testing Vaccines – Another Anti-vaccine Myth Requiring Debunking*. July 30, 2018. Accessing January 10, 2019. https://www.skepticalraptor.com/skepticalraptorblog.php/testing-vaccines-anti-vaccine-myth-debunking/.

36. Centers for Disease Control and Prevention. Vaccines for Children Program. https://www.cdc.gov/vaccines/programs/vfc/about/index.html. Updated May 25, 2018. Accessed January 10, 2019.

37. Centers for Disease Control and Prevention. Pertussis Frequently Asked Questions. https://www.cdc.gov/pertussis/about/faqs.html. Updated August 7, 2017. Accessed January 10, 2019.

38. Rasmussen SA, Jamieson DJ, Bresee JS. Pandemic influenza and pregnant women. *Emerg Infect Dis.* 2008;14(1):95-100. https://www.ncbi.nlm.nih.gov/pmc/articles/PMC2600164/.

39. Shakib JH, Korgenski K, Presson AP, et al. Influenza in infants born to women vaccinated during pregnancy. *Pediatrics*. 2016;137(6).

40. Grabenstein JD. What the world's religions teach, applied to vaccines and immune globulins. *Vaccine.* 2013;31(16):2011-2023. www.academia.edu/36360882/What_the_Worlds_religions_teach_applied_to_vaccines_and_immune_globulins.

41. The College of Physicians of Philadelphia. Human Cell Strains in Vaccine Development. https://www.historyofvaccines.org/content/articles/human-cell-strains-vaccine-development. Updated January 10, 2018. Accessed January 11, 2019.

42. National Catholic Bioethics Center. FAQ on the Use of Vaccines. https://www.ncbcenter.org/resources/frequently-asked-questions/use-vaccines/#refuseVacc. Accessed January 11, 2019.

43. Children's Hospital of Philadelphia. Vaccine Ingredients – Gelatin. Https://www.chop.edu/centers-programs/vaccine-education-center/vaccine-ingredients/gelatin. Accessed January 11, 2019.

44. U.S. Food and Drug Administration. Bovine Derived Materials Used in Vaccine Manufacturing Questions and Answers. https://www.fda.gov/biologicsbloodvaccines/vaccines/questionsaboutvaccines/ucm143521.htm. Updated March 23, 2018. Accessed January 11, 2019.

45. Heber D. When It's Null and Void: Understanding Batel Bshishim (One-Sixtieth). Spring 2011. https://www.star-k.org/articles/kashrut-kurrents/611/when-its-null-and-void-understanding-bagel-bshishim-one-sixtieth. Accessed January 11, 2019.

46. Gandhi MK. *An Autobiography: The Story of My Experiments With Truth.* Mineola, NY: Dover Publications; 1983.

47. The First Church of Christ. Scientist and Miscellany. Part 4: Youth and Young Manhood. https://mbeinstitute.org/Prose_Works/Miscellany_PartFour.html. Accessed January 11, 2019.

48. Hepatitis B – a silent killer. *Awake!* August 2010. https://www.jw.org/en/publications/magazines/g201008/Hepatitis-B-A-Silent-Killer/#?insight[search_id]=5ba85a88-2e95-4e1e-9f99-d495d64def24&insight[search_result_index]=3. Accessed January 11, 2019.

49. Questions From Readers. *The Watchtower – Study Edition.* June 15, 2000. https://www.jw.org/en/publications/magazines/w20000615/Questions-From-Readers/. Accessed January 11, 2019.

50. The College of Physicians of Philadelphia. Pneumococcal Disease. https://www.historyofvaccines.org/content/articles/pneumococcal-disease-0. Updated January 25, 2018. Accessed February 6, 2019.

51. Crawford C. *ACIP Recommends Routine PCV13 Immunization for Adults 65 and Older.* August 27, 2014. https://www.aafp.org/news/health-of-the-public/20140827pcv13vote.html. Accessed February 6, 2019.

52. Kobayashi M, Bennett NM, Gierke R, et al. Intervals between PCV13 and PPSV23 vaccines: recommendations of the Advisory Committee on Immunization Practices (ACIP). *MMWR.* 2015;64(34):944-947. https://www.cdc.gov/mmwr/preview/mmwrhtml/mm6434a4.htm.

53. American College of Rheumatology. *Press Releases: Methotrexate Drug holiday Improves Flu Vaccine Efficacy in Rheumatoid Arthritis Patients.* November 4, 2017. https://www.rheumatology.org/About-Us/Newsroom/Press-Releases/ID/838. Accessed January 11, 2019.

Influenza and HPV: A Closer Look at Two "Controversial" Vaccines— Point-Counterpoint, Part 3

> *In a controversy, the instant we feel angry, we have already ceased striving for truth, and begun striving for ourselves.*
>
> —Thomas Carlyle

In 1918, the world saw the worst influenza pandemic in its history. Called the Spanish flu for reports of its particular devastation in Spain, nearly 50 million people died worldwide. Nearly one-third of the world's population was infected and practically every family lost a loved one, or multiple loved ones **(Figure 11.1)**. This was before the development of the influenza vaccine, and it wouldn't be until 1933, when the influenza virus was isolated, that we would have some hope of protection against this devastating illness.

Until more recent times, cervical cancer was the leading cause of cancer deaths among women worldwide. This number was reduced in the 1950s when Dr. Georgios Papanikolaou developed a test (the Pap smear) to detect precancerous changes of the cervix. Through the use of this routine screening test, many cases of cervical cancer were averted. However, women of color and women of lower socioeconomic standing were still particularly affected. Lack of access to preventive care was a major barrier for many women. It wasn't until the 1980s that work on a human papillomavirus (HPV) vaccine began in earnest because of decades of work by a German virologist named Harald zur Hausen. He looked at HPV as a trigger for cancerous changes of the cervix, and finally concluded that HPV types 16 and 18 were highly oncogenic.[1] In 2006, a vaccine that protected against two strains of cancer-causing HPV and two strains of genital wart-causing HPV was licensed and first recommended for girls. Then, in 2011, as we increasingly recognized the role that HPV plays in male genital and throat cancers, the vaccine was also approved for use in boys.

Millions of deaths. Tens of thousands of cases of cancer. One would think that the public would clamor to get their hands on vaccines that can prevent the serious morbidity and mortality that accompany infection with these viruses. Yet, even though we have access to highly successful vaccines, rates of influenza vaccination and HPV vaccination are some of the lowest out there. During the 2016-2017 flu season, the influenza vaccine success rate in the United States was only 59% in children and 43.3% in adults.[2] That same year, even though all three vaccines (Tdap, meningococcal,

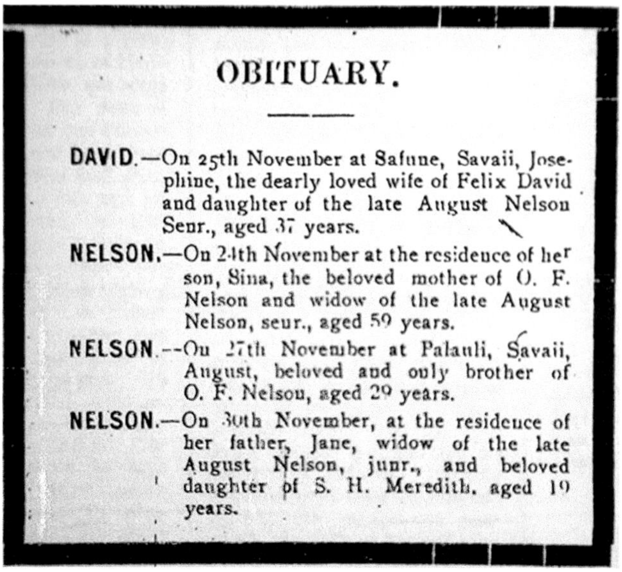

OBITUARY.

DAVID.—On 25th November at Safune, Savaii, Josephine, the dearly loved wife of Felix David and daughter of the late August Nelson Senr., aged 37 years.

NELSON.—On 24th November at the residence of her son, Sina, the beloved mother of O. F. Nelson and widow of the late August Nelson, seur., aged 59 years.

NELSON.—On 27th November at Palauli, Savaii, August, beloved and only brother of O. F. Nelson, aged 29 years.

NELSON.—On 30th November, at the residence of her father, Jane, widow of the late August Nelson, junr., and beloved daughter of S. H. Meredith, aged 19 years.

FIGURE 11.1 Obituary showing the toll on one family during the influenza pandemic. (Reprinted from the Samoan Times, 14-Dec-1918. 'Samoan influenza obituaries', https://nzhistory.govt.nz/media/photo/samoan-influenza-obituaries, (Ministry for Culture and Heritage), updated 20-Dec-2012. Licensed by Manatū Taonga for re-use under the Creative Commons Attribution-Non-Commercial 3.0 New Zealand License.)

and HPV) are recommended to be given at the same 11- to 12-year well-child visit, only 60% of boys and girls had received one of the HPV vaccine series and an even more dismal 43.4% were up-to-date with the full course of HPV vaccines. This compares to the 82% success rate for meningococcal meningitis and 88% success rate for Tdap administration.[3]

Where is the disconnect? What is it about these vaccines that makes them so much more difficult to convince people of than other vaccines? The remainder of this chapter will try to gain perspective on these questions by looking at the history of the influenza and HPV vaccines and their initially recommended target populations. We will address particular concerns voiced about each of these immunizations and highlight the statistics that should make our vaccination case for us (see Appendix B: Fast Facts about Vaccines for Patients and Clinic Staff for concise influenza and HPV vaccine talking points that can be provided to patients for their review).

◉ INFLUENZA

In 1933, influenza subtypes A and B (and rarely C) were first identified as the causative agents of the influenza illness. This led to production of the first influenza vaccine in 1938. In 1942, the Armed Forces Epidemiological Board developed a polyvalent vaccine, containing both A and B influenza strains. This vaccine was licensed in 1945 for use in the military and then in 1946 for general public use.[4] However, the vaccine proved ineffective in subsequent years and scientists eventually recognized influenza's capacity for rapid mutation. A process of observing the circulating, or active, flu strains from around the world began, and scientists started work to anticipate which strains would be affecting the United States in the coming season (see Appendix C: Vaccine Topics Explained for a video explaining how the flu vaccine is made). More than 100 countries conduct year-round surveillance for influenza and then send data to the World Health Organization, which makes yearly recommendations for strains to be included in the influenza vaccine. The Food and Drug Administration (FDA) is responsible for the final decision regarding which strains to include in each year's US-licensed influenza vaccines.[5] Let's look at the most common concerns voiced about the flu shot and how you can respond.

 1.   The flu shot doesn't work that well. What's the point if I'm still going to get the flu?

- As stated above, the flu shot represents a very educated guess about what strains of flu are going to be circulating that year. Some years' predictions are better than others. Consequently, people are keenly aware of the limitations of the flu shot. At its best, the influenza vaccine is about 60% effective.[6] As a result, people have received the flu shot and still gotten the flu or have known others to whom this has happened.

- We have good data to show, though, that a person vaccinated for influenza is significantly less likely to suffer severe consequences or death from an influenza illness than if they had not received the vaccine.

- Retrospective studies looking at deaths during each flu season show that, of those that died, typically greater than 80% had not received the flu shot.[7] The flu vaccine significantly reduces the risk of death from influenza.[8]

- Yes, many people may get the flu, feel temporarily unwell, and recover. However, despite our advances in medicine and technology, we still see an average of 140,000 to 720,000 hospitalizations and 12,000 to 56,000 deaths annually in the United States from influenza. The flu is not a mild illness (**Box 11.1**).

- The 2017-2018 flu season saw the greatest numbers of deaths in decades—80,000 people died, 185 of whom were children.[7] This influenza death rate is the equivalent of up to 152 crashes of a Boeing 747 jetliner (carrying an average of 524 passengers each).[10] Can you imagine the uproar that would occur if this were happening in our airline industry?

Box 11.1 Did You Know?

Our ability to fight off illness decreases as we age. Likewise, our ability to mount an immune response to vaccination decreases as we age. The elderly are at higher risk of complications from influenza (70%-85% of flu deaths occur in people older than 65 years), so it is important to make sure that they have a vaccine that is effective. There are a couple of different options for augmented vaccines for our senior population. The "high-dose" flu vaccine (a trivalent vaccine), approved in the United States since 2009, includes four times the amount of antigen as the regular flu shot in order to induce a stronger immune response. A clinical trial looking at 30,000 participants aged 65 and older showed a 24% greater reduction in influenza infections in seniors who received the high-dose vaccine compared with those that received the standard flu vaccine. The adjuvanted flu vaccine (a trivalent vaccine using the MF59 adjuvant to augment immune response) is another option for seniors. In a small study comparing the adjuvanted vaccine to regular-dose flu vaccine, the adjuvanted vaccine was 63% more effective. To date, we have no studies comparing the "high dose" to the "adjuvanted" vaccine. Each of these boosted vaccines may result in more frequent mild side effects (such as redness, swelling, malaise, etc.). Currently, the CDC and Advisory Committee on Immunization Practices do not recommend one flu vaccine over another for patients older than 65 years.[9]

- We need to change our expectations of the current flu vaccine. We need to start thinking of it as a way to decrease the severity of the illness and limit hospitalizations and death from influenza, not as a way to prevent the flu entirely.

2. **I'm healthy. I don't need to take the flu shot.**
    - The flu shot was originally advised only for the very young, the elderly, and the medically fragile (people thought to be at greatest risk of suffering from severe consequences of the flu). But in 2010, the Advisory Committee on Immunization Practices (ACIP) recommended use for *all* persons older than 6 months in order to better limit the spread of influenza.[11]
    - One of the difficulties in convincing questioning patients regarding the importance of the flu shot is that the majority of today's adults still remember when flu shots were *not* recommended annually. They remember being in the "low-risk" group and don't see what has changed that now requires them to get the influenza vaccine each year.
    - Not everyone who suffers severe consequences or death from the flu is in a high-risk group, however. A recent study in the journal *Pediatrics* looking at pediatric flu deaths in the United States from 2010 to 2016 noted that 50% of the children that died from influenza had no preexisting conditions. They were entirely healthy.[12] Those of us who are in good health may be at lower risk, but we are not immune to the possibility of severe consequences or death. And, what we can't predict is when the virus will mutate and create a particularly virulent and damaging strain from which we won't recover so easily.
    - Remember the 1918 influenza pandemic that we spoke of earlier? Nearly half of the people who died from that flu strain were in the healthy 20- to 40-year age range and the virus was so virulent that it sometimes killed within hours.[13] So, while researchers continue to search for a way to make a more universally effective influenza vaccine, we must stay vigilant.

3. **I got the flu from the flu shot. Why would I take a vaccine that could make me sick?**
    - First, make sure to clarify what kind of illness the person experienced after the vaccine. Many still believe that the flu shot protects against the "stomach flu," but it does not. The "stomach flu" is not influenza. Vomiting is a rare symptom of influenza and diarrhea is not typically part of the flu syndrome.
    - If an immune-compromised patient received the live-attenuated influenza vaccine administered intranasally, then this statement could well be true. Live-attenuated vaccines can make people sick whose immune systems are suppressed. However, the majority of people who make this claim are misunderstanding the way that the flu vaccine works.
    - The injectable influenza vaccine (the one most commonly given) is a killed virus vaccine. It has no live, or active, flu virus in it. It triggers the immune system to allow our bodies to recognize and fight off the flu. This sometimes makes us feel achy and tired or may give us a low-grade fever for a short time. This is just our immune system revving up and is an expected result of immunization, but it is not the flu. The actual flu is much worse.
    - When someone thinks they got the flu from the flu shot, the most likely explanation is that they got exposed to the flu either just before receiving the injection or during the first 2 weeks after receiving the injection, at which time the vaccine is not yet fully effective.
        - This is why it is important to get the flu shot before flu season begins, so we are fully protected from the flu by the time we may come into contact with it.

4. I have an allergy to eggs so I can't get the flu shot.

- Historically, we *did* caution people with egg allergies to avoid taking the flu shot. The influenza vaccine is most commonly produced in chicken eggs, though ongoing research is being done to develop non-egg means of production. However, for the 2016-2017 flu season, the ACIP changed its recommendations.

- Now, if reactions are mild or patients have difficulty eating only raw eggs, not cooked, then they can get a flu vaccine without concern. If the egg-allergy reaction is more severe (anaphylaxis, recurrent vomiting, etc.), the flu shot is still recommended, but it has to be given by a provider who can recognize and respond to a severe allergic reaction.[14] These recommendations are based on a large number of research studies showing no significant reaction in people allergic to eggs who received the injectable flu vaccine.[15] The risk of serious consequences of an influenza infection far outweighs the very small risk of serious reaction to a flu shot in this population of patients.

- If all else fails and egg-allergic patients still balk at the idea of getting a flu shot, there are currently two egg-free vaccines available, Flublok and Flucelvax. Both are indicated for use in people older than 18 years.

HUMAN PAPILLOMAVIRUS

HPV is a virus that causes tens of thousands of cases of cancer each year in the United States—cervical, vaginal, vulvar, penile, anal, rectal, oral, and throat cancers. It also causes genital warts and a less common condition called laryngeal papillomatosis. Because of its association with sexual activity, the HPV vaccine is an immunization that we have particular difficulty in getting parents to accept for their children. There are many myths and misunderstandings circulating that contribute to this issue and I will address these in turn. However, this is also one of the newest vaccines on the market and this, I believe, plays a large role in why these misunderstandings abound and why we see both patients, and sometimes even health care providers, being hesitant about its use.

The understanding of the role that HPV plays in the development of genital and oropharyngeal cancers is also relatively new in the field of medicine. Most practicing physicians have "grown up" during the era of the Pap smear. We get them. We perform them. We are very comfortable with and used to the procedure of screening for cervical cancer, and this test *has* gone a long way in early detection of changes so that cancer can be averted. What we are looking at now, however, is an attempt to prevent those precancerous and cancerous changes from happening in the first place. And with regard to the other cancers that HPV causes, there are no current screening exams that work to detect changes before they become a problem. The Pap smear continues to be of great help for women in the area of HPV detection and cervical cancer prevention, but it does nothing to help with the other cancers with which we are also concerned.

When the first HPV vaccine came out in 2006, I was a couple of years out of residency. I was a fledgling physician and was, and still am, exceedingly cautious, particularly when it comes to jumping on a bandwagon with respect to new medicines. I tend to like to use medicines that are tried and true, that are tested by history. I am not naïve to the fact that there are occasional adverse outcomes that come to light after large-scale use of a medicine that were not seen in premarketing studies. I was also uncertain as to why the original HPV vaccine was marketed only to girls and women. As a sexually transmitted infection, it is, by definition, transmitted through sexual contact between two people. Why were we not vaccinating boys? I certainly gave the vaccine, but did not push the issue if parents and patients expressed doubts. I was happy to rely on discussion of delaying sexual activity, keeping the number of sexual partners to a minimum, and on the success of the Pap smear screening exam.

Looking back, I wonder if this was the right choice. Around 2011, when the HPV immunization started being recommended for use in boys, I was gaining confidence in its use and effectiveness. Even though there were reports of fainting after the vaccine, I had only seen this once. I had seen no adverse outcomes following its use in my own patient population. At the same time, I was becoming increasingly aware of the successes that other countries, such as Australia, Sweden, and Finland, that were better at implementing widespread vaccination programs, were seeing in decreasing the incidence of genital warts, infections with the HPV vaccine-related strains, and HPV-related precancers[16-20] (see **Figure 11.2**).

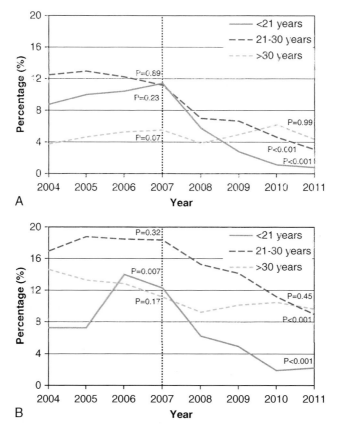

FIGURE 11.2 Following implementation of a nationally funded school–based HPV vaccination program in Australia in 2007, the percentage of young people diagnosed with genital warts decreased by a remarkable 88% in 4 y. It's important to note that this figure not only demonstrates this reduction in young women, who were the initial group targeted for vaccination in 2007, but also shows a sharp decline in the incidence of genital warts in young men, who did not themselves begin receiving the vaccine until 2011. This is an excellent demonstration of herd immunity in action, where vaccination of one group protects another, as yet unvaccinated, group. A, Australian-born women diagnosed with genital warts at first visit, broken down by age, 2004-2011. B, Australian-born heterosexual men diagnosed with genital warts at first visit, broken down by age, 2004-2011. As you can see, a significant decline in genital warts was seen after introduction of HPV vaccination programs—indicated by the vertical dotted line—in both females and males, even though males were not yet being vaccinated at that time. (Reproduced from Hammad A, Donovan B, Wand H, et al. Genital warts in young Australians five years into national human papillomavirus vaccination programme: national surveillance data. *BMJ*. 2013;346:f2032, with permission from BMJ Publishing Group Ltd.)

Even with our less-than-stellar track record for vaccinating against HPV in the United States, we are beginning to see reduction in the incidence of HPV infections and related precancers (cervical intraepithelial neoplasia [CIN]) here as well. In a recent study out of New Mexico looking at Pap Registry data from 2007 to 2014, involving nearly 100,000 women, a notable decreased incidence in cases was observed in women ages 15 to 19 (dropping from 3468.3 cases to 1590.6 cases of CIN1 per 100,000 women screened, from 896.4 to 414.9 for CIN2, and from 240.2 to 0 for CIN3). In women ages 20 to 24, the reduction in cases of CIN2 was also significant, dropping from 1027.7 to 627.1 cases. The decrease was greater than expected given the relatively low level of vaccine uptake in New Mexico (up to 40% over the years studied) and suggested a possible role of protection from partial vaccination, cross-protection against nonvaccine HPV types, and herd immunity.[21] The results of these data and other similar findings may someday inform a change in guidelines to begin screening for cervical cancer at a later age.

One of the greatest barriers to use of the HPV vaccine is in discussion of the virus' relation to sexual activity. The vaccine is licensed for use in ages 9 to 26, though has recently also been licensed for use in ages 27 to 45. ACIP recommendations regarding use in this later age group are still pending. Per current guidelines, we are recommending the HPV vaccine at the 11- to 12-year well-child check. This is typically a time when kids are unlikely to be having sex and the discussion at home and in schools about developing bodies and sexual activity is just beginning. The idea of having a conversation about this sexually transmitted infection and their child's future sexual activities makes many parents uncomfortable. How we approach this discussion is extremely important. In the following paragraph, I will lay out examples of how you might have this conversation with your patients and parents that will increase your chances of vaccination success.

As we discussed in chapter 6, the presumptive approach to vaccines is much more effective than a participatory approach. It assumes that the parents or child will be making the choice to vaccinate, and when it comes to introducing a newer vaccine, like HPV, it is helpful to recommend it in the same breath as we recommend the other "first adult" vaccines, with which families are more familiar. This method is called "bundling," or discussing the vaccines in "the same way on the same day," and has been recommended by the CDC to improve vaccine acceptance.[22] If we talk about the HPV vaccine as a separate topic, it introduces some small measure of doubt into parents' minds about its use at this age. Here's how the conversation should go…

"Mary, this year you are old enough to get your first adult vaccines—Tdap, the HPV vaccine, and the meningitis vaccine—to protect against tetanus, whooping cough, HPV cancers, and meningitis."

Contrast this with a discussion where the HPV vaccine is broken out…

"Jason, this year you are old enough to get your first adult vaccines—Tdap and the meningitis vaccine—to protect against tetanus, whooping cough, and meningitis. We also have the HPV vaccine to offer at this age."

It's not difficult to see how the first approach better "normalizes" the HPV vaccine and makes it seem like all the other important vaccines given at this age, which of course, it is. The other thing you will notice about these statements is that they both speak primarily to the patient and not to the parent. We, of course, want to address parental questions and concerns as they are the ones making the final decision about vaccines at this age. However, even if the parent opts against this vaccine or others, the child will eventually be old enough to make his or her own decisions. After age 18, kids can decide for themselves how they want to approach vaccines, and the HPV vaccine, though best if given earlier, can currently be given up through age 26. There is also a "mature minor rule" in some states, which allows children of a certain age to make independent decisions about anything regarding their sexual and mental health as well as issues related to substance use. These may vary state by state, so check your state's rules for specifics.[23]

Following the recommendation for these vaccines, some parents and kids are immediately on board. However, others will benefit from a discussion to get answers to questions and concerns they may have. We know that we will have greater success in getting kids and parents to accept the HPV vaccine if we discuss it as a cancer-prevention vaccine than if we discuss it as a vaccine to prevent a sexually transmitted infection (see **Table 11.1** showing the percentage of cancers caused by HPV). As previously stated, discussion of their child's sexual health can make parents uncomfortable, but who can't get behind an intervention that helps prevent their child from getting cancer?

TABLE 11.1 Percentage of Cancers Caused by HPV[24,25]

TYPE OF CANCER	% DUE TO HPV	STRAINS INVOLVED
Cervical	~91%-100%	70% caused by 16/18
Anal	~91%-95%	most caused by 16
Oropharyngeal	~70%	50% caused by 16
Vaginal	~65%-75%	most caused by 16
Vulvar	~50%-69%	most caused by 16
Penile	~35%-63%	most caused by 16

The following are concerns commonly encountered during counseling sessions with parents and teens about the HPV vaccine. If discussion of the sexual nature of transmission of HPV is unavoidable, there are several important points noted here that will help make your case for this lifesaving vaccine.

1. I'm worried that giving the HPV vaccine to my 11-year-old daughter will just give her permission to begin sexual activity at an earlier age.
    - There is no evidence to show that giving the HPV vaccine at age 11 or 12 will encourage earlier or riskier sexual activity. In fact, the opposite may be true.
    - A 2016 systematic review published in *Human Vaccines & Immunotherapeutics* demonstrated *no* earlier incidence of sexual activity–related outcomes (rates of sexually transmitted infection testing or diagnosis, pregnancy, contraceptive counseling, age of first sexual activity, or number of sexual partners) in individuals who received the HPV vaccine versus those that didn't.[26]
    - A recent study published in the *Canadian Medical Association Journal* looked at nearly 300,000 girls in British Columbia, which established a school-based HPV vaccination program in 2008. Researchers looked at markers of risky sexual activity both before and after vaccination

program implementation. The study found that sexual activity stayed the same or was *safer* in girls who had been vaccinated versus those that hadn't. The percentage of girls ever having had intercourse decreased from 21.3% to 18.3%, the percentage of girls having sex at an early age decreased from 14.3% to 10.2%, and the percentage of girls ever having been pregnant decreased from 5.9% to 3.4%. This trend was also seen in the use of illicit substances before intercourse, which decreased from 26.0% to 19.3%, and the use of condoms or birth control pills, which increased from 65.6% to 68.9% and from 45.1% to 54.5%, respectively. The percentage of girls with three or more sexual partners within the prior year remained unchanged.[27]

2. But why now? Why not wait until they are a little bit older to give them this vaccine?

   - We know from the study of immunology that our immune systems mount a better, more vigorous, response to vaccines when we are young.

   - Looking at antibody levels achieved in individuals given the HPV vaccine at ages 11 to 12 versus in later teen years, we see greater antibody levels developed in response to the vaccine at the younger age.[28] The vaccine will be more effective if we give it at the 11- to 12-year visit than if we wait until later adolescence or young adulthood.

   - Also, because the HPV vaccine is a prevention vaccine and does nothing for treatment of infection, we want to get the vaccine series completed *before* our kids become sexually active.

   - In 2016, the guidelines for administration of the vaccine changed. Now, if given before age 15, only two shots are required (given 6-12 months apart). However, if the series is started at age 15 or later, kids will still need the full three-shot series (given at 0, 2, and 6 months). The earlier they get it, the fewer shots are needed. (Observation: If the CDC and doctors were recommending vaccines just to make money, why would we decrease the number of vaccines recommended?)

   - Finally, if necessary, you can appeal to the pocketbook. For those who would qualify for the Vaccines for Children program, the vaccine series is fully covered up until age 19. After that, it is up to the parents or insurance to cover the cost of vaccines and each shot runs about $150.00. Getting the shot earlier is not only more effective, it is also potentially less expensive.

3. Isn't this vaccine just for at-risk teens? My kid is a good kid. He won't be engaging in any risky behavior.

   - The CDC estimates that there are currently 79 million Americans infected with the HPV virus, and 14 million people contract the virus each year. Nearly all of us will be exposed to the HPV virus at some point in our sexual lives. The fact that there are rarely any outward signs of the virus makes it extremely hard to avoid.

   - We may think we have the most responsible teen on the planet, but our teen can still be at risk. Our child may do everything right by delaying sexual activity and having only one sexual partner, but this virus is so common that it takes *no* high-risk activity to be exposed. A person could contract the virus the very first time they have sex. And in the case of genital warts, no actual intercourse is required. Skin-to-skin contact is all that is needed for transmission.

- We may have the greatest trust in our teen to do the right thing and make the right decisions, but do we want to stake their life on it? And do we want to put their fate in the hands of some future sexual partner with an unknown sexual history?
- We also have to remember what it was like to be a teenager. Think back to your own adolescence. Did you always share everything about your life with your parents? Did you ever do something as a teen that you look back on now and say to yourself, "What was I thinking?" Our kids will be no different.
- Finally, as much as we don't want to think about it, we must acknowledge that some of our children will suffer unwanted sexual contact. Shouldn't we help protect them as much as possible?

4. This vaccine is pretty new. I'm not sure I want to give my child something without an established safety record.
   - The HPV vaccine was licensed in the United States in 2006. Relative to all the other vaccines we recommend for kids, this one is new. And new is always a little scary.
   - But it is now 2019. This vaccine has been around for 13 years and is making great strides in decreasing the rates of genital warts and precancers (which now *won't* go on to develop into cancers).
   - Also important to note is that, before any vaccine comes to market, it is studied for safety and effectiveness for an average of 10 to 15 years (see chapter 5 for further discussion of vaccine development and monitoring) and monitoring continues after a vaccine is released to market. The HPV vaccine *does* have a well-established safety record.
   - Compared with other vaccine-preventable diseases for which we more readily vaccinate, HPV causes much more suffering and death. How often do we see someone dying from tetanus? Thankfully, very rarely—because we vaccinate. Tetanus is a terrible way to die. But so is cancer of your penis or cervix or throat.

5. Isn't this vaccine just for girls?
   - The HPV vaccine was originally marketed only to girls, but in 2011, it began being recommended to boys as well. This makes sense because boys can also contract HPV-related cancers (penile, anal, rectal, and oropharyngeal) and can transmit HPV to their sexual partners.

6. How effective is the vaccine if it doesn't cover all of the strains that cause cancer?
   - Our current 9-valent vaccine covers strains 6 and 11, which cause most cases of genital warts; strains 16 and 18, which cause the large majority of HPV-related cancers (approximately 70% of cervical cancer cases); and strains 31, 33, 45, 52, and 58, which can also cause HPV-related cancers (an additional 20% of cervical cancer cases are attributed to these strains).[29]
   - We still counsel teens to delay sexual activity and limit the number of sexual partners, but the 9-valent HPV vaccine is more than 90% effective at preventing the high-risk cancer-causing strains of HPV.

7. If we give the vaccine now, isn't it just going to wear off by the time they are sexually active?
   - HPV vaccines have been on the market for 13 years and postmarket analysis thus far shows no waning immunity, with further studies ongoing.[30,31]

8. I've heard that the HPV vaccine can actually cause cancer.

    - Although rates decreased in the younger age groups observed in the New Mexico Pap Registry study mentioned above, a rise in incidence of higher-grade dysplasia (CIN3)—not cancer—*was* seen in the older population studied (ages 25-29). Individuals studied were not divided with respect to vaccination status versus nonvaccination status. Researchers simply took a cohort of women pre- and post-vaccination era and looked at rates of CIN1, 2, and 3 by age group.[21] From this information, we cannot draw a correlation between the vaccine and rising rates of high-grade dysplasia. This age group may have had fewer people in it who had received the vaccine or may have included individuals who had lower-grade dysplasia to begin with (and we know that the HPV vaccine doesn't treat preexisting HPV infections) that progressed during the study timeframe. We simply don't know.

        - Given that the vaccine was licensed in 2006 and only began being offered in 2007, the older group would also not have received the vaccine until their late teen or early adult years. The ability of the vaccine to induce a robust immune response, as previously discussed, is not as great in later years as it would have been if the vaccine were given earlier.

        - These findings also likely reflect the changes in screening guidelines that occurred during the study timeframe, with longer screening intervals and increased HPV testing resulting in a greater number of referrals for colposcopy, and subsequent discovery of pathology, in this group.

        - A decrease in rates of CIN1 and CIN2 is the *most* important finding in this study, as this degree of cervical change is nearly a prerequisite for development of high-grade dysplasia or invasive cervical cancer. The cost, in terms of emotion, dollars, and patient morbidity, to evaluate and treat these lower-grade lesions is significant.

    - It most often takes decades to see the development of cervical and other HPV-related cancers, so only time will tell if the vaccine truly reduces cancer rates. But all available evidence to date, looking at decreasing rates of precancerous changes in people vaccinated against HPV, points to the likelihood that it will.

9. What about the girls who actually became infertile after getting the HPV vaccine?

    - Whenever a concern is voiced about any vaccine, scientists get to work to determine whether or not the concern is warranted. Is there any truth to the claim?

    - Multiple studies show *no* increased rates of premature ovarian insufficiency (POI) or failure in girls vaccinated versus those that are unvaccinated.

    - A recent study printed in the journal *Pediatrics* studied nearly 200,000 girls receiving their 11- to 12-year vaccines (HPV, Tdap, MenACWY) and found only one case of POI following HPV vaccination. In that case, the delayed menstrual period was not noted until 23 months after the patient received the vaccine.[32] This is hardly proof that the vaccine caused the delayed period or produced infertility.

    - What *can* lead to fertility problems is the HPV infection itself. If a woman develops cervical precancer or cancer from HPV, partial removal of the cervix or full hysterectomy may be necessary. The procedures that are required to treat the serious effects of HPV infection could most certainly affect pregnancy outcomes.

10. But what about the illnesses that people are reporting after the HPV vaccine?

- Vaccine skeptics claim numerous other serious health effects caused by the HPV vaccine. Though case reports have been made for a variety of conditions, such as postural orthostatic tachycardia syndrome (POTS), chronic fatigue, complex regional pain syndrome (CRPS), and various autoimmune diseases, it is highly difficult to establish causation in these instances because of small sample sizes and lack of a control population.[33]

  › POTS—A study published in the *Journal of Adolescent Health* looked at the incidence of POTS following HPV vaccination. Researchers, studying cases reported to the Vaccine Adverse Event Reporting System (VAERS) between 2006 and 2015, detected no safety signals for POTS and HPV vaccination. In fact, their findings found report of only one case of POTS per 6.5 million HPV vaccine doses given in the United States.[34] I wouldn't call this a strong association.

  › Chronic fatigue—A large study from Norway, looking at approximately 175,000 girls who were offered the quadrivalent HPV vaccine in the 7th grade, found no increased incidence of chronic fatigue syndrome in individuals who had received the vaccine compared with those who hadn't.[35]

  › CRPS—A 2015 study examined case reports of CRPS from Japan and the United Kingdom. Of the 17 cases noted, only 5 met criteria for the diagnosis of CRPS. The study noted that the incidence of CRPS following vaccination for HPV 16 and 18 was "statistically significantly below expected rates."[36] Another study, reviewing VAERS data, noted only 22 cases of CRPS reported between 2006 and 2015, a timeframe during which 67 million doses of HPV vaccination were given. Additionally, a 35% increase in reports to VAERS was noted following a Japanese media report of CRPS after HPV vaccination, demonstrating how VAERS reports are potentially impacted by media attention.[37]

  › Autoimmune diseases—Multiple studies looking at rates of development of a variety of autoimmune conditions following HPV vaccination suggest no association between the two. Diseases, such as lupus, rheumatoid arthritis, Sjögren disease, multiple sclerosis, type 1 diabetes, Graves disease, Hashimoto thyroiditis, and others, do not occur more commonly in those vaccinated against HPV than they do in the baseline population.[38-40] A particularly powerful study from France[40] looked at over 2 million girls ages 13 to 16 between the years 2008 and 2012 (37% of whom received the HPV vaccine). Researchers found *no* association with 12 of the 14 studied autoimmune diseases. There was a mild increase in incidence of Guillain-Barré syndrome noted in the first 2 months following vaccination, the finding of which, authors note, has not reliably been found in other studies.[41-43] A weak association was also found with inflammatory bowel disease (IBD). However, this association did not persist with further time from vaccination, leading researchers to conclude that "our results do not support a causal association between HPV vaccination and IBD"[42] (see Appendix E: Journal Articles Addressing Specific Vaccine Concerns for a list of studies related to vaccines and autoimmune disease).

Universal influenza immunization and HPV vaccination recommendations are relatively new, and this lack of familiarity contributes to the public's uncertainty about vaccine effectiveness and safety. However, these vaccines have now been around for decades. Scientists continue to search for any signals of significant adverse effects following immunization and none have been reproducibly found. These vaccines have the potential to save tens of thousands of US lives each year and hundreds of thousands of lives worldwide. Despite this, we are far from our Healthy People 2020 goals for immunization with these vaccines (70% influenza vaccination in adults older than 18 years and 80% HPV vaccination of females by age 15).[44] Strong recommendations from patients' primary care providers can go a long way toward improving uptake of these lifesaving vaccines. And don't forget that one of the most influential arguments you can make for influenza and HPV immunization, or for any immunization, is that you give it to yourself and to your children. It means a great deal to patients to know that their medical provider is confident enough in the effectiveness and safety of vaccines to give them to their loved ones.

References

1. Nour NM. Cervical cancer: a preventable death. *Rev Obstet Gynecol*. 2009;2(4):240-244.
2. Centers for Disease Control and Prevention. Flu Vaccination Coverage, United States, 2016-17 Influenza Season. https://www.cdc.gov/flu/fluvaxview/coverage-1617estimates.htm. Updated September 28, 2017. Accessed January 12, 2019.
3. Walker TY, Elam-Evans LD, Singleton JA, et al. National, regional, state, and selected local area vaccination coverage among adolescents aged 13-17 Years – United States, 2016. *MMWR (Morb Mortal Wkly Rep)*. 2017;66(33):874-882.
4. Barberis I, Myles P, Ault SK, et al. History and evolution of influenza control through vaccination: from the first monovalent vaccine to universal vaccines. *J Prev Med Hyg*. 2016;57(3):E115-E120.
5. Centers for Disease Control and Prevention. Selecting Viruses for the Seasonal Influenza Vaccine. https://www.cdc.gov/flu/about/season/vaccine-selection.htm. Updated September 4, 2018. Accessed January 12, 2019.
6. Centers for Disease Control and Prevention. Seasonal Influenza Vaccine Effectiveness, 2004-2018. https://www.cdc.gov/flu/professionals/vaccination/effectiveness-studies.htm. Updated November 15, 2018. Accessed January 12, 2019.
7. Centers for Disease Control and Prevention. Summary of the 2017-2018 Influenza Season. https://www.cdc.gov/flu/about/season/flu-season-2017-2018.htm. Updated November 2, 2018. Accessed January 12, 2019.
8. Centers for Disease Control and Prevention. CDC Study Finds Flu Vaccine Saves Children's Lives. https://www.cdc.gov/media/releases/2017/p0403-flu-vaccine.html. Accessed January 12, 2019.
9. Centers for Disease Control and Prevention. Fluzone High-Dose Seasonal Influenza Vaccine. https://www.cdc.gov/flu/protect/vaccine/qa_fluzone.htm. Updated October 19, 2018. Accessed February 6, 2019.
10. Duddu P. *The Biggest Passenger Airplanes in the World*. Aerospace Technology; August 23, 2013. https://www.aerospace-technology.com/features/feature-biggest-passenger-airplanes-in-the-world/. Accessed January 12, 2019.
11. The College of Physicians of Philadelphia. *Flu Vaccine Recommended for All Adults*. March 15, 2010. https://www.historyofvaccines.org/content/blog/flu-vaccine-recommended-all-adults. Accessed January 12, 2019.
12. Shang M, Blanton L, Brammer L, et al. Influenza-associated pediatric deaths in the United States, 2010-2016. *Pediatrics*. 2018;141(4):e20172918.
13. Taubenberger JK, Morens DM. 1918 Influenza: the mother of all pandemics. *Emerg Infect Dis*. 2006;12(1):15-22.
14. Centers for Disease Control and Prevention. Flu Vaccine and People With Egg Allergies. https://www.cdc.gov/flu/protect/vaccine/egg-allergies.htm. Updated December 28, 2017. Accessed January 12, 2019.

15. Greenhawt M, Turner PJ, Kelso JM. Administration of influenza vaccines to egg allergic recipients: a practice parameter update 2017. *Ann Allergy Asthma Immunol*. 2018;120:49-52.

16. Read TR, Hocking JS, Chen MY, et al. The near disappearance of genital warts in young women 4 years after commencing a national human papillomavirus (HPV) vaccination programme. *Sex Transm Infect*. 2011;87(7):544-547.

17. Brotherton JM, Fridman M, May CL, et al. Early effect of the HPV programme on cervical abnormalities in Victoria, Australia: an ecological study. *Lancet*. 2011;377(9783):2085-2092.

18. Leval A, Herweijer E, Ploner A, et al. Quadrivalent human papillomavirus vaccine effectiveness: a Swedish national cohort study. *J Natl Cancer Inst*. 2013;105(7):469-474.

19. Rana MM, Huhtala H, Apter D, et al. Understanding long-term protection of human papillomavirus vaccination against cervical carcinoma: cancer registry-based follow-up. *Int J Cancer*. 2013;132(12):2833-2838.

20. Garland SM, Kjaer SK, Munoz N, et al. Impact and effectiveness of the quadrivalent human papillomavirus vaccine: a systematic review of 10 years of real-world experience. *Clin Infect Dis*. 2016;63(4):519-527.

21. Benard VB, Castle PE, Jenison SA, et al. Population-based incidence rates of cervical intraepithelial neoplasia in the human papillomavirus era. *JAMA Oncol*. 2017;3(6):833-837.

22. Centers for Disease Control and Prevention. Talking to Parents About HPV Vaccine. https://www.cdc.gov/hpv/hcp/for-hcp-tipsheet-hpv.html. Updated May 2018. Accessed January 12, 2019.

23. King County. The Mature Minor Rule. https://www.kingcounty.gov/depts/health/locations/family-planning/health-care-providers/mature-minor-rule.aspx. Updated January 3, 2019. Accessed January 12, 2019.

24. National Cancer Institute. HPV and Cancer. Accessed February 13, 2019. https://www.cancer.gov/about-cancer/causes-prevention/risk/infectious-agents/hpv-fact-sheet.

25. Centers for Disease Control and Prevention. How Many Cancers are Linked With HPV Each Year? https://www.cdc.gov/cancer/HPV/statistics/cases.htm#5. Accessed February 13, 2019.

26. Kasting ML, Shapiro GK, Rosberger Z, et al. Tempest in a teapot: a systematic review of HPV vaccination and risk compensation research. *Hum Vaccin Immunother*. 2016;12(6):1435-1450.

27. Ogilvie GS, Phan F, Pedersen HN, et al. Population-level sexual behaviors in adolescent girls before and after introduction of the human papillomavirus vaccine (2003-2013). *CMAJ (Can Med Assoc J)*. 2018;190(41):e1221-e1226.

28. Schuchat A, Brady MT. *HPV Vaccine Can't Wait*. AAP News; August 31, 2012. www.aappublications.org/content/early/2012/08/31/aapnews.20120831-1. Accessed January 12, 2019.

29. Joura EA, Giuliano AR, Iversen OE, et al. A 9-valentine HPV vaccine against infection and intraepithelial neoplasia in women. *N Engl J Med*. 2015;372:711-723.

30. De Vincenzo R, Conte C, Ricci C, et al. Long-term efficacy and safety of human papillomavirus vaccination. *Int J Womens Health*. 2014;6:999-1010.

31. Centers for Disease Control and Prevention. HPV Vaccine Information for Young Women. https://www.cdc.gov/std/hpv/stdfact-hpv-vaccine-young-women.htm. Accessed January 12, 2019.

32. Naleway AL, Mittendorf KF, Irving SA, et al. Primary ovarian insufficiency and adolescent vaccination. *Pediatrics*. 2018;142(3):e20180943.

33. Butts BN, Fischer PR, Mack KJ. Human papillomavirus vaccine and postural orthostatic tachycardia syndrome: a review of current literature. *J Child Neurol*. 2017;32(11):956-965.

34. Arana J, Mba-Jonas A, Jankosky C, et al. Reports of postural orthostatic tachycardia syndrome after human papillomavirus vaccination in the vaccine adverse event reporting system. *J Adolescent Health*. 2017;61(5):577-582.

35. Feiring B, Laake I, Bakken IJ, et al. HPV vaccination and risk of chronic fatigue syndrome/myalgic encephalomyelitis: a nationwide register-based study from Norway. *Vaccine*. 2017;35(33):4203-4212.

36. Huygen F, Verschueren K, McCabe C, et al. Investigating reports of complex regional pain syndrome: an analysis of HPV-16/18-adjuvanted vaccine post-licensure data. *EBioMedicine*. 2015;2(9):1114-1121.

37. Weinbaum CM, Cano M. HPV vaccination and complex regional pain syndrome: lack of evidence. *EBioMedicine*. 2015;2(9):1014-1015.

38. Liu EY, Smith LM, Ellis AK, et al. Quadrivalent human papillomavirus vaccination in girls and the risk of autoimmune disorders: the Ontario Grade 8 HPV Vaccine Cohort Study. *CMAJ (Can Med Assoc J)*. 2018;190(21):E648-E655.

39. Genovese C, La Fauci V, Squeri A, et al. HPV vaccine and autoimmune diseases: systematic review and meta-analysis of the literature. *J Prev Med Hyg*. 2018;59(3):E194-E199.

40. Miranda S, Chaignot C, Collin C. Human papillomavirus vaccination and risk of autoimmune diseases: a large cohort study of over 2 million young girls in France. *Vaccine.* 2017;35(36):4761-4768.

41. Andrews N, Stowe J, Miller E. No increased risk of Guillain-Barré syndrome after human papilloma virus vaccine: a self-controlled case-series study in England. *Vaccine.* 2017;35(13):1729-1732.

42. Gee J, Sukumaran L, Weintraub E, et al. Risk of Guillain-Barré syndrome following quadrivalent human papillomavirus vaccine in the Vaccine Safety Datalink. *Vaccine.* 2017;35(43):5756-5758.

43. Arnheim-Dahlström L, Pasternak B, Svanström H, et al. Autoimmune, neurological, and venous thromboembolic adverse events after immunisation of adolescent girls with quadrivalent human papillomavirus vaccine in Denmark and Sweden: cohort study. *BMJ.* 2013;347:f5906.

44. Office of Disease Prevention and Health Promotion. Immunization and Infectious Diseases. HealthPeople. gov. https://www.healthypeople.gov/2020/topics-objectives/topic/immunization-and-infectious-diseases/national-snapshot. Accessed January 12, 2019.

Vaccine Ingredients—What Is All That Stuff Anyway?

All things are poison, and nothing is without poison. The dosage alone makes it so a thing is not a poison.

—Paracelsus

There's little that worries vaccine-hesitant patients more than the "stuff" that is in vaccines. They have heard that vaccine ingredients are "toxic." They have heard that there is aborted fetal tissue and that there are monkey cells in our vaccines. The substances listed in the package inserts often have long and unusual-sounding chemical names that are not easily recognizable. It is easy to see why vaccine ingredients could be concerning for some people. However, the reality of what's in vaccines is much less frightening. Unlike lists of food ingredients, vaccine ingredients must include products used in the process of manufacturing a vaccine, even if none of that substance, or only trace amounts of that substance, remain in the final product. Moreover, many of the ingredients found in vaccines or used in production of vaccines actually already exist in the human body (for example, sodium, potassium, urea, histidine, and formaldehyde) or are in foods we consume every day (such as sucrose, dextrose, lactose, vitamins, yeast, and eggs).

This chapter will take you through the steps of vaccine production, highlighting the substances used along the way (known as excipients). In learning the process of making a vaccine and the purpose of the ingredients used in the manufacturing and final production of a vaccine, we can hopefully make that "stuff" that is in vaccines seem much less scary.

Let's start from the beginning. First, the bacteria or viruses that we are using to build an immunity to through vaccination have to be grown and replicated.

Growth of Viruses and Bacteria. Viruses and bacteria are the active ingredients in a vaccine. Some vaccines contain whole viruses or bacteria that are either live but weakened, or are killed and fully inactivated. Other vaccines contain only pieces of viruses or bacteria (usually proteins or sugars from the surface of the organism), which trigger the immune response but do not cause disease.

1. **Human and animal cells**—Viruses will only grow in human or animal cells. Cells are the "manufacturing plants" for viruses and bacteria. Within the cells, these organisms can grow and replicate, later to be separated from their cellular "homes" and purified multiple times over. DNA is not stable when exposed to chemicals and is, therefore, denatured or broken down so much that exceedingly tiny amounts (on the order of trillions of a gram) of DNA, if any, remain in the final vaccine product. Any DNA that does remain is highly fragmented and could not create a whole protein. In such a state, it is practically impossible for any DNA from the vaccine manufacturing process to incorporate itself into the DNA of the person getting the vaccine. If this *could* occur, gene therapy would be much easier than it has turned out to be.[1]

   - Human cell strains—As discussed in chapter 10, there are two human cell lines (WI-38 and MRC-5) used in vaccine production.
   - Animal cell strains—A variety of animal cells are also used in viral vaccine production, including Vero cells (derived from cells of an African green monkey), embryonic chick and duck cells, Madin-Darby canine kidney cells (derived from cells of an adult cocker spaniel), insect cells, and embryonic guinea pig cells.[2,3]
   - Genetically modified organisms—Use of genetically modified cells or genetic material (DNA or RNA) within those cells is a promising method of vaccine production under study. A virus itself may be genetically altered, rendering it noninfectious but retaining the ability to stimulate an immune response. Or, DNA that codes a part of an infectious organism can be placed into another organism for mass production to later be used for vaccine manufacture.[4]
     - Recombinant DNA technology—This is a type of genetic modification technology. Recombinant vaccines are made when small pieces of DNA from the organism we want to protect against are put into bacterial or yeast cells to produce large quantities of an active ingredient for manufacture of the vaccine. In the case of the hepatitis B vaccine, for example, yeast cells are used to produce a hepatitis B surface protein.[5]

2. **Growth media**—Some bacteria do not need to be grown in human or animal cells but can instead be grown on cultures using nutrient-rich media to foster growth. There are numerous brands of growth media used in vaccine production, including, Eagle's medium, Stainer-Scholte medium, Medium 199, and others.[6] Media ingredients typically include proteins (for example, soy peptone and bovine casein), amino acids (for example, L-cysteine and L-histamine), vitamins (for example, ferric nitrate and magnesium sulfate), carbohydrates (for example, dextrose and galactose), and salts (for example, potassium chloride and sodium pyruvate). These and other ingredients are used at this stage of the production process to provide an optimal growth environment for the active vaccine ingredients.[7]

Next, the desirable viruses or bacteria or pieces of viruses or bacteria that are needed for vaccine production have to be processed and purified.

Processing and Purification. Substances used in production of vaccines may or may not have any residual presence in the finished product. If there is any substance remaining, it is usually only in trace amounts. The following are the various substances used in processing and purifying the vaccine.

1. **Antibiotics:** These are used only during manufacturing to prevent bacteria from growing in and contaminating the vaccine. Antibiotics that commonly cause allergic reactions (such as sulfa- and penicillin-containing antibiotics) are not used. Less commonly allergenic antibiotics (such as neomycin and polymyxin B) are used for production of vaccines. There may be tiny amounts of antibiotic remaining in the final vaccine product, but, depending on the type of allergic reaction, people with mild allergies could still receive vaccines that use the antibiotic in production. This should be discussed with a medical provider first, however.

2. **Inactivating agents:** These are used to inactivate viruses and bacteria so that they can't induce the illness against which they are meant to protect. These agents are diluted significantly and very little remain in the final vaccine product. These include formaldehyde (a pear has 50 times more formaldehyde than any vaccine),[5] glutaraldehyde (the amount remaining in any vaccine is <50 ng, which is one *billionth* of a gram),[8] and *beta*-propriolactone (which is present only in the anthrax vaccine and, after placement in solution with water, is fully broken down and harmless).[9]

3. **Protein purifiers:** The purpose of protein purification is to separate out or isolate one or a few proteins of interest from a complex mixture of process-related impurities (such as those used in growing a virus or bacterium). The goal is to retain the largest amount of protein with the fewest amount of contaminants. Some of the substances used in the purification process include ammonium sulfate, cetyltrimethylammonium bromide, hexadecyl-trimethylammonium bromide, and sodium taurodeoxycholate.[10]

Then, the purified virus, bacterium, or particle has to be "packaged" in a solution for administration to patients.

Making the Final Product. Other than the virus or bacterium itself, the substances that make up the ultimate components of a vaccine are those that enhance immunogenicity (or ability to induce an immune response), allow the viral and bacterial proteins and other ingredients to remain in solution, and enable stability of the vaccine over time and across changes in temperature, acidity, light, and humidity.

1. **Adjuvants**—These are used to "strengthen and lengthen" the immune response to a vaccine. They also absorb protein that helps keep the vaccine components from sticking to the walls of the container during storage.[5] They are only used in inactivated virus vaccines.
   - **Aluminum:** Aluminum hydroxide, aluminum phosphate, potassium aluminum phosphate, potassium aluminum sulfate, and amorphous aluminum hydroxyphosphate sulfate.

> Also found in most naturally occurring foods, water, breast milk, formula, breads, cakes, antacids, food packaging products, and more
> Vaccines with aluminum are more likely to cause redness and hardness at the injection site and rarely cause a granuloma (localized mass of granulation tissue), which is not dangerous but can last for months to years

- **MF59 (squalene oil):** MF59 comes from highly purified fish oil. It is only used in Fluad, an influenza vaccine, which is used in people older than 65 years of age.
    > Also found in naturally occurring oil found in humans, plants, and animals
    > Common side effects related to MF59 are injection site pain, swelling, redness, low-grade temperature, headache, malaise, fatigue, and shivering[5]

- **MPL (3-O-desacyl-4'-monophosphoryl lipid A):** This form of lipid A molecule induces a strong immune response but is 100-fold less toxic than other forms, such as lipopolysaccharide.[11] It is currently only a component of the bivalent HPV vaccine, which is no longer commonly recommended, given availability of the nine-valent vaccine.

- **Xanthan:** This is traditionally used as a thickening agent and stabilizer. It is present in the rotavirus diluent, but it is also being studied and holds promise as an adjuvant to improve the immune response to vaccines.[12]
    > Also found in toothpaste, medicines, gluten-free foods, yogurt, ice cream, and other commonly used products

- **QS-21:** This compound is derived from the Chilean soapbark tree (*Quillaja saponaria*) and is used as an adjuvant in the Shingrix vaccine to enhance immune response. It is also under investigation for use in HIV, malaria, and cancer vaccines.[13]

- **CpG motifs:** These are synthetic adjuvants used in the newly released Heplisav-B vaccine, a 2-dose vaccine series licensed for prevention of hepatitis B infection in adults age 18 years and older. In studies, they proved safe at levels used in vaccines and showed no long-term increase in autoantibody levels, suggesting no role in triggering autoimmune disease.[14]

2. **Preservatives**—These are used to prevent bacteria and fungi from contaminating vaccines when a multiuse vial is opened. It is not necessary in single-dose vials. Multidose vials are used for illnesses that see possible epidemics (such as the flu) because they are less expensive to make than single-dose vials (think about all the packaging necessary to make individual doses) and because they can be made quickly in large quantities in case of emergency need.

- **Thimerosal:** This is an ethyl mercury–based preservative that is now present only in the multidose flu vials.

- **2-Phenoxyethanol:** This compound has very little toxicity in humans and is broken down and excreted through exhalation, urine, and stool.
    > Also found in cosmetics, baby care products, and eye and ear drops[15]

- **Phenol:** Phenol is an aromatic alcohol frequently used as a preservative in vaccines.[15]

- **Benzethonium chloride:** This compound has anti-infective, antiseptic, and surfactant properties. It is currently only used in the anthrax vaccine, which is not a routine vaccination.
    > Also found in hand and body washes[16]

◦ **EDTA (ethylenediaminetetracetic acid sodium):** In vaccines, this compound is used as a preservative but also has use as a chelating agent (it binds minerals and metals in order to remove them from the body).

⟩ Also found in shampoos, contact lens cleansers, cosmetics, and more; intravenous EDTA used to treat lead poisoning, radiation exposure, and significant elevations of blood calcium; and used to fortify the grain supply with iron for nutritional enhancement[17]

3. **Stabilizers**—Stabilizers help keep the vaccine from breaking down when exposed to heat, humidity, acidity, and light. They help a vaccine maintain its potency over time.

◦ **Gelatin (porcine or bovine):** In its use in vaccines, gelatin is usually derived from pigs. It is highly purified and hydrolyzed (broken down by water), so much so that DNA testing on vaccines is unable to identify the original source of the gelatin.[5]

◦ **Human serum albumin:** This is the most common protein found in human blood. It comes from human blood donors whose blood has been screened. The manufacturing process removes any risk of passing on viruses from the serum, and there have never been any viral diseases linked to use of human serum albumin in vaccines.[5]

◦ **Recombinant human serum albumin:** This does not contain any human or animal products. It is produced by taking the gene for human albumin and inserting it into cells (such as yeast cells), which can then generate large quantities of human albumin without having to take it from human blood.[5]

◦ **Bovine calf and fetal serum albumin/protein:** This type of protein is derived from cow blood.

◦ **Bovine extract and casamino acid:** Casein and whey are the main components of milk. Casein is separated out and hydrolyzed from bovine milk to produce one of the most nutrient-rich milk proteins. In combination with other supplemented ingredients, casein is used to make casamino acids, which act as stabilizers in vaccine production.[18]

◦ **Sorbitol:** A naturally occurring substance in the human body and in fruit and berries, sorbitol is often used as a sweetener in food and drinks. Note: Sorbitol is usually harmless, but people with an allergy to sorbitol or with rare hereditary fructose intolerance[a] may have concerns about its presence in vaccines.[19]

◦ **Others:** There are multiple other stabilizers that may be used in small amounts in vaccines (for example, urea, glycerol, and monosodium glutamate).[5]

---

[a]Hereditary fructose intolerance (HFI)—This is not the same as dietary fructose intolerance or fructose malabsorption. HFI is a rare (1:20,000 to 30,000) autosomal recessive deficit in an enzyme responsible for metabolism of fructose in the liver. Because sorbitol is converted to fructose, people with HFI also do not tolerate sorbitol consumption. Patients with HFI will typically have vomiting after eating foods containing fructose or sorbitol and may suffer failure to thrive until the condition is diagnosed. Cautions are provided for IV infusion of products containing fructose or sorbitol, where the natural defense mechanism (vomiting) to rid the body of these sugars is bypassed and where reactions can be severe. However, in the European Medicines Agency's *Information for the package leaflet regarding fructose and sorbitol used as excipients for medicinal products in human use* (October 9, 2017), vaccines using sorbitol as an excipient "have been administered for a long time without any known incidence of severe events due to HFI, in particular vaccines recommended for children below 2 years of age (MMR, VZV). Therefore the warning for those products should differ from the warning for products administered intravenously."[19]

4. **Buffers**—These are substances that are used to preserve the pH (acid-base balance) of vaccines. This is particularly important to ensuring the effectiveness of oral vaccines that encounter the acidic environment of the digestive tract. They can also decrease side effects such as gas and bloating.[20] These most commonly include salts (such as sodium chloride—table salt—and potassium chloride) and substances you may recognize as ingredients in antacids (such as sodium bicarbonate and calcium carbonate).

5. **Emulsifiers**—Also listed as surfactants, these are used to hold other vaccine ingredients together that might normally separate out (such as oil and water), to keep them in suspension.
   - **Polysorbate 80 (also called TWEEN 80):** This is a common food additive that is used in very small amounts in vaccines compared with its use in foods.
     - Also found in ice cream, salad dressings, sauces, and more
     - The amount of polysorbate 80 in the HPV vaccine is small at only 50 mg; compared to the 170,000 mg in a ½ cup of ice cream[21]
   - **Polysorbate 20 (also called TWEEN 20):**
     - Also used in cosmetics, lotions, sunscreens, deodorant, baby oil, etc.
     - Listed on the CleanIngredients.org database, which lists products that meet the EPA's Safer Choice Standard, designed to safeguard human and environmental health[22]
   - **Sorbitan trioleate:**
     - Also used in skin care and skin cleansing products, moisturizers, and makeup[23]
   - **Nonylphenol ethoxylate:** This compound is used as a detergent and emulsifier. If allowed to accumulate in the environment, it can be toxic to animals, particularly aquatic species. Although, there is "little evidence for any significant effects of exposure to nonylphenol ethoxylate on human health."[24]
   - **Triton X-100 (octoxynol-10 or octophenol ethoxylate):** This is *not* the same thing as octoxynol-9, which is used as a vaginal spermicide. They are chemically different substances (10 repeating ethoxy groups instead of 9) and therefore, have different biochemical actions. It is also used in the influenza vaccine to lyse (break down) cell membranes.[25]

6. **Residual proteins**—Though very little of the substances used for growth and production remain in the vaccine end product, there are a couple of components that deserve mention as they have the rare potential to cause allergic reactions. In the processing and purification section, we discussed the very minute amounts of residual antibiotics that may remain in vaccines and the need for caution with use in people who have allergy to those antibiotics. Residual proteins may remain from the growth phase of vaccine production that people with egg or yeast allergies need to be aware of and may have questions or concerns about.
   - Egg (ovalbumin) protein: Several vaccines (see below) are or have been grown in fertilized hen's eggs or on a culture that contains chick embryo cells. Although egg-free methods of production are being developed, no contraindications currently exist to getting *routinely* recommended vaccines for those with egg allergy.
     - Influenza—In 2016, the Advisory Committee on Immunization Practices (ACIP) changed the recommendation against flu vaccination for those with egg allergy
       - If reactions are mild or one can eat cooked eggs without difficulty, routine vaccination is recommended.

❏   If reactions are severe (anaphylaxis, recurrent vomiting, etc.), the flu vaccine can still be given but must be given in a setting and by a clinician who can recognize and treat a severe allergic reaction.[26]

›   MMR—This vaccine is only grown on a culture with chick embryo cells. Because it is not produced in chicken eggs, there is so little egg protein present in the vaccine that it poses no threat to those with an egg allergy[5] (**Box 12.1**)

›   Yellow Fever—This vaccine is not a routinely recommended immunization. As it also may contain egg protein, this vaccine, unlike the others listed above, still retains a caution about use in those with an egg allergy[28]

❏   If reactions are mild, consider skin testing to check for reactivity before administering this vaccine.

❏   If reactions are severe, but immunization is required for travel to a high-risk area, consider referral to an allergist for desensitization.

Box 12.1   Did You Know?

In 1963, Maurice Hilleman, working with Merck Co. to develop a mumps vaccine, cultured the mumps virus from the throat of his daughter, Jeryl Lynn Hilleman. In 1966, using the attenuated Jeryl Lynn strain, a mumps vaccine was produced and replaced the previously used killed virus mumps vaccine in 1978. Later studies on the Jeryl Lynn strain discovered that it actually contained two distinct substrains of the virus. JL1 grows best in Vero and chick embryo fibroblast cell cultures, whereas JL2 prefers growth in embryonated chicken eggs. The heterogeneity of substrains is likely partially responsible for the high efficacy of the vaccine. JL1 is the major substrain and JL2 the minor substrain in the vaccine. Monitoring of the substrain ratio can be used as part of the quality control ensuring vaccine consistency.[27]

Yeast protein: Yeast is used in production of the HPV vaccine and the hepatitis B vaccine. There is little yeast protein remaining in these vaccines and severe allergic reactions are very rare. Nevertheless, current recommendations indicate an avoidance of these vaccines if there is a prior severe allergic reaction to the vaccine itself or to any component of the vaccine (which includes yeast).[29,30]

7.   **Taste improvers**—These are used only in oral vaccines. For example, the rotavirus vaccine contains 1 g of sugar (sucrose) to give it a more pleasant taste.

8.   **Latex**—Latex is not present in the vaccine itself but is used in the packaging of certain vaccines (some vials or syringes may contain natural rubber latex). The ACIP General Best Practice Guidelines for Immunization states that "immediate-type allergic reactions due to latex allergy have been described

after vaccination, but such reactions are rare. If a person reports a severe anaphylactic allergy to latex, vaccines supplied in vials or syringes that contain natural rubber latex should be avoided if possible."[31] If the vaccine is still given, the health care provider should be ready to treat any possible latex-induced allergic reactions, including anaphylaxis. The statement also explains that "for patients with a history of contact allergy to latex, vaccines supplied in vials or syringes that contain dry natural rubber or natural rubber latex may be administered."[31]

Additional Resources

If you are interested in finding out every ingredient in a particular vaccine or would like to know how much of each ingredient remains in each vaccine, check out the following websites.

- https://www.cdc.gov/vaccines/pubs/pinkbook/downloads/appendices/B/excipient-table-2.pdf
- www.vaccinesafety.edu/components-Excipients.htm

References

1. Children's Hospital of Philadelphia. Vaccine Ingredients – DNA. https://www.chop.edu/centers-programs/vaccine-education-center/vaccine-ingredients/dna. Accessed January 15, 2019.
2. Animal Cell Technology Industrial Platform. Vaccines and Animal Cell Technology. http://www.actip.org/library/vaccines-and-animal-cell-technology/. Updated June 2013. Accessed January 15, 2019.
3. Florida State University. Madin-Darby Canine Kidney Epithelial Cells (MDCK Line). https://micro.magnet.fsu.edu/primer/techniques/fluorescence/gallery/cells/mdck/mdckcells.html. Updated November 15, 2015. Accessed January 15, 2019.
4. 7.24A: Genetically engineered vaccines. In: *Biology LebreTexts*. https://bio.libretexts.org/Bookshelves/Microbiology/Book%3A_Microbiology_(Boundless)/7%3A_Microbial_Genetics/7.24%3A_Transgenic_Organisms/7.24A%3A_Genetically_Engineered_Vaccines. Updated January 9, 2018. Accessed January 15, 2019.
5. Oxford Vaccine Group. Vaccine Ingredients. University of Oxford Vaccine Knowledge Project. http://vk.ovg.ox.ac.uk/vaccine-ingredients. Updated January 3, 2019. Accessed January 15, 2019.
6. Vaccine ingredients and manufacturer information. ProCon.org. https://vaccines.procon.org/view.resource.php?resourceID=005206#bovine. Updated September 19, 2016. Accessed January 15, 2019.
7. Johns Hopkins Bloomberg School of Public Health. Vaccine Excipients per 0.5 mL dose. Institute for Vaccine Safety. www.vaccinesafety.edu/components-Excipients.htm. Updated December 21, 2018. Accessed January 15, 2019.
8. Herlihy SM, Hagood EA. *Your Baby's Best Shot: Why Vaccines are Safe and Save Lives*. Rowman and Littleflied, Inc. Lanham, MD; 2012:40:chap 4.
9. National Institute of Allergy and Infectious Diseases. Other Vaccine Ingredients. https://www.niaid.nih.gov/research/other-vaccine-ingredients. Accessed January 15, 2019.
10. Labombe. Protein purification. https://www.labome.com/method/Protein-Purification.html. Updated January 7, 2019. Accessed January 15, 2019.

11. Cluff CW. Monophosphoryl lipid A (MPL) as an adjuvant for anti-cancer vaccines: Clinical results. In: Madame Curie Bioscience Database. https://www.ncbi.nlm.nih.gov/books/NBK7284/. Accessed January 16, 2019.

12. Schuch RA, Oliveira TL, Collares TF, et al. The use of xanthan gum as vaccine adjuvant: an evaluation of immunostimulatory potential in BALB/c mice and cytotoxicity in vitro. *BioMed Res Int.* 2017;2017:9. 3925024.

13. Zhu D, Tuo W. QS-21: a potent vaccine adjuvant. *Nat Prod Chem Res.* 2016;3(4):e113.

14. Scheiermann J, Klinman DM. Clinical evaluation of CpG oligonucleotides as adjuvants for vaccines targeting infectious diseases and cancer. *Vaccine.* 2014;32(48):6377-6389.

15. The Immunisation Advisory Center. Vaccine Components. www.immune.org.nz/vaccines/vaccine-development/vaccine-components. Updated November 2017. Accessed January 16, 2019.

16. U.S. Food & Drug Administration. Thimerosal and Vaccines. https://www.fda.gov/biologicsbloodvaccines/safetyavailability/vaccinesafety/ucm096228. Updated February 2, 2018. Accessed January 16, 2019.

17. WebMD. EDTA. https://www.webmd.com/vitamins/ai/ingredientmono-1032/edta. Accessed January 16, 2019.

18. Animal-origin peptones: casein and whey peptones. In: BD Bionutrients Technical Manual. 4th ed. http://www.bdbiosciences.com/ds/ab/others/Casamino_Acids.pdf. Accessed January 16, 2019.

19. *Fructose and Sorbital Used as Excipients in Medicinal Products for Human Use [package insert].* Canary Wharf, London, UK: European Medicines Agency; 2017.

20. Lal M, Jarrahian C. Presentation matters: buffers, packaging and delivery devices for new, oral enteric vaccines for infants. *Hum Vaccin Immunother.* 2016;13(1):46-49.

21. Children's Hospital of Philadelphia. Vaccine Ingredients. https://www.chop.edu/centers-programs/vaccine-education-center/vaccine-ingredients. Accessed January 16, 2019.

22. Oxiteno. What is polysorbate? – Polysorbate 20 vs. 60 vs. 80 Uses. June 12, 2018. https://www.oxiteno.us/what-is-polysorbate-20-vs-60-vs-80-uses. Accessed January 16, 2019.

23. Prospector. Sorbitan Trioleate (SPA85). https://www.ulprospector.com/en/na/PersonalCare/Detail/4230/122885/Sorbitan-Trioleate-SPA85. Accessed January 16, 2019.

24. Scottish Enviornmental Protection Agency. Scottish Pollutant Release Inventory: Nonylphenol Ethoxylates. http://apps.sepa.org.uk/spripa/pages/substanceinformation.aspx?pid=154. Accessed January 16, 2019.

25. Iannelli V. *Does the Flu Shot Contain a Vaginal Spermicide?* Vaxopedia; October 18, 2017. https://vaxopedia.org/tag/triton-x-100/. Accessed January 16, 2019.

26. Centers for Disease Control and Prevention. Flu Vaccine and People With Egg Allergies. https://www.cdc.gov/flu/protect/vaccine/egg-allergies.htm. Updated December 28, 2017. Accessed January 16, 2019.

27. Amexis G, Rubin S, Chizhikov V, et al. Sequence diversity of Jeryl Lynn strain of mumps virus: quantitative mutant analysis for vaccine quality control. *Virology.* 2002;300:171-179.

28. Centers for Disease Control and Prevention. Contraindications for Administering Yellow Fever Vaccine. https://www.cdc.gov/travel-training/local/HistoryEpidemiologyandVaccination/contraindications-administering-yellow-fever-vaccine.pdf. Accessed January 16, 2019.

29. Centers for Disease Control and Prevention. HPV (Human Papillomavirus) VIS. https://www.cdc.gov/vaccines/hcp/vis/vis-statements/hpv.html. Updated December 2, 2016. Accessed January 16. 2019.

30. More D. Vaccines and Food Allergies. Verywell Health. https://www.verywellhealth.com/vaccines-and-food-allergy-83069. Updated October 9, 2018. Accessed January 16, 2019.

31. Centers for Disease Control and Prevention. Latex in vaccine packaging. In: Atkinson W, Wolfe S, Hamborsky J, McIntyre L, eds. *Epidemiology and Prevention of Vaccine-Preventable Diseases.* 13th ed. Washington, DC: Public Health Foundation; 2015. https://www.cdc.gov/vaccines/pubs/pinkbook/downloads/appendices/B/latex-table.pdf. Updated April 2015. Accessed January 16, 2019.

It's a Jungle Out There: Navigating Vaccine Advice in the News and on the World Wide Web

The greatest enemy of knowledge is not ignorance, it is the illusion of knowledge.

—DANIEL J. BOORSTIN

As discussed briefly in chapter 2, Genesis of the Anti-vaccine Movement, the primary difference between the anti-vaccine movement of old and that seen today is the advent of the World Wide Web. For better or for worse, information now travels with lightning speed and anyone with a will and a bit of tech savvy can set up shop on the Internet and dispense information. Data are a few keystrokes away, and the scientific studies and health research that were previously largely the purview of doctors and scientists are now available to all. For the most part, this is a good thing. We want patients to be knowledgeable about their health. However, for those without the training to differentiate good information from bad, or likely conditions from unlikely, the information encountered on the Web can be confusing and scary.

Medical practitioners have a love-hate relationship with Dr. Google, as we affectionately call our Internet search engine colleague. When it comes to very rare conditions, having patients now be able to research their symptoms and contribute to the diagnostic process can be advantageous. Many of us have had encounters with patients who have diagnosed themselves accurately even before setting foot in our offices. Access to a wealth of health information and to technology that allows people to track health data facilitates patient engagement, and patients have become more active participants in their health as a result. However, more often than not, we see the downside of Internet searches. We see patients who are overwhelmed and made anxious by the information they have encountered online.

This chapter will delve into the role that the Internet and news and social media play in the vaccine discussion. It will highlight what our patients are encountering in their foray into web-based health advice, with particular attention paid to the individuals and sites that make up the online anti-vaccine community. It will discuss the tactics used by those individuals and sites to instill doubt into the minds of unsuspecting patients and parents, who are just trying to get more information to make informed health decisions. Finally, the chapter will offer ways in which you can help guide your patients in interpreting information they find online, to determine whether or not it is worth their trust and confidence.

THE ROLE OF MEDIA IN THE VACCINE DISCUSSION

Many would argue that the media have been complicit in perpetuating the concern over the safety of vaccines. Both traditional news media outlets, such as CNN and CNBC, and more popular media programs, such as *The Oprah Winfrey Show* and *The Dr. Oz Show* have given voice over the years to anti-vaccine activists and conspiracy theorists, such as Jenny McCarthy and Robert F. Kennedy Jr. (**Box 13.1**). We have seen nationally broadcast "documentaries," such as Lea Thompson's 1982 *Vaccine Roulette* and PBS Frontline's 2015 *The Vaccine War*, fan the flames of fear and confusion about the safety and efficacy of vaccines. This type of media coverage suggests to the public that there is a "debate" about vaccine safety. Though there may be discussion about vaccines, there is no "debate." Vaccines have been proven safe and effective time and again and have saved the lives of millions of people.

 Box 13.1   Did You Know?

The anti-vaccine movement is organized, well-funded, and is making its way into a political arena near you. Andrew Wakefield and others are throwing their weight behind political action committees that support anti-vaccine, anti-science candidates. Texans for Vaccine Choice, whose mission is to help elect anti-vaccine politicians, is one such group that Wakefield supports.[1] The anti-vaccine movement is also active in deploying their most noted spokespersons to testify at House and Senate hearings in various states seeking to limit philosophical and religious exemptions to vaccines. These "experts," such as Robert F. Kennedy, Jr. and Del Bigtree, like to tout their support for "choice," "medical freedom," and "parental rights," appealing to those independent-minded people who want to keep "government" out of their health care. Yet, one-off health decisions do not a successful public health program make. Should we be concerned? Yes. The pro-vaccine, pro-science community needs to become as vocal and politically active as our anti-vaccine, anti-science counterparts, or we can expect them to gain the ear of even greater numbers of political representatives in the future.

In her article for *Forbes*, analyzing the Frontline documentary *The Vaccine War*, Tara Haelle describes the problem with giving equal airtime to the anti-vaccine movement in the name of "balanced reporting." She states, "False balance is presenting 'both sides' of an issue in a way that makes it appear as though both are weighted equally, when, in fact, one side carries the heft of all the scientific research behind it and the other carries only anecdotes and cherry-picked, non-replicated studies and case studies in lousy medical journals. I'm certainly not the only one who has pointed out the negative impact of false balance in vaccine reporting. A feature in Columbia Journalism Review by Curtis Brainard in mid-2013 placed substantial responsibility for vaccine fears squarely on the shoulders of an irresponsible press."[2]

Having faulty or misleading information heavily covered in the news, and then having this information retracted, also leads to a lessening in the public's confidence in news outlets. If the major news outlets, whom we trust to do thorough investigative journalism and to present us with facts and the truth, cannot be trusted to provide accurate information, then where do we turn to get our news? This issue is increasingly seen when it comes to political discussions; when news organizations such as Fox are so blatantly right-leaning and stories are spun to put the best light on a situation, but not necessarily to reflect the facts of the story; when MSNBC, which some would argue goes too far in the other direction, parades their eternal panels of liberal commentators across the screen; when there is no "news," when there is only hype; when we can no longer trust the "experts," it puts all of us who *are* experts in our field in an unfavorable light. Perhaps we, too, are as easily swayed or influenced as others. When it comes to news reports about vaccines and vaccine-preventable disease, we must demand accountability to the facts and not sensationalism. The health of our people depends on it.

INTERNET AND SOCIAL MEDIA IMPACT ON THE VACCINE DISCUSSION

A 2011 study looking at the use of Twitter to track disease activity during the H1N1 influenza pandemic noted that "an estimated 113 million people in the United States use the Internet to find health-related information with up to 8 million people searching for health-related information on a typical day."[3] Another study, published by the *Journal of Medical Internet Research* in 2016, looked at the number of tweets between February 1 and March 9 of 2015 (in the setting of a measles outbreak) using the word "vaccination" and its common derivatives (for example, "vaccines" and "vax"). In that short timeframe, 669,136 vaccine-related tweets were identified from around the globe. Vaccines and vaccine-preventable disease are most certainly being discussed on social media.[4]

Researchers in that same study also found that residents of Oregon and Vermont, the two states with the highest rates of nonmedical exemptions to school-entry vaccination nationwide, had the greatest social media engagement on the topic and contributed the most to vaccine discussions on Twitter. Furthermore, results demonstrated a greater impact of vaccine-related stories contributed by news organizations compared with those of tweets by health organizations in communicating health-related information. This suggests that people with the medical and scientific backgrounds to be discussing these issues are not the ones contributing the most to the conversation.[4] The anti-vaccine movement on the Internet and social media is vocal, and false or misleading information is easy to find. Consequently, it is vital that the online presence of physicians, other medical professionals, and scientists, as purveyors of truth and reason, grows and expands. See chapter 15: A Call to Action, for further discussion.

Search engine optimization (SEO) is defined by the *Oxford English Dictionary* as "the process of maximizing the number of visitors to a particular website by ensuring that the site appears high on the list of results returned by a search engine."[5] There are multiple ways to maximize SEO that this author does not claim to fully understand, but anti-vaccination activists seem to be experts at use of this tactic to drive traffic to their websites. A study analyzing YouTube videos discussing immunizations found that 32% opposed vaccination and that anti-vaccine videos had more reviews and higher ratings than pro-vaccine videos. Researchers examining Canadian Internet users and their sharing of influenza vaccine information on networks, such as Twitter, Facebook, YouTube, and Digg found that 60% promoted anti-vaccine sentiment.[6] Another study examined the top 10 results found on seven leading search engines, using the search terms "vaccination" and "immunization" and found that 43% of the top search results were anti-vaccine, including all top 10 on Google.[7] Patients' use of the Internet to find health information is not going away. The pro-vaccine camp has got to get better at marketing itself and using techniques, such as SEO, to our advantage to ensure that factual information is rising to the top of Internet searches. The good news is that it seems we are making some positive strides in this direction.

In the process of writing this book, which has been in production (either in the research or writing phase for the last several years), I have noticed a shift. Lately, when typing in search terms aimed at looking into anti-vaccine claims, the sites that rise to the top of the search tend to be sites providing factual information, debunking the myths that are propagated so easily by anti-vaccine websites. Sites such as the Centers for Disease Control and Prevention (CDC), National Institutes of Health (NIH), Immunize. org, and others are now at the top of this list. One of the most active anti-vaccine sites, the National Vaccine Information Center (NVIC), which should more accurately be called the National Vaccination *Mis*information Center, acknowledges this trend in its December 2018 post titled "The new Internet police protecting you from freedom of thought and speech." They liken the "policing" of fake news and misinformation to an "electronic burning of books."[8] However, if the information being put forward on their site as truth and fact is indeed truthful and factual, then they should have no worries that attempts to rank sites based on these criteria will decrease their searchability. The move by search engines and social media giants to hold those with an online presence accountable to the truth and to responsible reporting gives me hope that, going forward, our patients will less often be bombarded with false and manipulative information that leads them away from making good health choices.

THE ECHO CHAMBER

Another byproduct of social media marketing and advertising, in feeding us what we want to see or learn about, is the creation of what is commonly referred to as an "echo chamber." Many of us have undoubtedly seen this at work when it comes to the marketing of products. For example, if my 15-year-old son searches for new basketball shoes on my home computer, my Facebook feed is suddenly inundated with adds from Nike and Adidas. However, the same can happen in the marketing of ideas. In this regard, the term echo chamber refers to a situation in which "certain ideas, beliefs or data points are reinforced through repetition of a closed system that does not allow for the free movement of alternative or competing ideas or concepts."[9] Social media echo chambers, as described in a 2016 *Washington Post* piece on the topic, allow people to amplify or "promote their favorite narratives, form polarized groups, and resist information that doesn't conform to their beliefs."[10] A 2016 study analyzing 376 million Facebook users' interactions with over 900 news outlets found that people often seek news information from only a few sites, resulting in "major segregation and growing polarization in online news consumption."[11] Essentially, people tend to "seek information that aligns with their views."[12] This feeds our *confirmation bias* which, as discussed in chapter 3 (Psychology of the Anti-vaccine Movement), is the tendency to embrace information that confirms our preestablished beliefs while rejecting information that casts doubt on those beliefs.

The echo chamber also lulls us into the false sense that "everything" we are reading on our feeds supports a particular notion and that "everyone" feels the same way we do. So, in the case of anti-vaccine sentiment, if a patient searches the terms "toxins in vaccines" and happens upon the NVIC website, they are more likely to receive further articles on their Facebook feed going forward that would call into question the safety of vaccines. Or, if they post something that supports an anti-vaccine point of view, and they are part of a like-minded group, they will receive "likes" for that viewpoint that furthers the sense that theirs is a commonly-held belief, because that like-minded group is unlikely to be offering up the opposing point of view. Certainly, people on both sides of any debate can fall victim to the echo chamber effect. However, it is helpful for us, as medical providers, to be able to discuss this possibility with our patients so that they can recognize when it may be impacting their medical decision-making.

TACTICS AND TROPES

Merriam-Webster defines a trope as a "common or overused theme or device."[13] Tactics used by the anti-vaccine movement are rife with tropes that are used to introduce doubt and fear into patients' minds, leading them to question the efficacy and safety of vaccines. It is important to be familiar with these as we discuss vaccine information with our patients and as we move forward in our fight against misinformation and pseudoscience. In addition to reviewing their most common tactics, we will also look at the most influential people in the anti-vaccine movement. As stated by Sun Tzu, a Chinese military strategist and Taoist philosopher from the 6th century BCE,[14] "Know thy self, know thy enemy. A thousand battles, a thousand victories."[15] Only in knowing the tactics and faces of our anti-vaccine "enemy" can we truly hope to win the battle to keep our patients healthy and safe.

The 2016 word of the year by *Oxford Dictionaries* was "post-truth." It is defined as "relative to or denoting circumstances in which objective facts are less influential in shaping public opinion than appeals to emotion and personal belief."[16] This appeal to emotion and personal belief occurs *all the time* in the vaccine discussion and is partly why the anti-vaccine movement has been so successful in attracting unsuspecting parents to their cause. KO, in chapter 4, There and Back Again: How Anti-vaxxers Change Their Minds, sums it up beautifully when she says "Fear is a powerful motivator, and when I was trying to find information about the safety of vaccines, I came across some pretty scary stories online about children who were allegedly injured by vaccines. We assume that parents know their children deeply, and when a parent claims their child changed drastically and immediately after a series of immunizations, I think our instinct is to believe that parent."

There are numerous other tactics and tropes used by the anti-vaccine movement to sway people to their way of thinking. An article by Davies, Chapman, and Leask titled "Antivaccination Activists on the World Wide Web" categorizes these as *Rhetorical Appeals*, which include "evidence of authority and scientific rigour," "emotive appeals," and "evidence of conspiracy, search for truth" and *Explicit Claims*.[7] These are described in detail in **Box 13.2**, where each type of appeal or claim is highlighted and examples given.

Now that we know what tactics and tropes are used to try to convince people that vaccines are unnecessary and unsafe, let's look at the prominent figures in the movement. I have chosen to discuss those most commonly encountered during my research. Certainly, there are many others that you may come across, locally or online. However, the individuals described below are those with the deepest pockets and the greatest sphere of influence, both nationally and internationally (**Box 13.3**).

 Box 13.2   Anti-vaccine Tropes and Tactics

Adapted from Antivaccination Activists on the World Wide Web by Davies P, Chapman S, Leask J. in *Archives of Disease in Childhood*.[7]

Rhetorical Appeals
1.   Evidence of authority and scientific rigor:
   - *Quasi official:* organizations with names implying authority or official status
     - The National Vaccine Information Center (NVIC)
   - *"Scientific" references:* reference literature from established medical journals (frequently with cherry-picked data to support their claims), alternative health literature, and works published by anti-vaccination "experts"
     - "Flu vaccines are killing senior citizens, study warns"[17]
   - *Both sides:* claim to present "both sides" of the vaccine "debate" for readers to judge (Despite the claim, a mere 15% of sites studied by Davies, Chapman, and Leask actually presented pro-vaccine information.)[7]
     - Video series by Ty Bollinger *The Truth About Vaccines*
   - *Actually present both sides*: provide arguments for and against vaccination
     - 10% of anti-vaccine websites discussed the benefits of immunization compared with 20% of pro-vaccine websites that discuss the potential serious complications caused by vaccines[18]
   - *Links to pro-vaccination groups:* links to government and other health agencies supporting vaccination
     - 25% of anti-vaccination websites link to further pro-vaccination websites[18]
2.   Emotive appeals:
   - *Personal testimony:* personal accounts of illness/harm felt to be because of vaccination or stories of persecution for anti-vaccine beliefs
     - "First They Came for the Anti-Vaxxers"[19]
   - *Responsible parenting:* deciding not to vaccinate is in the best interests of the child, and parents who refuse vaccines are acting responsibly in accordance with their parental instincts
     - "I know my child better than anyone and his immune system is strong enough to handle these illnesses."
   - *"Us" versus "Them"*: anti-vaccinationists are caring, concerned allies to loving parents, together they will stand firm against the corrupt interests of uncaring doctors and government
     - "Gone are the days when you could blindly follow your doctor's recommendations or count on your health plan or some government agency to put your best interest first."[20]
   - *Back to nature:* "natural" methods of preventing disease are preferable to the "artificial" practice of vaccination; "natural" lifestyles will protect from disease and make vaccination unnecessary
     - "Natural health activist Brittney Kara shares...why we don't need vaccines to protect our children from infections."[21]

3. Conspiracy/search for truth
    - *Cover up:* information about the health hazards of vaccination is being covered up or purposefully withheld from the public
      - "The Truth is Out: Gardasil Vaccine Coverup Exposed"[22]
    - *Excavation of the facts:* presenting allegedly reliable but previously hidden or neglected information that calls into question the accepted wisdom about the safety of vaccines
      - "Thompson explained they simply eliminated the incriminating data, thereby vanishing the link."[23]
    - *Free and informed choice:* informed decisions by parents can only be made free from the "coercion" of doctors and after learning the "facts" as presented by anti-vaccinationists
      - "My main goal today in continuing to research vaccines is to provide families with evidence of vaccine safety and efficacy defects—information they are unlikely to hear from their doctors—so that truly informed decisions can be made."—Neil Z. Miller[24]
    - *Foolish doctors:* medical orthodoxy is ill-informed and outdated against the enlightened and compassionate anti-vaccinationists; doctors don't get taught much about vaccines and are too afraid to go against the grain to acknowledge the truth
      - "The idea that there are 'medical experts' who, by virtue of the MD initials placed after their names, automatically know more than anyone else about vaccines is pervasive. This commonly held belief persists, despite overwhelming evidence that doctors are taught almost nothing about vaccines in medical school."[25]
    - *Rebel doctors:* thoughtful and enlightened doctors (with real MDs after their names) have broken with the medical orthodoxy and are now questioning vaccines
      - "A must-watch video from the brave Dr. Moss, a university-affiliated medical doctor, explaining the deaths from measles and from the measles vaccine"[26]
    - *Unholy alliance for profit:* vaccine promotion by doctors, pharmaceutical companies, researchers, and public health bureaucrats is motivated by monetary gain and for the extension of government control over civil liberties
      - "…some doctors do not want families who do not vaccinate in their practice, not because of health concerns for their patients, but because accepting patients who do not vaccinate disqualifies these doctors from receiving thousands of dollars in bonuses from insurance companies."[27]

Explicit Claims
- *Trivial diseases:* Vaccine-preventable diseases are not as dangerous as doctors say they are. I had chickenpox and I was just fine.
- *Poisons:* Vaccines are made from poisons and other unnatural products that are "toxic" to our health.

Continued

- *Vaccines are harmful:* Vaccines cause various diseases such as cancers and asthma.
- *Vaccines weaken the immune system:* There are too many shots given at once and this overwhelms the immune system.
- *Idiopathic concerns:* Vaccines cause all sorts of behavioral and medical problems of uncertain cause.
- *Vaccines don't work:* Vaccines aren't that effective. The flu shot was only 20% effective against the flu this year.
- *Alternative health treatments are superior:* Homeopathy and naturopathy are safer and more natural alternatives to vaccination.
- *A natural lifestyle will keep me healthy:* If someone gets sick from a vaccine-preventable disease, then they had an unnatural lifestyle.
- *Diseases were declining before vaccines:* Improvements in hygiene and sanitation are really what caused a drop in disease rates, not vaccines.

(Adapted from Davies P, Chapman S, Leask J .Antivaccination activists on the world wide web. *Arch Dis Child.* 2002;87(1):22-25. https://adc.bmj.com/content/87/1/22. The examples cited have been added and did not appear in Davies' original article.)

Box 13.3   Who's Who in the Anti-vaccine Movement

1. Andrew Wakefield—A discredited British physician, author, film producer, and anti-vaccine media sensation who published the now-retracted paper suggesting a link between the MMR vaccine and autism. Despite this, many in the anti-vaccine community still regard him as a hero.

2. Robert F. Kennedy, Jr.—A once disbarred but reinstated lawyer, environmental activist, author, syndicated talk show host, cofounder of a bottled water company called Tear of the Clouds, LLC., and founder of Waterkeeper Alliance (an umbrella group that supports efforts of environmental organizations to protect their local bodies of water) and the World Mercury Project. He is known for his continued belief in the disproven link between vaccines and autism, believing there to be a government cover-up regarding the "damaging" effects of thimerosal on children.[28]

3. Barbara Loe Fisher—Cofounder of Dissatisfied Parents Together (DPT), which later became known as the NVIC, of which she is now president. She coauthored the book *DPT: A Shot in the Dark*, suggesting a link between the whole-cell pertussis vaccine and autism. She worked with the US Congress to develop the National Childhood Vaccination Injury Act of 1986.[29] She is active in the fight against any legislation that would limit nonmedical exemptions to vaccinations for school enrollment.

4. Joseph Mercola, DO—Joseph Mercola is an osteopathic physician by train-
    ing and founder of the alternative medicine website mercola.com where
    he touts often-disproved medical claims (including many anti-vaccine
    assertions) and markets a variety of controversial medical devices and
    dietary supplements. He is listed by the mediabiasfactcheck.com site as
    low in conspiracy theory but high in quackery.[30]
5. Paul Thomas, MD—Paul Thomas is an integrative medicine pediatri-
    cian currently practicing in Portland, Oregon. He is founding director
    of the organization Physicians for Informed Consent and co-chair for
    Oregonians for Medical Freedom. He is also coauthor of the book *The
    Vaccine-Friendly Plan*, the title of which is misleading as he is not very
    vaccine-friendly. He recommends an alternate schedule or eliminating
    certain vaccines altogether (including polio, which he claims is unnec-
    essary because it is "not infectious," and any vaccine in pregnancy
    because of the risk of "toxins").[31] His site claims to bring you "the best
    and most important research, information, products, vitamins and nutri-
    tional supplements, books, videos, blogs, and other recommendations
    from Dr. Paul Thomas."[31]
6. Robert Sears, MD—Of Dr. Sears' Alternative Vaccine Schedule fame,
    Robert Sears is a pediatrician whose book *The Vaccine Handbook: Making
    the Right Decision for your Child* has led parents astray in making healthy
    vaccine decisions since the date of its first publication in 2007. He even
    goes so far in his book as to encourage parents to keep their decisions
    not to vaccinate to themselves and to hide among the herd. Most
    recently, following passage of California bill SB277, which banned non-
    medical vaccine exemptions, he has come under fire with the Medical
    Board of California for demonstrating "gross negligence" in supplying
    a nonevidence-based letter for medical exemption from vaccines for a
    two-year-old patient.[32] On July 27, 2018, his license was revoked. He is
    only eligible for reinstatement after a prolonged probationary period and
    if he complies with the Board's requirements for continuing medical and
    ethical education.[33]
7. Mayer Eisenstein, MD—Mayer Eisenstein was a physician, anti-vaccine
    guru, and owner of the Chicago-based holistic medicine practice
    Homefirst, which ultimately dissolved following the clinic's multimil-
    lion dollar loss in a wrongful death suit. He was also founder of the
    Autism Recovery Clinic where he treated autistic children with leuprolide
    (Lupron) (a treatment dismissed as junk science by endocrinologists and
    autism experts) and pedaled the use of supplements to prevent autism
    and the swine flu. He was, conveniently, married to the owner of a natu-
    ral pharmaceutical company.[34] He coauthored the book *Make an Informed
    Vaccine Decision for the Health of Your Child,* written in conjunction with
    Neil Z. Miller (see discussion below) and was on the Board of Directors
    for the Medical Voices Vaccine Information Center. He passed away in
    2014.[35]

Continued

8. Sherri Tenpenny, DO—There is not a lot of information available about Sherri Tenpenny that isn't of her own writing. She is an Osteopathic physician practicing in Ohio and is the author of four books opposing vaccination. She is a staunch anti-vaccine proponent, pushing the debunked myth linking vaccines and autism. According to skepticalraptor.com, she does not believe in the germ theory of disease, instead believing that infection comes from microbes populating damaged tissue caused by "toxins."[36]

9. Suzanne Humphries, MD—Nephrologist turned homeopath, Suzanne Humphries claimed that her views of vaccines were forever changed in 2009 after encountering several cases of kidney failure following influenza vaccination. Respectfulinsolence.com discusses her denial of any benefit to vaccines and quotes her claims that doctors who support vaccination have a "stake in upholding false paradigms" and are "indebted to the government for hundreds of thousands of dollars," which apparently impacts their ability to see the "truth" about vaccines. In reference to the eradication of smallpox, she claims that it was not eradicated by vaccines and that doctors "say this out of conditioning rather than out of understanding the history or science."[37]

10. Toni Bark, MD—Once a traditionally trained physician, Toni Bark traded in her stethoscope for homeopathy. She runs The Center for Disease Prevention and Reversal, which offers procedures such as lipodissolve and whole-body vibration, as well as products through her online store called Skin and Chocolate. Her site states that she is "an athlete and a dancer and works intimately with other movers and shakers."[38] She is commonly found on discussion panels with other anti-vaccine promoters and is featured in the online video series referenced in chapter 2 called *The Truth about Vaccines.* She is the primary voice in the movie "Bought" which claims vaccines to be ineffective and the cause of autism.

11. Neil Z. Miller—Miller is a medical research journalist and director of the ThinkTwice Global Vaccine Institute. Despite the lack of scientific training to lend credence to his work, he has managed to publish several articles in conjunction with partner-in-crime Gary S. Goldman, a computer scientist affiliated with the World Association for Vaccine Education, and publish several books, including *Vaccine Roulette: Gambling With Your Child's Life.*[39]

12. Jennifer Margulis—Jennifer Margulis is a journalist and author, cowriting books with Dr. Paul Thomas and penning her own books such as *The Business of Baby.* A *New York Times* review of the book suggested that, in focusing on a "largely bygone 1950s dynamic between women and doctors, in fact, Margulis has missed the real problem for today's patients: too much information and too few reliable intermediaries who can sort fact from rumor. Margulis herself proves unfit for this role in a shockingly irresponsible chapter on vaccines. All of her favorite conceits are here: the money-hungry pharmaceutical companies; the pediatricians who schedule

routine immunizations simply to collect insurance reimbursements; the health care workers who patronize and bully women who refuse vaccinations for their children; and the brave parents who 'decide that they do not want to intramuscularly inject their child with something that is not part of the natural course of life."[40] She has been featured in Ty Bollinger's *The Truth about Vaccines* video and makes such unsubstantiated claims, there and in other arenas, as (I will paraphrase) "most doctors don't vaccinate their own children according to the CDC schedule." She is careful to call herself not "anti-vaccine" but "pro-questions"[41] and peppers into her anti-vaccine rhetoric important questions about birth complications and mortality rates in the United States that, unfortunately, lend her other more fringe ideas legitimacy.

13. J. B. Handley—Devout follower of Andrew Wakefield and cofounder of the group Generation Rescue, which has claimed that autism spectrum disorders are a misdiagnosis of mercury poisoning. He is still vocal on the Internet but less in the spotlight these days as Generation Rescue is now spearheaded by actress Jenny McCarthy.[42]

14. Jenny McCarthy—Actress, model, and now board member and "celebrity influencer" for the anti-vaccine organization Generation Rescue. She became vocal in the anti-vaccine community after her son was diagnosed with autism following receipt of his MMR vaccine. She was cosponsor with Jim Carrey of the "Green Our Vaccines" rally in Washington, D.C. in 2008. Her celebrity status has given her a wide audience with appearances on Oprah, Frontline, CNN, CNBC, and more. Generation Rescue lists its goal as working toward "recovery" for kids with autism.[43]

15. Michael "The Health Ranger" Adams—Founder of naturalnews.com, a "conspiracy-minded alternative website" that has "roughly 7 million unique visitors each month."[44] He is anti-vaccine, anti-GMO (genetically modified organism), and an AIDS denialist who has been featured on *The Dr. Oz Show* (Mehmet Oz himself is a thorn in the side of the science community). *Natural News* has been described by David Gorski, MD of the website Science-Based Medicine as a one-stop shop for "virtually every quackery known to humankind, slathered with a heaping helping of unrelenting hostility to science-based medicine and science in general."[45] His website and videos have been intermittently blacklisted by Google and YouTube. The McGill University Office for Science and Society notes that naturalnews.com is just the "tip of a very large iceberg" with over 50 sites attributed to Mr. Adams pushing "fear of medicine and science…, anti-left and pro-freedom hype…, and doomsday prep advice."[46]

16. Del Bigtree—Vaxxedthemovie.com touts Del Bigtree as a filmmaker and investigative medical journalist whose "further investigation into the wrongful destruction of Andrew Wakefield's career orchestrated by Big Pharma and the UK Department of Health inspired him to focus all of his attention on what he believes to be the most crucial documentary of the year."[47]

WHAT IS AN UNSUSPECTING PATIENT TO DO?

As stated in the title, it's a jungle out there. Dissecting all the conflicting information that we, and our patients, are bombarded with is getting more complicated and time-consuming. I truly believe that one of the reasons those in the anti-vaccine movement have been so successful in spreading their message is that they have the funds and the time to devote to creating compelling online content. They are a marketing machine. Whereas we, your average boots-on-the-ground physician or advanced practice provider, are just trying to take good care of people, get through our harried days, and find time to spend with family and friends. We have not devoted, in any organized way, nearly as much man power and time in creating content that is concise, patient-friendly, and educational. So how can we, with our desire to help our patients not fall victim to fearmongering and misleading content, help patients navigate the information they are finding online? In addition to letting patients know of the tropes and tactics they may encounter on anti-vaccine websites and blogs (making use of *inoculation theory* as discussed in chapter 3, Psychology of the Anti-vaccine Movement), consider providing these tips to help them determine good information from bad, or reputable sources from questionable (See Appendix F: Navigating Information on the Internet and Social Media for a patient checklist of the tips below.).

1. Know your source.
   - Look for articles published in scientific journals. However, keep in mind that not all journals are created equal. Some open-access journals have less rigorous admission standards, and publication of minimally edited articles allows for the appearance of legitimacy when it is not always warranted.
     - Google Scholar is a search engine that will bring research articles to the top of your search. However, keep the above advice in mind as not all journals are equally reputable.
     - Government-funded, not-for-profit, and university sites tend to be trustworthy.
       - Such as the CDC, NIH, the Mayo Clinic, etc.
     - Disease-specific sites are also typically reliable sources (with some exceptions, such as Age of Autism).
       - These include sources such as The American Cancer Society and The American Diabetes Association.
   - Research the author. You can often find bios and critiques that will tell you if their work is considered mainstream or fringe.
     - Consider whether they have a background that allows them to speak with authority on the topic.
   - Check their references. Do their references come from legitimate sources?
     - If their references tend to link back to articles they wrote themselves or to journals or articles that have not followed rigorous research standards, move on.
2. Fact Check.
   - For articles written on blogs or in newslike fashion, dig deeper into their claims. You can use various fact-checking sites to help in this endeavor.
     - Snopes.com
     - Politifact.com

> *The Washington Post* Fact Checker
> FactCheck.org, which includes a feature called SciCheck
> NPR.fact check
> Especiales.univision.com/detector-de-mentiras (Lie Detector, Spanish language)
> Facebook fact checking[48]
> Sciencebasedmedicine.org

3. Get up-to-date information.
   - Science is constantly changing and we need to know whether the information we are working with is up-to-date.
     > Check the dates of the articles you are reading or the dates of the most recent update for the site you are working with.

4. Don't put all of your eggs in one basket.
   - Discovering scientific "truth" takes time and repeated testing. We can't rely on one study to give the whole picture.
     > If a study claims a particular finding, don't just stop there. Read other studies on the same topic. Only if multiple other studies come to the same conclusion, if the totality of evidence points in the same direction, can we put our faith in the finding.

5. Check for conflict of interest.
   - As much as possible, we want to look for sources of information that are non-biased.
     > If a site is trying to sell you something, there is more likely to be inherent bias in their recommendations (for example, "Don't get vaccines! Instead, use this AMAZING supplement to boost your immunity. You can buy it on my site for the low price of $39.99!") If the site is trying to sell you something, it's time to move on.

6. If it sounds too good to be true, it probably is.
   - In desperation, we sometimes search for a miracle; that essential oil that will take away our anxiety or the ionized water treatment to cure cancer.
     > If there were a miracle cure for cancer, science wouldn't be hiding it from you.
     > If there were a miracle cure for anything, the pharmaceutical industry would be all over it and you wouldn't have to find it from an obscure online salesman.
     > If you are wondering if something you read online is legitimate, ask your doctor or clinician. They can help.

WHAT'S THE UPSIDE?

It may seem that there is very little upside to the Internet and social media when it comes to vaccines and other health discussions. However, in the same way that it can be a thorn in our sides, it can be used to amplify our message, to give voice to facts and reason, and to provide a resource for patients who are looking for legitimate sources of health information. Many physicians are already using it as a bullhorn to provide sound health advice and to refute anti-science and pseudoscience claims. A relatively young group, organized by New York physician Dr. Dana (pronounced "Donna") Corriel, is beginning to make headway. Doctors on Social Media

(#SoMeDocs, @SoMeDocs) are a group of concerned physicians who are taking their message of health and responsible information sharing to the "streets" of the Internet. Moreover, it's not just individuals who are venturing into this unchartered territory of the World Wide Web. Medical institutions, both academic and private, are also beginning to establish social media departments and strategies to provide education, improve health communication with patients, and garner feedback for the improvement of patient care.

Social media is now also being used to try to improve the health of the population. For example, some are taking advantage of its data collection possibilities to track global discussions and predict illness outbreaks. In his article, "Trending Now: Using Social Media to Predict and Track Disease Outbreaks," Charles W. Schmidt explains, "social media, cell phones, and other communication modes have opened up a two-way street in health research, supplying not just a portal for delivering information to the public but also a channel by which people reveal their concerns, locations, and physical movements from one place to another. That two-way street is transforming disease surveillance and the way that health officials respond to disasters and pandemics."[49] For example, scientists looking at the use of Twitter to track disease activity and public concern during the H1N1 influenza pandemic found that "Twitter traffic can be used…to estimate disease activity in real time, ie, 1 to 2 weeks faster than current practice allows."[3]

There is certainly the Good, the Bad, and the Ugly of the Internet. As it is increasingly used as a health resource, it is our job as clinicians to help our patients navigate and sort through the information they are encountering. It can seem a herculean task, but armed with the information and advice given above, hopefully it will become a less onerous one going forward. Helping to improve our patients' Internet savvy when it comes to online health information, ultimately increasing their health literacy, will undoubtedly pay dividends for health outcomes in the future.

References

1. Berezow A. *Andrew Wakefield Helps Elect Anti-Vaccine Politicians in Texas*. February 21, 2109. Accessed February 26, 2019. https://www.acsh.org/news/2019/02/21/andrew-wakefield-helps-elect-anti-vaccine-politicians-texas-13830.

2. Haelle T. *The Vaccine War': What You Should Know After You Watch PBS Frontline's Special*. Forbes. March 25, 2015. Accessed January 11, 2019. https://www.forbes.com/sites/tarahaelle/2015/03/25/the-vaccine-war-what-you-should-know-after-you-watch-pbs-frontlines-special/#1f1f2f1a7b66.

3. Signorini A, Segre AM, Polgreen PM. The use of Twitter to track levels of disease activity and public concern in the U.S. during the influenza A H1N1 pandemic. *PLoS One*. 2011;6(5):e19467. https://www.ncbi.nlm.nih.gov/pmc/articles/PMC3087759/?report=reader.

4. Radzikowski J, Stefanidis A, Jacobsen KH, et al. The measles vaccination narrative in Twitter: a quantitative analysis. *JMIR Public Health Surveill*. 2016;2(1):e1. https://publichealth.jmir.org/2016/1/e1/pdf.

5. Search engine optimization. In: English Oxford Living Dictionaries. Accessed January 11, 2019. https://en.oxforddictionaries.com/definition/search_engine_optimization.

6. Husain A, Ali S, Ahmed M, et al. The anti-vaccination movement: a regression in modern medicine. *Cureus*. 2018;10(7):e2919. https://www.ncbi.nlm.nih.gov/pmc/articles/PMC6122668/#!po=35.7143.

7. Davies P, Chapman S, Leask J. Antivaccination activists on the world wide web. *Arch Dis Child*. 2002;87(1):22-25. https://www.ncbi.nlm.nih.gov/pmc/articles/PMC1751143/pdf/v087p00022.pdf.

8. Loe Fisher B. *The New Internet Police Protecting You From freedom of Thought and Speech*. National Vaccine Information Center; December 3, 2018. Accessed January 11, 2019. https://www.nvic.org/NVIC-Vaccine-News/December-2018/internet-police-protect-you-from-freedom-of-speech.aspx.

9. Echo chamber. In: Techopedia. Accessed January 11, 2019. https://www.techopedia.com/definition/23423/echo-chamber.

10. Emba C. *Confirmed Echo Chambers Exist on Social Media But What Can We Do About Them?* Washington Post; July 14, 2016. Accessed January 11, 2019. https://www.washingtonpost.com/news/in-theory/we/2016/07/14/confirmed-echo-chambers-exist-on-social-media-but-what-can-we-do-about-them/?utm_term=.f1f38d1cf3fc.

11. Schmidt AL, Zollo F, Del Vicario M, et al. Anatomy of news consumption on Facebook. *Proc Natl Acad Sci USA*. 2017;114(12):3035-3039. https://www.pnas.org/content/pnas/114/12/3035.full.pdf.

12. Anderson J, Rainie L. *The Future of Truth and Misinformation Online*. Pew Research Center Web site; October 19, 2017. Accessed January 11, 2019. www.pewinternet.org/2017/10/19/the-future-of-truth-and-misinformation-online/.

13. Trope. In: Merriam-Webster Dictionary. Accessed January 11, 2019. https://www.merriam-webster.com/dictionary/trope.

14. Mark JJ. *Sun-Tzu, definition*. In: *Ancient History Encyclopedia*. January 4, 2013. Accessed January 11, 2019. https://www.ancient.eu/Sun-Tzu.

15. Sun-Tzu Quotes; Brainy Quote Web site. Accessed January 11, 2019. https://www.brainyquote.com/quotes/sun_tzu_384112.

16. Word of the year: post-truth. In: English Oxford Living Dictionaries. Accessed January 11, 2019. https://en.oxforddictionaries.com/word-of-the-year/word-of-the-year-2016.

17. Adl-Tabatabai S. *Flu Vaccines Are Killing Senior Citizens, Study Warns*. News Punch Web site; November 17, 2017. Accessed January 11, 2019. https://newspunch.com/flu-vaccines-killing-senior-citizens/.

18. Sak G, Diviani N, Allam A, et al. Comparing the quality of pro- and anti-vaccination online information: a content analysis of vaccination-related webpages. *BMC Public Health*. 2016;16:38. https://www.ncbi.nlm.nih.gov/pmc/articles/PMC4714533/.

19. Shaffer B. First They Came for the Anti-Vaxxers. Kelly Brogan, MD Web site. Accessed January 12, 2019. https://kellybroganmd.com/first-came-anti-vaxxers/.

20. Thomas P, Margulis J. *The Addiction Spectrum: A Compassionate, Holistic Approach to Recovery*. New York, NY: HarperOne; 2018.

21. Cook L. *A Vaccine Free Lifestyle Is A Healthy Lifestyle*. Stop Mandatory Vaccination Web site; July 20, 2016. Accessed January 12, 2019. http://www.stopmandatoryvaccination.com/vaccine-free/a-vaccine-free-lifestyle-is-a-healthy-lifestyle/.

22. Brogan K. The Truth is Out: Gardasil Vaccine Coverup Exposed. Kelly Brogan, MD Web site. Accessed January 12, 2019. https://kellybroganmd.com/truth-out-gardasil-coverup-documents-exposed/.

23. Mercola J. *"Vaxxed" — the Hidden Story of How Vaccine Safety Has Been Undermined and Suppressed*. Mercola Web site; October 13, 2018. Accessed January 12, 2019. https://articles.mercola.com/sites/articles/archive/2018/10/13/vaxxed-film-on-vaccine-safety.aspx.

24. Miller NZ. *Make An Informed Vaccine Decision*; 2013. Accessed January 12, 2019. http://thinktwice.com/Make_an_Informed_Vaccine_Decision.pdf.

25. Cáceres M. *What Doctors Learn in Medical School About Vaccines*. The Vaccine Reaction Web site; July 27, 2018. Accessed January 12, 2019. https://thevaccinereaction.org/2018/07/what-doctors-learn-in-medical-school-about-vaccines/#_edn11.

26. Learn the Risk. *127 Deaths from the Measles Vaccine in the Last 15 Years*. Learn the Risk Web site; June 8, 2018. Accessed January 12, 2019. https://www.learntherisk.org/doctors/.

27. Fluegge M. *8 Reasons Why Your Child's Doctor Pushes Vaccines*. Vaccine Truth Web site; August 6, 2016. Accessed January 12, 2019. https://vactruth.com/2016/08/06/8-reasons-doctors-push-vaccines/.

28. Robert F. Kennedy, Jr. Biography. Biography Web site. Updated April 28, 2017. Accessed January 12, 2019. https://www.biography.com/people/robert-f-kennedy-jr-20832775.

29. Barbara Loe Fisher Biography. ProCon.org Web site. Updated February 3, 2010. Accessed January 12, 2019. https://vaccines.procon.org/view.source.php?sourceID=009411.

30. Conspiracy-Pseudoscience. Media/Bias Fact Check Web site. Updated November 24, 2018. Accessed January 12, 2019. https://mediabiasfactcheck.com/mercola/.

31. Gorski D [Orac]. *Dr. Paul Thomas: A Rising star in the Antivaccine Movement*. Respectful Insolence Web site; March 9, 2018. Accessed January 12, 2019. https://respectfulinsolence.com/2018/03/09/dr-paul-thomas-newest-antivaccine-pediatrician-making-name-himself/.

32. Gorski D [Orac]. *Antivaccine Pediatrician Dr. Bob Sears Finally Faces Discipline from the Medical Board of California*. Respectful Insolence Web site; June 29, 2018. Accessed January 12, 2019. https://respectfulinsolence.com/2018/06/29/dr-bob-sears-finally-faces-discipline/.

33. Accusation against: Robert William Sears, MD. Medical Board of California. June 27, 2018. Case No. 800-2015-012268. Accessed January 12, 2019. http://www2.mbc.ca.gov/BreezePDL/document.aspx-?path=%5CDIDOCS%5C20180627%5CDMRAAAGL14%5C&did=AAAGL180627201150927.DID.

34. Callahan P, Tsouderos T. *Autism Doctor: Troubling Record Trails Doctor Treating Autism*. Chicago Tribune; May 22, 2009. Accessed January 12, 2019. https://www.chicagotribune.com/news/chi-autism-doctor-eisenstein-may22-story.html.

35. Mayer Eisenstein. In: *Encyclopedia of American Loons*. July 28, 2013. Accessed January 12, 2019. http://americanloons.blogspot.com/2013/07/645-mayer-eisenstein.html?m=1.

36. Tenpenny S. *Why Do I Call it the "Anti-Vaccine Religion"? Let Me Explain*. Skeptical Raptor Web site; April 5, 2018. Accessed January 12, 2019. https://www.skepticalraptor.com/skepticalraptorblog.php/tag/sherri-tenpenny/.

37. Gorski D [Orac]. *Dr. Suzanne Humphries and the International Medical Council on Vaccination: Antivaccine to the Core*. Respectful Insolence Web site; February 16, 2011. Accessed January 12, 2019. https://respectfulinsolence.com/2011/02/16/dr-suzanne-humphries-and-the-internation/.

38. Bark T. About Us. Disease Reversal Web site. Accessed January 12, 2019. http://disease-reversal.com/about-us/.

39. Neil Z. Miller & Gary S. Goldman. *Encyclopedia of American Loons*. March 11, 2014. Accessed January 12, 2019. http://americanloons.blogspot.com/2014/03/950-neil-z-miller-gary-s-goldman.html?m=1.

40. Paul AM. *Bad News for Baby*. New York Times; May 10, 2013. Accessed January 12, 2019. https://www.nytimes.com/2013/05/12/books/review/the-business-of-baby-by-jennifer-margulis.html.

41. Palfreman J. (Director). The vaccine war. [Television series episode] In: Sullivan MR (Producer), *Frontline*. Boston, MA: Central Broadcasting Service; April 27, 2010. http://www.pbs.org/wgbh/pages//frontline/vaccines/etc/margulis.html.

42. Gorski D [Orac]. *The return of J. B. Handley*. January 14, 2015. Respectful Insolence Web site. Accessed January 12, 2019. https://respectfulinsolence.com/2015/01/14/the-return-of-j-b-handley/.

43. Generation Rescue. Who We Are. Accessed January 12, 2019. http://www.generationrescue.org/who-we-are/.

44. Blake M. *Popular Anti-Science Site Likens Journalists to "Nazi Collaborators" Over GMO Coverage*. Mother Jones; July 25, 2014. Accessed January 12, 2019. https://www.motherjones.com/kevin-drum/2014/07/popular-conspiracy-site-likens-pro-gmo-journalists-nazi-collaborators/.

45. Gorski D. *Mike Adams on Dr. Mehmet Oz's colon Polyps: "Spontaneous" Disease?* Science-Based Medicine Web site; September 6, 2010. Accessed January 12, 2019. https://sciencebasedmedicine.org/mike-adams-on-dr-mehmet-ozs-colon-polyps-spontaneous-disease/.

46. Jarry J. *Mike Adams Is Building An Alternate Reality Online*. McGill University; February 15, 2018. Accessed January 12, 2019. https://www.mcgill.ca/oss/article/quackery/mike-Adams-building-alternate-reality-online.

47. Vaxxed. Filmmaker Biographies. Vaxxed the Movie Web site. Accessed January 12, 2019. http://vaxxedthemovie.com/filmmaker-biographies/.

48. Lyons T. *Hard Questions: How Is Facebook's Fact-Checking Program Working?* Facebook's Newsroom Web site; June 14, 2018. Accessed January 12, 2019. https://newsroom.fb.com/news/2018/06/hard-questions-fact-checking.

49. Schmidt CW. Trending now: using social media to predict and track disease outbreaks. *Environ Health Perspect*. 2012;120(1):a30-a33. https://www.ncbi.nlm.nih.gov/pmc/articles/PMC3261963/.

Making Your Clinic a Lean, Mean, Vaccinating Machine

Alone we can do so little; together we can do so much.

—Helen Keller

We, as clinicians, can do everything right. We can educate ourselves regarding the science behind vaccines, we can use every encounter to offer vaccines, and we can encourage patients to voice their questions and concerns so that they know we are open to honest discussion about vaccines. But, what if we can't even get the patients to come into the office? What if the patient is there, but in the process of rooming, the medical assistant says, "Gosh, I waited to get my child vaccinated for HPV. I didn't want my daughter thinking she could start having sex right away." (You may wonder if this truly ever happens, but unfortunately it does). What if you have the patient in the room, they are ready to have the vaccine, and it turns out the clinic ran out of the vaccine a week ago. I can't tell you how frustrating it is to spend time and energy convincing a vaccine-hesitant patient to get a vaccine, only to not have the vaccine available to give! We're forced to send them out the door to return later. What are the chances that that person is going to come back?

Not only do we need to educate ourselves about vaccine science and fact, we need to educate our staff, those who are on the frontlines speaking with patients more often than we do. We also need to create organizational efficiencies that will bring patients into the clinic, will convey a strong and consistent message about the importance of vaccines, will facilitate the follow-up necessary for vaccine series so patients' care doesn't fall through the cracks, and will make sure we have the tools and supplies we need to do our jobs effectively.

This chapter provides a list of organizational interventions that will help you increase your success rates in getting your patients vaccinated and help take some of the pressure off of you as the only person responsible for success or failure of your clinic's vaccine program.

1. Participate in your community's vaccine registry and encourage other medical providers and pharmacies to participate as well. These state-run Immunization Information Systems (IIS) are "confidential, population-based, computerized databases that record all immunization doses administered by participating providers to persons residing within a given geopolitical area."[1] At an individual level, the IIS help us to keep patients on schedule with vaccines and decrease

the chances that they will get unnecessary repeat doses. At the population level, they can be used for surveillance and in guiding public health initiatives. Your regional public health department can put you in touch with your local IIS so that you can become enrolled as a participating provider (**Box 14.1**).

Box 14.1   Immunization Information Systems

State by State Immunization Information System Contact Information—https://www.cdc.gov/vaccines/programs/iis/contacts-locate-records.html.

2. Get your clinic involved in the Vaccines for Children (VFC) program. The VFC program is a "federally funded program that provides vaccines at no cost to children who might not otherwise be vaccinated because of inability to pay." This includes children younger than 19 years of age who are Medicaid-eligible, Alaskan Native, American Indian, uninsured, or underinsured.[2] The VFC program allows you to provide government-purchased vaccines for your eligible patient population with reduced out-of-pocket costs for you, thus increasing vaccination rates and decreasing burden of disease in this at-risk population. To become involved, you will need to contact your state VFC program coordinator and ask for a Provider Enrollment Package to be mailed out. When this is completed, you will need to prepare for a site visit to go over the administrative requirements of the program and to ensure proper storage and handling of the VFC vaccines (**Box 14.2**). Then, let the vaccinating begin!

Box 14.2   Becoming a VFC Provider

Why and How to Become a VFC Provider—https://www.cdc.gov/vaccines/programs/vfc/providers/questions/qa-join.html.

3. Get the patients in the door. Use mailings, use robocalls, or use health coaches or medical assistants to make vaccine stats a "vital sign," something we review on every patient at every encounter (office visit, telephone call, etc.). Thinking about vaccines needs to become second nature for us and for our medical assistants. In looking at our vaccination successes and where we have room for improvement at the local level, it seems we sometimes miss out on getting our preteens and teens in for their well-child checks. Our percentages for getting kids up-to-date on their Tdap, meningitis, and HPV vaccines, as a result, are not where they should be. In 2017, the national average for adolescent vaccine coverage was best for Tdap at 88.7%, MenACWY coverage for one dose was 85.1% but only 44.3% for both recommended doses, and HPV coverage was 65.5% for one dose and a mere 48.6% for completion of the series.[3] We all know how life gets in the way of doing things to take care of ourselves. Sometimes we need a gentle nudge or reminder. Perhaps we could query our patient databases

on a monthly basis and send out "Happy Birthday" cards to all of our kids turning 11, reminding them to return to clinic for their wellness visit and to get caught up on these very important vaccines. This is just one idea. There is no one specific way to tackle this effort. Each clinic or health system may have their own unique approaches to making this work. But we do need to put our heads together to make sure that patients are getting in. We can't vaccinate them if they are not in front of us.

4. Educate your staff—everyone from the front office to schedulers to medical assistants to your fellow providers. Everyone needs to know the facts and the recommendations about vaccines so that we can all be offering the same message. Nothing is more confusing to patients than having one person tell them one thing and someone else giving conflicting advice. We need to be on the same page. This approach helps to address any vaccine hesitancy in your staff, as well. There are always staff who initially refuse to get their annual flu vaccine, but with a bit of education, and a requirement to wear a mask for the entirety of the flu season if they continue to opt against vaccination, we can often get staff to change their minds. At the end of the book, you will find educational resources for patients and staff. You can use these to create a talk for your clinic. Schedule a morning or lunchtime meeting and go over immunization recommendations and facts about vaccines with your staff. Give them talking points that they can use when working with patients. Moreover, set universal expectations for review of patients' vaccine histories (for example, when patients call in for refills on medications, have the medical assistants check to see if they are up-to-date and bring them in if they are due). In my clinic, we have handed out information about vaccines that addresses commonly voiced concerns (see Appendix B: Fast Facts about Vaccines for Patients and Clinic Staff) and have given each staff member a button to wear stating our commitment to vaccinating. We also hold a drawing where staff put responses to vaccine questions (For example, "True or False: The flu shot protects against the stomach flu") in a box and, once a week, we draw a winner for a Starbucks gift card. Again, use your creativity developing your own ideas. Let's try to make vaccine education fun and engaging!

5. Use standing orders for vaccines.[4] If we train our staff well and we trust and expect that they will follow the proper guidelines for giving vaccines, we can allow them to give vaccines per protocol without us having to sign off on every single shot. We can review the protocols and sign off once. This suffices for "giving an order" for vaccines and takes up less of our time having to enter individual orders or sign off on each vaccine (**Box 14.3**). This allows our staff to work to the limits of their training and demonstrates our trust in them to provide quality care for our patients. When staff are involved directly with patient care, they feel more a part of the team. Vaccination rates go up and staff engagement improves. It is a win-win situation.

 Box 14.3   Standing Orders for Vaccines

Standing Orders for Administering Vaccines: How to Get Started—www.immunize. org/standing-orders.

6. Don't just wait for well visits.[5] Use every opportunity to discuss vaccines. As we know, some of our patients don't come in for routine preventive care unless required. Many patients only come in for acute issues. However, even the acute care visit for a sprained ankle or a migraine or for pain management can be an excellent opportunity to get patients caught up on vaccines. "Amber, I know that you are here to discuss your migraines," we might say, "but it looks like you are due to get your final HPV shot—let's go ahead and get that done while you're here." This will take a bit of preplanning, having either the provider or the medical assistant review the vaccination history to look for any gaps before the patient arrives, but it is a relatively simple way to capture those patients who may otherwise not come in on a routine basis. Moreover, usually, patients appreciate the opportunity to get as much done at one encounter as possible **(Box 14.4)**.

Box 14.4 Did You Know?

If your patient knows they started a vaccine series (hepatitis B, for example) but never finished it, you do not need to restart the series. It doesn't matter how long it has been since the last part of the series was given, the patient only needs to complete the series. If the patient is certain that they never completed the series but cannot remember how many shots in the series they received, you can always give a booster and then check an antibody titer 4 to 8 weeks later[6] to see if full immunity has developed (in the case of hepatitis B, you would check an HBsAb level). If patients are just delayed in starting their vaccine series, check the Centers for Disease Control and Prevention's website for catch-up schedules.[7]

7. Schedule their next shot before leaving. When a vaccine requires a series of shots (hepatitis A, HPV, and the new shingles vaccine, for example), have the patient schedule to return for the next shot in the series before they leave the building. They can be provided with an appointment card (which patients are more likely to honor than if just told to "come back in 6 months"). For many electronic medical records, an "appointment" will also generate a reminder call a few days prior. Each of these interventions increases the chance that the patient will return to complete the vaccine series.

8. Use wait times to your advantage. Why not give patients something to occupy their time while they wait to be seen? If you have televisions in your waiting room, instead of the news or cartoons, set up a rotation of informational videos that can educate patients while they wait. This would be exceedingly helpful for introducing vaccine information but can be used to address other health care topics as well. We could even offer video games for the kids that teach them about general and vaccine health[8] all while "playing a game." In our examination rooms, have pamphlets or posters (aesthetically presented of course—people will look past information that appears cluttered and disorganized) for patients to peruse while they wait.

9. Engage your staff. During vaccine "seasons" (back-to-school and influenza season), get your whole clinic excited and onboard for promoting vaccines. Have staff wear T-shirts that say "vaccines save lives" or some other pro-vaccine message. Put the names of staff members who are wearing their shirts in a pot and

draw for a weekly prize. Have clinic-wide competitions to see which clinics can get the highest percentage of staff vaccinated. Then have those vaccinated staff members wear a sticker or button that says "I got my flu shot!" If patients see that providers and clinics think it is important enough to get their entire clinic vaccinated, they may just find it important enough to vaccinate themselves.

10. Chip away at anti-vaccine sentiment. It is rare that an entire visit can be devoted to the discussion of vaccines. But it often takes a visit's worth of time or more to cover all of the questions and concerns that patients have. Discuss what you can, when you can. Use every opportunity to engage patients and encourage vaccines. But if you don't have a lot of time to devote to the issue, have resources that you can give patients for further reading (See the Appendix for useful handouts to guide patients in their education about vaccines). Let them know that they can reach out at any time with questions and that they can return at any time to get caught up on their immunizations. If we tackle the issue little by little, we can often find a crack in the anti-vaccine armor and will do so in a way that is not overwhelming to us or to our patients.

11. Have a clinic vaccine champion (or two)—someone who is well versed in the schedule, knows requirements for storage and administration, and knows indications for vaccines outside the normal schedule and contraindications for vaccines in certain patient populations. Support these people with dedicated time and finances to participate in periodic vaccine training.

12. Have a go-to resource or resources that anyone in clinic can use to answer questions about vaccines in the moment. I highly recommend that each clinic have a copy of what are commonly known as "The Pink Book" and "The Purple Book." These texts have everything you need to know to manage, administer, and educate about vaccines during the day-to-day workings of your clinic (**Box 14.5**).

Box 14.5   Vaccine Resources for Day-to-Day Clinical Practice

- "The Pink Book"
Hamborsky J, Kroger A, Wolfe C. (2015). *Epidemiology and Prevention of Vaccine-Preventable Diseases* (13th ed.). Washington, D.C.: Public Health Foundation.
  Or access it online at: https://www.cdc.gov/vaccines/pubs/pinkbook/index.html
- "The Purple Book"
Marshall, G. (2018). *The Vaccine Handbook: A Practical Guide for Clinicians.* (7th ed.). West Islip, NY: Professional Communications Inc.

13. Make vaccine ordering an ongoing and seamless process. As every clinic and every clinic population is different, I don't have an exact formula to lay out for you for success in vaccine ordering. But working with your vaccine champion and your purchasing department to adequately estimate the number of vaccines and to have continuous influx of vaccines during high-use times (flu season, for example) is extremely important. That way we can avoid that frustrating encounter where we have convinced the patient to get their immunization, but then don't have the immunization to give.

14.   Work with your specialists to create a coordinated approach to vaccines. Although vaccinating is often delegated to the primary care provider, many subspecialists deal with the consequences of vaccine-preventable disease. Gynecologists have known the consequences of congenital rubella syndrome and are keenly aware of the havoc that influenza can wreak on a pregnancy, which is a relatively immune-compromised state. They see cervical, vaginal, and vulvar cancers and precancers. Urologists deal with penile cancer. Colorectal surgeons treat anal and rectal cancer. Dentists and ENTs encounter and treat head and neck cancers. Neurologists see the consequences of meningococcal meningitis and influenza-induced Guillain-Barré syndrome. Imagine the successes we could have in vaccinating if all providers, not just primary care, recommended immunizations. It is sometimes more impactful if the specialist, whom patients don't generally think of as concerned with vaccines, makes a strong statement about the importance of getting vaccinated. For example, patients may think, "If my urologist is recommending the flu shot, it must be important!" Vaccination is a team sport, and subspecialists can have a vital role to play if we just engage them. All hands on deck!

15.   Consider expanding sites at which your patients can receive vaccines. This works particularly well at increasing our rates of influenza vaccination. Have cardiology or pulmonology or oncology offices, among others, carry the flu shot, and take advantage of the opportunity to vaccinate when the patient is in the office. Making health care convenient to patients will increase our immunization success rates. This will require that all nursing staff and medical assistants, some who may have gotten out of the habit of giving vaccines, are offered a refresher on shot administration. But most folks went into the profession because they enjoy working one-on-one with patients, so they will likely appreciate the retraining and enjoy the ability to participate in patient care.

16.   Consider incentivizing vaccinations.[4] This works particularly well for young people. At college health fairs, we could advertise a raffle for an Amazon gift card, for example, and students can put their name in the drawing after getting their flu shot. Likewise, offering food or transportation vouchers, baby products, or gift cards can incentivize parents to get their children or themselves vaccinated.

17.   Make regular updates about changes in the vaccine schedule a routine part of department meetings, so that everyone is onboard with the most up-to-date recommendations.

18.   Use your electronic health record (EHR) to promote vaccination.[5] A study published in *JAMA Network Open* in September of 2018 found that adding a "best practices" prompt for medical assistants in the EHR to ask about and order flu vaccinations during the rooming process significantly increased influenza vaccination rates in the practices studied.[9]

19.   Produce analytics to provide each clinic and each provider with granular data about how they are doing with their vaccination efforts. We medical professionals tend to be competitive people. If we see that we are not meeting standards, or that our numbers fall significantly below those of our partners, most of us will be chomping at the bit to get those numbers up.

20.   With adult vaccines, consider targeting high-risk populations; people older than 65 years of age who are due for pneumococcal vaccines and influenza, people who are immune compromised, and people with chronic lung or cardiac disease, for example. When these patients get sick, they have a tendency

to get very sick and a large number of our health care dollars are spent on hospitalizations in the elderly and medically complex. Most electronic medical records can search patients based on diagnosis codes that would identify them as higher risk. This list can then be cross-referenced with the immunization database to see who is up-to-date and who merits intervention through an outreach program (such as, e-mails, mailings, and phone calls).

21. Consider offering immunization clinics—separate days (for my clinic, we have 2 to 3 Saturdays in the autumn months) where we staff the clinic only for quick check-in and flu shot administration. These shots can be billed for existing patients or payed out of pocket for nonestablished patients. This allows you to vaccinate multiple patients at once and to capture some of their family members and other community members as well. If feeling particularly motivated, you could even research the vaccine histories of everyone signed up for the clinic and offer them other vaccines that they may be due for. These "flu clinics" are a service much appreciated by the community as it makes it more convenient for them to get their care.

22. Finally, if approved by your risk manager, take your services on the road! Clinics at nursing homes, schools, and college campuses can help get preventive care to some of our more vulnerable or poorly compliant patients.

The 2017-2018 American Academy of Family Physicians (AAFP) Adolescent Immunization Awards recently recognized eight residency programs which successfully put these approaches into action. These programs studied techniques for boosting immunization rates for influenza, Tdap, HPV, and meningitis vaccines. "The techniques used include creating a team approach, strongly recommending all vaccines, implementing standing orders, trying new technologies, understanding electronic medical record capabilities, leveraging community outreach and offering incentives.... By implementing their projects, six of the residencies raised the rates for most or all of the recommended vaccines—sometimes spectacularly—while the other two residencies increased rates for a few vaccines."[10] In looking at measures that we can use to increase our vaccination rates, it's not just about putting data in front of the patient. Though the science *is* very important, the "art" of medicine and community health is where we may make the biggest difference. We've got to get creative in our approach to accessing patients and engaging our clinical and community partners.

It sometimes feels like we are alone on this journey to get patients vaccinated but there is much that our clinics and organizations can do to help. Work with your clinic management and administrators to develop a coordinated approach to the immunization process and both you and your patients will benefit.

References

1. Centers for Disease Control and Prevention. About Immunization Information Systems. https://www.cdc.gov/vaccines/programs/iis/about.html. Updated May 15, 2012. Accessed December 23, 2018.
2. Centers for Disease Control and Prevention. Vaccines for Children Program. https://www.cdc.gov/vaccines/programs/vfc/index.html. Updated April 17, 2018. Accessed December 23, 2018.
3. Walker T, Elam-Evans L, Yankey D, et al. National, regional, state, and selected local area vaccination coverage among adolescents aged 13-17 years – United States, 2017. *MMWR Morb Mortal Wkly Rep.* 2018;67:909-991.
4. Dube E, Gagnon D, MacDonald N. Strategies intended to address vaccine hesitancy: review of published reviews. *Vaccine.* 2015;33(34):4191-4203.
5. Ventola C. Immunization in the United States: recommendations, barriers, and measures to improve compliance. *Pharm Ther.* 2016;41(7):426-436.

6. Hepatitis B Foundation. *The 3-shot Hepatitis B Vaccine–Do I Need to Restart the Series If I am off the Recommended Schedule?* October 25, 2017. www.hepb.org/blog/the-3-shot-HBV-vaccine-do-i-need-to-restart-the-series-if-i-am-off-the-recommended-schedule/. Accessed February 7, 2019.

7. Centers for Disease Control and Prevention. Table 2. Catch-up Immunization Schedule for Persons Aged 4 Months–18 Years Who Start Late or Who are More Than 1 Month Behind, United States, 2019. https://www.cdc.gov/vaccines/schedules/hcp/imz/catchup.html. Accessed February 7, 2019.

8. The Immunization Partnership. *How to Have Fun Learning About Vaccines.* September 20, 2018. https://www.immunizeusa.org/blog/2018/September/20/tip-vaccine-games/. Accessed December 26, 2018.

9. Kim R, Day S, Small D, et al. Variations in influenza vaccination by clinic appointment time and an active choice intervention in the electronic health record to increase influenza vaccination. *JAMA Netw Open.* 2018;1(5):e181770. https://jamanetwork.com/journals/jamanetworkopen/articlepdf/2702210/kim_2018_oi_180107.pdf.

10. Haas P. *Try These Techniques to Boost Adolescent Immunizations.* American Acad Fam Physicians; August 3, 2018. https://www.aafp.org/news/health-of-the-public/20180803fdaimmunawards.html. Accessed December 23, 2018.

15

A Call to Action

There are risks and costs to a program of action. But they are far less than the long-range risks and costs of comfortable inaction.

—John F. Kennedy

Y̶ou will hear those who study science denial and other social psychology phenomena discuss the role of the Dunning-Kruger effect in contributing to a person's ability to believe in, as H. L. Mencken stated, "the palpably not true." How can people believe so confidently in an idea that has an overwhelming amount of evidence against it (that the Earth is flat, that climate change isn't real, that vaccines cause autism)? The Dunning-Kruger effect is an effect that both those with little knowledge and those with a considerable amount of knowledge fall victim to. Essentially, it is the observation that people with little expertise or ability often evaluate themselves as having *superior* expertise or ability. They "don't have enough knowledge to know they don't have enough knowledge."[1] Moreover, the opposite can be true for people with superior ability and expertise. They tend to *underestimate* their ability and expertise because they have enough knowledge to know that there is a lot they don't know.

This effect is at play when we or our colleagues suffer from *imposter syndrome*, where we undervalue our competency and feel like a fraud. As physicians and advanced practice providers, scientists, and other health officials, we know a great deal about our fields of study, but we also recognize how much there is that we don't know. This can cause us to doubt ourselves. "If there's so much that we don't know, how can we feel confident in what we say and in the advice that we give?" we may wonder. We often feel at risk of being "found out," that somehow someone is going to figure out that we really don't know what we are talking about. This syndrome can lead us to avoid speaking up and speaking out for fear of being "discovered."

Prior to reading this book, you may have doubted your expertise and lacked confidence in your ability to speak with authority about the safety and efficacy of vaccines. You may have shied away from encouraging your vaccine-hesitant patients to have discussions about their concerns. You may have defaulted to the "just let it slide" approach with patients who have previously declined vaccinations. In this book, I have provided tools to help you through these challenges. I have reviewed the history of vaccines, vaccine-preventable diseases, anti-vaccine sentiment, the psychology at play in the anti-vaccine movement, and the robust system of checks and balances designed to ensure vaccine safety and efficacy. I am hopeful that, with this new knowledge, you have gained further trust in our vaccine recommendations as they stand. I have also offered proven interviewing techniques and data-driven responses to the many questions and concerns that you get from patients, as well as information you can use to help your patients better interpret what they are reading online.

183

This information should grant you greater confidence in your expertise and ability to educate your patients with accurate information, while maintaining a strong relationship and feeling that you are "on the same team," even if you ultimately have to agree to disagree.

It's important to remember that the old adage, "If at first you don't succeed, try, try again," still stands as sound advice. You may not change your patients' mind the first time you have the conversation, or the seventh time. But eventually, with persistence and an honest expression of caring and concern for your patients' well-being, at least some of those who initially decline vaccines will come around. Douglas Opel et al. studied a group of pediatricians during vaccine counseling interactions with parents of 1- to 19-month-old children who were being seen for health supervision visits. Of parents counseled about vaccines who initially declined immunizations for their child, 47% of parents eventually agreed to vaccination if their provider persisted with a strong recommendation.[2] It goes to show that if we have confidence in our ability to make an impact, and we continue to educate, counsel, and offer strong encouragement for immunization, we will find greater successes in getting our patients vaccinated (**Box 15.1**).

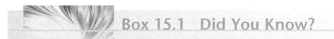 Box 15.1 Did You Know?

We all know that vaccines are an excellent way to prevent viral and bacterial infections, but have you ever thought about the fact that, in preventing these infections, we are also decreasing the incidence of antimicrobial resistance? If someone can avoid getting the flu and the subsequent bacterial pneumonia that sets in on top of it, they won't need antibiotics. If we prevent recurrent ear infections and bronchitis by immunizing against *Haemophilus influenzae* type b and pneumococcal disease, kids won't need as many antibiotics. Moreover, with fewer antibiotics comes a decrease in the development of antibiotic resistance! Yet another reason to strongly support and encourage immunization.

Physicians and other health care providers are traditionally nose-to-the-grindstone sort of people. We go to work early; we try to take good care of our patients and to get patients seen on time; we work hard to get our charting done; we come home late, and, somewhere in there, we try to fit in time with our loved ones. Our jobs can be quite rewarding but are also often physically and emotionally draining. Many providers have little energy left for advocacy and involvement on a larger scale. But the rapid dissemination of information via the Internet has created inroads for easy access to faulty information, and our patients are falling victim to it. Those of us with knowledge and expertise should be the ones leading the way in online health education and advice. If we don't, you can guess who will pick up the slack. It will be the Mike "The Health Ranger" Adams and J. B. Handleys of the world, who are *not* experts in the field, who will use the Internet bullhorn to spread the misinformation and pseudoscience that we so desperately want our patients to avoid.

We must, as a group, bring our experience and caregiving talents to where the community is, and the community is on the Internet and social media. Though we may be more comfortable educating in the sphere of our clinics than we are with public speaking and broadcasting our medical opinions over the airwaves, the fastest way to get the facts out to a large group of people is through speaking up and making our voices heard across media channels (news, radio, Facebook, Twitter, etc.). We know that the number one driver of a patient's decision to vaccinate is a strong recommendation from their provider. Imagine the successes we could have if those strong recommendations from respected health care providers drowned out the doubts cast by the anti-vaccine movement.

In joining the online or media conversation, we may worry that putting our opinions out there publicly could alienate some of our patients, particularly if our opinions have to do with more controversial topics such as vaccinations. But in dedicating our careers to medicine and healing, we promised to advocate for the health of our patients and communities. That advocacy does not end once we leave the examination room. Our patients need trustworthy health advice now more than ever. They are searching for it on the Web, and physicians, scientists, and researchers need to be the ones providing that reliable content.

In speaking up, we may also worry about liability issues—if we are felt to be offering medical advice without an established relationship with the patient, for example. We do have to be cautious about this, making sure to offer qualifications to our recommendations and encouraging patients to seek counsel from their own medical providers who know them personally. If you are an employed provider or are a partner in a multiprovider group, consider discussing your social media presence with your risk manager to make sure you are not bringing any liability upon your clinic or partners. If you are an independent clinician, discuss your social media voice with your lawyer in order to mitigate any risk.

As we venture into this world of social media, we need to remember that, just as our approach matters in that one-on-one interaction in our offices, it matters to the online vaccine discussion as well. If we hope to make positive strides in getting patients onboard with science and fact, it is important to bring the same level of compassion and empathy to the social media discussion that we bring to our clinic visits. Because of its more impersonal nature, Internet discussions have the propensity to devolve into unhelpful back-and-forth jabs at the other person. We have to remember to take the moral high ground. Our online interactions are important. Losing our cool doesn't just impact the person we may be having a disagreement with but also the countless others observing the discussion. Just as criticizing or speaking down to a patient for their views would be unlikely to garner praise or change that person's opinion, so too would it have the potential to alienate and anger some of your Twitter followers or Facebook "friends."

We also need to go into our online interactions with eyes wide open about the encounters we may have there. We should prepare ourselves for things to get occasionally uncomfortable. Given the false sense of anonymity that some people feel in their social media interactions, the rare person will feel justified in bad behavior; they may attack not only our views but our character and motivations; they may try to engage us in a "shouting match," encouraging us to give in to our baser instincts to defend ourselves or to go on the offensive. Moreover, some anti-vaccine activists can be downright mean, going on the attack and trying to discredit those who speak up for vaccines. However, giving voice to Internet trolls by taking part in back-and-forth engagement will only serve to put *their* misguided and misinformed ideas forward into the broader consciousness. We must keep in mind what we learned in chapter 3, Psychology of the Anti-vaccine Movement. We only want to amplify correct information and facts, not add fuel to the anti-vaccine fire.

Whether the issue we are passionate about is vaccination, or the importance of cardiovascular exercise, or promoting child safety—if we want to make a larger impact, we have to consider looking beyond our one-on-one interactions to educate in a more public forum. Here are just a few ways you can get involved:

- Become a vaccine advocate or champion for your clinic.
- Work with your administrators to support pro-vaccine initiatives.
- Share pro-vaccine and pro-science content with your family and friends on Facebook.
- Spread the word about outbreaks in your community and elsewhere.
- Post a picture of yourself and your children getting your flu shot.
- Become part of the social media vaccine conversation. Introduce your own content or comment in support of other pro-vaccine messages.

- Contribute articles to your local paper or write for online or print magazines.
- Be available to your local news stations for stories about local outbreaks or the current season's flu vaccine.
- Give talks at churches, schools, community centers, and others.
- Speak to your local political representatives about the importance of vaccines and pro-vaccine legislation.
- Get involved with your local public health department.
- Run for office.
- Write a book.

We may have to tiptoe out of our comfort zones to get our message across, but we can do it. We must do it. The rise in anti-science sentiment, particularly anti-vaccine sentiment, is having real-world implications in a profoundly negative way. With every percentage point drop in herd immunity, more and more lives are at risk. There are numerous ways, both big and small, that we can begin to make our voices heard. If we are willing to get involved, speak up, and educate on a larger stage, the entire world can be our classroom.

References

1. Azarian B. *The Dunning-Kruger Effect May Help Explain Trump's Support.* August 22, 2018. https://www.google.com/amp/s/www.psychologytoday.com/us/blog/mind-in-the-machine/201808/the-dunning-kruger-effect-may-help-explain-trumps-support%3famp. Accessed January 13, 2019.
2. Opel DJ, Heritage J, Taylor JA, et al. The architecture of provider-parent vaccine discussions at health supervision visits. *Pediatrics.* 2013;132(6):1037-1046. http://pediatrics.aappublications.org/content/132/6/1037.

Vaccine-Preventable Diseases Information

VARICELLA ZOSTER VIRUS (CHICKENPOX) (FIGURE A1)

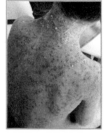

FIGURE A1
Chickenpox rash caused by varicella zoster virus. (*Courtesy of Gzzz.* https://commons.wikimedia.org/wiki/File:Severe_chickenpox.jpg. CC-BY-SA-4.0.)

- **Common symptoms**
    1. Fever
    2. Fatigue
    3. Loss of appetite
    4. Headache
    5. Rash (itchy, fluid-filled blisters that commonly start on the face, chest, and back, then spread to the rest of the body)

- **Complications**
    1. Bacterial skin and soft-tissue infections
    2. Pneumonia
    3. Brain infection/inflammation (called encephalitis)
    4. Bloodstream infection (called sepsis)
    5. Bleeding problems
    6. Dehydration
    7. Death (Note: Chickenpox is much more serious if contracted as an adult or by immune-compromised persons.)

- **Transmission/contagion**
    1. Transmission is through respiratory secretions/droplets or through direct contact with fluid from blisters.
    2. A person infected with chickenpox is highly contagious from 1 to 2 days before rash appears until all lesions have formed crusts (typically 10 to 14 days)—guidelines recommend isolation until no new lesions appear within a 24-hour period.

- **Vaccine information**
    1. The varicella zoster vaccine was licensed for use in the United States in 1995.
    2. It is a live-attenuated virus vaccine, so should not be given to someone with a compromised immune system.
    3. It's a two-dose series—first dose recommended at age 12 to 15 months with a second dose given at age 4 to 6 years.
    4. The vaccine is estimated to be about 94% effective after two doses.

- **Impact of chickenpox before vaccine was available[a]**
    1. Cases—In the early 1990s, there were approximately 4 million cases each year.
    2. Hospitalizations—Rates of hospitalization ranged from 8000 to 18,000 each year.
    3. Deaths—There were 100 to 150 deaths reported each year.

- **Reduction in disease/complications after vaccine was available[a]**
    1. Cases—From 2000 to 2010, rates of chickenpox declined by 79%.
    2. Deaths—From 2008 to 2011, deaths from chickenpox declined by 87%.[1]

---

[a]All data reflect US statistics unless otherwise indicated.

DIPHTHERIA (FIGURE A2)

- **Common symptoms**
  1. Weakness
  2. Sore throat
  3. Fever
  4. Swollen glands in the neck

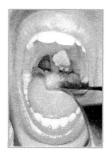

- **Complications**
  1. The "pseudomembrane" shown in the picture forms a covering, which can block the airway, causing trouble breathing and swallowing
  2. Damage to the heart muscle (called myocarditis)
  3. Damage to the nerves (called polyneuropathy)
  4. Loss of the ability to move (called paralysis)
  5. Lung infections, causing pneumonia and respiratory failure
  6. Death (even with treatment, about 1 in 10 patients will die)

- **Transmission/contagion**
  1. Transmission is most common through the respiratory tract.
  2. Without treatment, illness is contagious for approximately 2 to 4 weeks.

- **Vaccine information**
  1. Vaccine became available in the 1940s when it was added to tetanus toxoid and pertussis vaccine (DTP)—we now use DTaP and Tdap or DT or Td.
  2. Individual diphtheria vaccine is not available.
  3. Diphtheria is a killed/inactivated virus vaccine.
  4. DTaP is recommended to be given at ages 2, 4, and 6 months, at age 15 to 18 months, and then again at 4 to 5 years old. The adult form (Tdap) is recommended at the age of 11 to 12 years and every 10 years thereafter.
  5. Effectiveness is estimated at approximately 97% after three or more doses.

- **Impact of diphtheria before vaccine was available[a]**
  1. Cases—In 1921, there were 206,000 recorded cases.
  2. Deaths—In 1921, there were 15,520 recorded deaths.[2]

- **Reduction in disease/complications after vaccine was available[a]**
  1. Cases—From 2004 to 2015, there were two recorded cases.
  2. Deaths—The last reported death in the United States was in 2003.[3]

---

[a]All data reflect US statistics unless otherwise indicated.

HAEMOPHILUS INFLUENZAE B (HiB) (FIGURE A3)

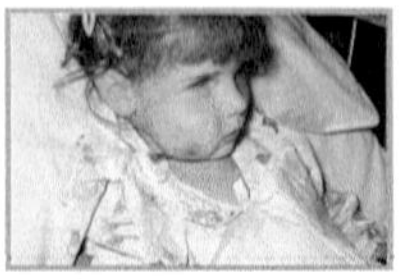

FIGURE A3
Facial swelling in a patient because of *Haemophilus Influenza* B. (*Courtesy of Children's Minnesota/Infection Prevention.* http://www.immunize.org/photos/hib-photos.asp.)

- **Common symptoms**
  1. Symptoms depend on location of infection and can range from mild to severe
  2. Ear infections in children—restlessness, ear pain, fever
  3. Bronchitis in adults—cough, shortness of breath, fever

- **Complications**
  1. Pneumonia
  2. Blood infection (called bacteremia), which can result in loss of limbs
  3. Infection of the covering of the brain and spinal cord (called meningitis), which can cause brain damage, vision loss, or hearing loss (suffered by 15% to 30% of survivors)
  4. Swelling in the throat (called epiglottitis)
  5. Skin infections (called cellulitis)
  6. Inflammation of the joint (called infectious arthritis)
  7. Death—3% to 6% of children with meningitis from HiB will die from the disease

- **Transmission/contagion**
  1. Transmission is through respiratory droplets spread by coughing/sneezing.
  2. *Haemophilus* bacteria can live in nasal/respiratory passages without causing infection. It can spread as long as the bacteria are present and until the patient is treated with 24 to 48 hours of appropriate antibiotic therapy.

- **Vaccine information**
  1. Conjugate vaccine was licensed in 1987.
  2. The Hib vaccine is a killed/inactivated vaccine.
  3. The Hib vaccine is recommended to be given at ages 2, 4, and 6 months, and age 12 to 15 months.
  4. It is estimated to be between 95% and 100% effective in fully vaccinated individuals.[4]

- **Impact of Hib before vaccine was available[a]**
  1. Cases—Approximately 20,000 children younger than 5 years of age got severe Hib disease annually.
  2. Deaths—About 1000 children died per year.

- **Reduction in disease/complications after vaccine was available[a]**
  1. Cases—Now, less than 1 case per 100,000 occurs in children younger than 5 years of age.[5]
  2. Deaths—The last deaths reported by the CDC, totaling 4, were in 2010. No death reports are available since that time.

---

[a]All data reflect US statistics unless otherwise indicated.

HEPATITIS A (FIGURE A4)

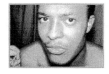

FIGURE A4 Jaundice caused by hepatitis A. (*Courtesy of Centers for Disease Control and Prevention.* http://www.immunize.org/photos/hepatitis-a-photos.asp.)

- **Common symptoms**
  1. Fever
  2. Tiredness
  3. Loss of appetite
  4. Nausea/vomiting
  5. Abdominal pain
  6. Dark urine
  7. Jaundice or yellowing of the skin

- **Complications**
  1. Dehydration
  2. Liver failure, which can require liver transplant in 10% to 20% of patients
  3. Death

- **Transmission/contagion**
  1. Transmission is through the fecal-oral (stool to mouth) route. In the United States, transmission is most common during travel to areas where there are poor sanitary conditions or from food workers following improper hand washing before food preparation.
  2. A person with hepatitis A is contagious from 2 weeks prior to showing symptoms. Contagion decreases over time but can last 1 week or more after symptoms develop.

- **Vaccine information**
  1. The hepatitis A vaccine was licensed in the United States in 1995, first recommended only for high-risk groups. Universal childhood vaccination was recommended in 2006.
  2. The hepatitis A vaccine is a killed/inactivated virus vaccine.
  3. It is a series of two shots—the first dose is given to all children starting at the age of 1 year and the second dose is recommended 6 months later. It is also recommended for food handlers.
  4. The vaccine is 94% effective after one dose[6] and 100% effective after two doses.

- **Impact of hepatitis A before vaccine was available[a]**
  1. Cases—Approximately 59,606 cases were reported in 1971.
  2. Deaths—Before vaccine was available, there were an average of 96 deaths per year, greater with increasing age at infection and greater in men than women.

- **Reduction in disease/complications after vaccine was available[a]**
  1. Cases—In 2014, there were 1239 recorded cases.[3]
  2. Deaths—In 2014, there were 26 recorded deaths from hepatitis A.[3]

---

[a]All data reflect US statistics unless otherwise indicated.

HEPATITIS B (FIGURE A5)

- **Common symptoms**

  1. Acute hepatitis B—Fever, fatigue, loss of appetite, abdominal pain, nausea/vomiting, dark urine, clay-colored bowel movements, joint pain, and yellowing of the skin/eyes (called jaundice)
  2. Chronic hepatitis B—Few symptoms until the virus causes chronic liver disease, then symptoms can be similar to those listed above but are due to liver failure

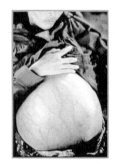

FIGURE A5
Liver failure caused by hepatitis B. (*Courtesy of Centers for Disease Control and Prevention.* http://www.immunize.org/photos/hepatitis-b-photos.asp.)

- **Complications**

  1. Chronic hepatitis B—liver damage, liver failure, liver cancer, and death.

- **Transmission/contagion**

  1. Hepatitis B is transmitted through blood or body fluids (from an infected mother to her baby during birth, sharing needles or other drug preparation equipment, sex with an infected partner, direct contact with blood or open sores—toothbrushes, razors, shared glucose meters, blood transfusions before the blood supply was screened, needle sticks, and exposure to tears or saliva).[7]
  2. In acute infection, persons are contagious from 1 to 2 months before and after symptoms develop. Chronically infected persons are always contagious.

- **Vaccine information**

  1. Currently used recombinant hepatitis B virus vaccines were licensed in 1986 and 1989.
  2. The hepatitis B vaccine is a killed virus vaccine with no live/infectious particles.
  3. Hepatitis B vaccine is recommended at birth, and ages 2 and 6 months. A three-dose series is also recommended for all medical/dental workers and other high-risk groups.
  4. The hepatitis B vaccine is approximately 95% effective following the full series.[8]

- **Impact of hepatitis B before vaccine was available**[a]

  1. Cases—In the mid-1980s, there averaged 26,000 cases of acute hepatitis B per year.
  2. Deaths—If exposed during childhood, one in four will become chronically infected and 15% of those will eventually die of liver disease. Of those 26,000 acute cases, that is 975 deaths from chronic hepatitis B.

- **Reduction in disease/complications after vaccine was available**[a]

  1. Cases—After vaccination efforts began, the incidence of *acute* hepatitis B dropped by 75%, the greatest decline seen in children and teens (94%).[8]
  2. Deaths—We are still dealing with consequences of *chronic* hepatitis B acquired before vaccines were available. Currently, there are anywhere from 800,000 to 1.4 million people with chronic hepatitis B virus infection. Approximately 3000 people in the United States die from hepatitis B infection each year.

---

[a]All data reflect US statistics unless otherwise indicated.

HUMAN PAPILLOMAVIRUS (HPV) (FIGURES A6 AND A7)

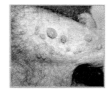

- **Common symptoms**
  1. Genital warts, which one might be able to see or feel but generally don't cause any symptoms (such as itching or pain)
  2. Causes cancer, but there are typically no symptoms of this until changes are further advanced, at which time one might notice bleeding, pain, nonhealing lesions, difficulty swallowing, or change in voice character

- **Complications**
  1. Cancer—cervical, vaginal, vulvar, anal, rectal, penile, and throat/mouth
     a. Treatment of these cancers can require surgical removal of the lesions (resulting in potential disfigurement and fertility issues if the cervix or uterus has to be removed). Chemotherapy and/or radiation therapy may also be required.

  2. Laryngeal papillomatosis (warts in the throat)
     a. Can require multiple surgical excisions (they tend to recur) or even tracheostomy if warts are large or numerous enough to affect breathing.
  3. Death

- **Transmission/contagion**
  1. Transmission is through skin-to-skin contact. Friction/rubbing alone can transmit genital warts (no penetration is required). Transmission is most common during vaginal, oral, and anal sex. Rarely, warts can be transmitted from mother to baby during delivery through an infected birth canal.
     a. There are currently 79 million Americans infected with HPV.
     b. There are 14 million new HPV infections each year.
     c. Most all of us will come in contact with HPV at some point in our sexual lives.
  2. Contagion—HPV is highly contagious, primarily because there are often no outward signs or symptoms of infection, thus making it hard to avoid.

- **Vaccine information**
  1. The HPV vaccine was licensed for use in girls in 2006 and for boys in 2011.
  2. Initially, vaccine options covered only two strains (2-valent) of cancer-causing HPV, or four strains (4-valent), two cancer-causing and two wart-causing strains. Now we universally use a 9-valent vaccine (seven cancer-causing and two wart-causing strains).
  3. The HPV vaccine is a killed virus vaccine.

Continued

4. It is recommended to be given anywhere from the age of 9 to 26 years, but preferably at the age of 11 or 12 years. If started before the age of 15 years, only two shots are given 6 to 12 months apart. If started after the age of 15 years (and in select high-risk groups), three shots are given at 0-, 2-, and 6-month intervals.

5. It has recently been approved for use by the Food and Drug Administration (FDA) in people aged 27 to 45 but has not yet been recommended routinely by the Advisory Committee on Immunization Practices.

6. The HPV vaccine is nearly 100% effective against the most common cancer-causing and wart-causing strains of HPV.[9]

- **Impact of HPV before vaccine was available**[a]

  1. Cases—

     a. Genital Warts—Up to 360,000 cases were reported per year in the United States.[10]

     b. Cancers—Estimates range from 31,000 to 41,000 cases of HPV-related cancers diagnosed yearly in the United States. HPV causes about 3% of all cancers in women and 2% of all cancers in men.

- **Reduction in disease/complications after vaccine was available**[a]

  (**Note:** 1. The United States has not been as successful as other countries at vaccinating against HPV. Therefore, our statistics are less impressive than countries where HPV vaccination is greater. To see the largest impact, postvaccination statistics are taken from studies out of Australia where HPV vaccination is more universal.

  2. It takes many years to develop cancer. The vaccine has not been out long enough to see a large drop in cancer rates. However, we do see a significant decrease in rates of genital warts and precancers.)

  1. Cases—

     a. Genital warts—A 92% reduction in genital warts was seen after introduction of the 4-valent HPV vaccine.

     b. Cancers—

        i. In Australia, a 34% reduction in low-grade precancerous changes and 47% reduction in high-grade precancerous changes have been seen since introduction of the vaccine.[11]

        ii. Predictive models suggest that, with high rates of vaccination, we could see 90% to 93% reduction in rates of cervical cancer.

        iii. In the United States, 31,000 cases of HPV-related cancers are still diagnosed each year.

---

[a]All data reflect US statistics unless otherwise indicated.

INFLUENZA (FIGURE A8)

- **Common symptoms**
  1. Body aches
  2. Fatigue
  3. Fever
  4. Sore throat
  5. Headache
  6. Cough

- **Complications**
  1. Pneumonia
  2. Respiratory failure
  3. Inflammation of the brain (called encephalitis)
  4. Inflammation of the cardiovascular system, resulting in higher rates of heart attack and stroke
  5. Death

- **Transmission/contagion**
  1. Transmission is via respiratory droplets
  2. Contagious from 1 to 2 days before the onset of symptoms until fever breaks

- **Vaccine information**
  1. The influenza virus was isolated in 1933 and the first multivalent vaccine (containing more than one strain) was introduced in 1942. In the early 1970s, it became known that the influenza virus mutates. The World Health Organization began a surveillance program, which recommends yearly changes to the components of the vaccine, depending on the strains most commonly circulating that year.
  2. The flu injection is a killed virus vaccine. The flu nasal spray is a live-attenuated/weakened virus vaccine.
  3. The influenza vaccine is recommended to be given to everyone older than 6 months of age. The very first immunization given in early childhood is two vaccines spread apart by a month. After that, the vaccine is given only once yearly.
  4. At its best, the influenza vaccine is approximately 60% effective in preventing the flu. However, it is significantly more effective in preventing hospitalizations and death (of people that die from the flu, 80% to 90% did *not* have the flu vaccine).

- **Impact of influenza before vaccine was available[a]**
  1. Cases—Information wasn't recorded until 1900. The number of cases was highly variable depending on the year.
  2. Deaths—The worst pandemic in history (The Spanish Flu of 1918) saw one-third of the world's population infected and 50 million deaths in a single year. The average rate of deaths pre-vaccine was around 10.2/100,000.[12]

---

[a]All data reflect US statistics unless otherwise indicated.

Continued

- **Reduction in disease/complications after vaccine was available**[a]

  (**Note:** We have not been very effective at widely administering the flu vaccine in the United States. Therefore, we still see significant cost, in both lives and dollars, from yearly influenza outbreaks.)

  1. Cases—Influenza causes between 9.2 million and 35.6 million illnesses and between 140,000 and 710,000 hospitalizations each year.[13]
  2. Deaths—In a given year, we still see 12,000 to 56,000 deaths annually (though in 2017-2018 we had 80,000 deaths) from influenza in the United States. The average influenza death rate is now down to an average of 0.56/100,000.

---

[a]All data reflect US statistics unless otherwise indicated.

MEASLES (FIGURE A9)

- **Common symptoms**
  1. High fever
  2. Cough
  3. Runny nose
  4. Watery, red eyes
  5. Tiny white spots (Koplik spots) may appear in the mouth a few days after symptoms begin
  6. Rash, which breaks out 3 to 5 days after symptoms begin, usually starting at the face and spreading downward

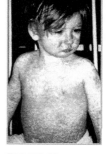

FIGURE A9
Measles rash on a child. (*Courtesy of Centers for Disease Control and Prevention.* http://www. vaccineinformation.org/photos/ measiac004.jpg.)

- **Complications**
  1. Ear infections, which can result in permanent hearing loss
  2. Diarrhea, which can cause dehydration
  3. Pneumonia
  4. Swelling/inflammation of the brain (called encephalitis)—this can lead to seizures and can leave children deaf or with intellectual disabilities
  5. Long-term complication called subacute sclerosing panencephalitis, which is a rare but fatal disease of the nervous system that develops 7 to 10 years after infection[14]
  6. Death

- **Transmission/contagion**
  1. Transmission is through respiratory droplets—it can live for up to 2 hours in a space where an infected person coughed/sneezed.
  2. Contagion—highly contagious—approximately 90% of nonimmune people who come in contact with an infected person will contract the illness. Measles is contagious from 4 days before to 4 days after the rash appears.[15]

- **Vaccine information**
  1. The measles vaccine was licensed in 1963. It is offered in the combined measles, mumps, and rubella (MMR) vaccine.
  2. The MMR vaccine is a live-attenuated virus vaccine. It should not be given to patients with immune suppression but is safe for everyone with a healthy immune system.
  3. The first dose of the MMR vaccine is recommended at age 12 to 15 months with the second dose given at 4 to 6 years of age. A third dose is recommended as a booster for at-risk persons during outbreaks. If you were born before 1957, it is presumed that you have natural immunity to measles.[16]
  4. Two doses of MMR vaccine are 97% effective against measles.

Continued

MEASLES *(Continued)*

- **Impact of measles before vaccine was available**[a]

  1. Cases—3 to 4 million people in the United States were infected each year.
  2. Hospitalizations—Approximately, 48,000 people were hospitalized each year.
  3. Deaths—400 to 500 people died each year, and an additional 1000/y suffered from encephalitis.

- **Reduction in disease/complications after vaccine was available**[a]

  1. Cases—Thanks to vaccination, measles was declared eliminated in the United States in 2000. However, owing to decreased immunization rates, we are seeing a reemergence of this vaccine-preventable disease. In 2014, we saw a record number of 667 cases, the majority of whom were unvaccinated. Of those infected, 1 in 4 will require hospitalization, 1 in 1000 will develop encephalitis, and 1 to 2 in 1000 will die from the disease.
  2. Death—The last measles death occurred in the United States in 2015. However, measles outbreaks in Europe in 2018 have resulted in more than 70 deaths.

---

[a]All data reflect US statistics unless otherwise indicated.

MENINGOCOCCAL DISEASE (MENINGOCOCCAL MENINGITIS AND MENINGOCOCCAL SEPTICEMIA) (FIGURE A10)

- **Common symptoms**
  1. Can begin as a flulike illness (fever, fatigue, headache, etc)
  2. Stiff neck
  3. Nausea/vomiting/diarrhea
  4. Pain with light in the eyes (called photophobia)
  5. Confusion
  6. Severe aches/pains in the joints, muscles, abdomen, or chest
  7. Cold hands/feet and chills
  8. Rapid breathing
  9. Later stages show a dark purplish rash

- **Complications**
  1. Deafness
  2. Seizures and other nervous system problems
  3. Brain damage
  4. Loss of limbs
  5. Death—rapid treatment with appropriate antibiotics is vital as this disease can kill quickly

- **Transmission/contagion**
  1. Transmission is via spread of respiratory and throat secretions (saliva).
  2. Contagion—It takes close or prolonged exposure to contract a meningococcal infection (kissing, sharing utensils, coughing). These bacteria live no more than a few minutes outside the body, so disease is not spread as easily as colds or flu. It is generally contagious from 2 to 10 days before, to about 14 days after symptoms develop (though it could be contagious much longer if the person becomes a carrier).[17] Those exposed to meningococcal disease should receive prophylaxis (preventative antibiotics) as this disease is so dangerous.

- **Vaccine information**
  1. The first meningococcal vaccine was approved in 1978. The current conjugate vaccine (MenACWY) was approved in 2005. The MenB vaccines were licensed in 2014 and 2015.
  2. The meningococcal vaccine contains no active bacteria, therefore it cannot cause meningococcal disease.
  3. The first dose of the conjugate vaccine is recommended at age 11 to 12 years with a booster 5 years later. The conjugate vaccine is also recommended for anyone over 2 months old with certain immune system disorders or who has a damaged or missing spleen, persons with HIV,[18] those working with meningococcal bacteria in laboratories, and those traveling to parts of the world considered part of the "meningitis belt." The MenB vaccine is optional for those ages 16 to 23 years and is recommended for at-risk individuals as outlined above.[19]
  4. The conjugate vaccine is at least 85% effective. The MenB vaccine is 63% to 88% effective.

Continued

- **Impact of meningococcus before vaccine was available[a]**

  1. Cases—Incidence peaked around 1980 when there were approximately 1.50/100,000 cases of meningococcal disease. When the conjugate vaccine was introduced in 2005,[20] there were an average of 0.42/100,000 cases per year.

  2. Deaths—If we use the US census numbers of approximately 226.5 million people in 1980 and if we assume a 15% mortality (see below), the total deaths from meningococcus would be approximately 510 people.

- **Reduction in disease/complications after vaccine was available[a]**

  1. Cases—As of 2016, the case rate was 0.12/100,000. There are rare outbreaks each year, more commonly in dormitory settings. According to immunize.org, in 2016 there were 315 total cases reported.[18]

  2. Death—Of that 2016 group, there were 49 deaths. Without treatment, invasive meningococcal disease is nearly 50% fatal. Even with treatment, 10% to 15% will die from this infection and, of those that survive, 20% will have permanent injury, such as loss of limb, hearing loss, or brain damage.

---

[a]All data reflect US statistics unless otherwise indicated.

MUMPS (FIGURE A11)

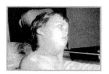

FIGURE A11
Child with mumps. (*Courtesy of Centers for Disease Control and Prevention.* http://www.immunize.org/photos/mumps-photos.asp.)

- **Common symptoms**
    1. Fever
    2. Muscle pain
    3. Fatigue
    4. Headache
    5. Loss of appetite
    6. Swollen and tender salivary glands under the ears on one or both sides (called parotitis)

- **Complications**
    1. Inflammation of the testicles in postpubertal males (called orchitis), which can rarely result in infertility
    2. Inflammation of the covering of the brain and spinal cord (called meningitis)
    3. Inflammation of the brain (called encephalitis)
    4. Inflammation of the ovaries (called oophoritis) and breast tissue (called mastitis)
    5. Higher rates of miscarriage if contracted during pregnancy
    6. Deafness
    7. Death (rare)

- **Transmission/contagion**
    1. Transmission is from saliva or mucous from the mouth, nose, or throat. An infected person can spread the virus by sneezing, coughing, talking, sharing utensils/cups, kissing, or by touching a surface that is then touched by others. People in close quarters (college dorms, prisons, close-knit communities) or with prolonged exposure to someone with mumps is at higher risk for contracting the virus.
    2. Mumps is contagious from a few days prior to 5 days after the glands begin to swell. People diagnosed with mumps are recommended to be isolated for up to 5 days after onset of parotid gland swelling.

- **Vaccine information**
    1. The mumps vaccine first became available in 1963. An improved vaccine was introduced in 1968. In 1971, the mumps vaccine was combined with measles and rubella immunizations in the MMR vaccine.
    2. The MMR vaccine is a live-attenuated virus vaccine. It is safe for people with a healthy immune system but should not be given to those who have immune compromise.
    3. The MMR vaccine is recommended to be given at ages 12 to 15 months and again at 4 to 6 years of age. High-risk groups may receive a booster during outbreaks.
    4. One dose of the mumps vaccine is 78% effective and two doses are approximately 88% effective.

Continued

MUMPS *(Continued)*

- **Impact of mumps before vaccine was available**[a]
  1. Cases—Before the mumps vaccine, there were approximately 186,000 cases reported annually with many more that went unreported.[21]
  2. Death—Luckily, death is very rare, but up to 25% of people will have permanent damage (such as deafness) from a mumps infection.

- **Reduction in disease/complications after vaccine was available**[a]
  1. Cases—Since vaccine, mumps incidence has decreased by 99% but has not been eliminated. There have been periodic outbreaks, largely in communities that are unvaccinated or under-vaccinated and in which there is close and prolonged contact.[22]
  2. Deaths—There have been no reported deaths during recent outbreaks.

---

[a]All data reflect US statistics unless otherwise indicated.

PERTUSSIS (WHOOPING COUGH) (FIGURE A12)

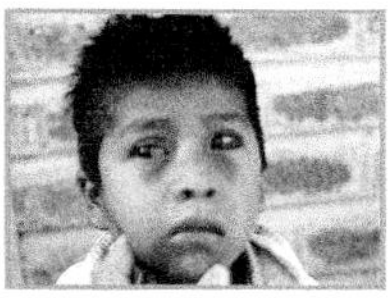

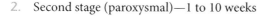

FIGURE A12
Child with pertussis. Note the bruising on the face and broken vessels in the eyes from coughing. (*Courtesy of Centers for Disease Control and Prevention.* http://www.immunize.org/photos/pertussis-photos.asp.)

- **Common symptoms**
  1. First stage (catarrhal)—1 to 2 weeks
     a. Low-grade fever
     b. Runny nose
     c. Mild cough
     d. Apnea (short periods of stopping breathing, primarily seen in infants)
  2. Second stage (paroxysmal)—1 to 10 weeks
     a. Fits of rapid/numerous coughs followed by a "whoop" sound
     b. Vomiting after coughing
     c. Exhaustion from coughing fits
  3. Third stage (convalescent)—weeks to months
     a. Chronic cough

- **Complications**
  1. Respiratory distress/apnea/secondary bacterial pneumonias/pneumothorax
  2. Dehydration/decreased eating (called anorexia)
  3. Nose bleeds, bruising around the eyes/face from forceful coughing
  4. Fractured ribs
  5. Urinary incontinence, rectal prolapse, hernias
  6. Brain bleeding (called a subdural hematoma), seizures, encephalopathy
  7. Death—most deaths occur in infants under 3 months of age

- **Transmission/contagion**
  1. Transmission is via respiratory droplets.
  2. Pertussis is highly contagious: 75% to 100% of unimmunized household contacts of someone with pertussis will contract the infection.[23] It is contagious from 7 days after exposure to the bacteria until 3 weeks after the onset of coughing spasms. People are most contagious during the first (catarrhal) stage of the illness. Initially thought a disease of childhood, studies show that adults represent 25% of all cases. Symptoms are milder and often go undiagnosed, leading to easier spread to infants/children if the illness is not treated.

- **Vaccine information**
  1. The first pertussis inactivated toxoid was developed in 1921 but not widely used until the 1930s. The first pertussis vaccine was developed in the 1930s but not widely used until the 1940s when it was combined with the diphtheria and tetanus vaccines in the DTP vaccine.[24]
  2. The pertussis (in the combined DTaP or Tdap) is a killed virus vaccine.
  3. The DTaP is recommended at ages 2, 4, and 6 months, and at 15 to 18 months. The first Tdap is recommended at the age of 11 to 12 years. Pregnant women should receive Tdap with every pregnancy (preferably between 27 and 36 weeks' gestation). Tdap is also recommended for those who will be in close contact with infants.

Continued

4. The pertussis vaccine is about 80% to 90% effective. However, it has fairly rapidly waning immunity such that by 4 years after the vaccine, only 3 to 4 out of 10 people will still be protected. Keeping up-to-date with the recommended vaccine schedule is the best way to protect our loved ones and ourselves.[25]

- **Impact of pertussis before vaccine was available**[a]

  1. Cases—Prior to vaccine, there were more than 200,000 cases each year in the United States.[26]
  2. Deaths—About 9,000 children died yearly in the United States from pertussis.

- **Reduction in disease/complications after vaccine was available**[a]

  1. Cases—After vaccine, the case rate dropped to less than 3000 per year in the 1980s. However, we are seeing resurgence with approximately 48,000 cases in 2012, 24,000 cases in 2013, and 33,000 cases in 2014.
  2. Deaths—2017 estimates show 15,808 reported cases with 13 deaths.[27]

---

[a]All data reflect US statistics unless otherwise indicated.

PNEUMOCOCCAL DISEASE (FIGURE A13)

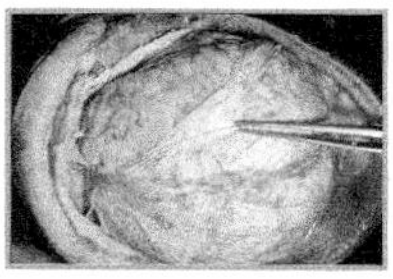

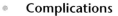

FIGURE A13
Pneumococcal meningitis. (© *World Health Organization. Found at* http://www.immunize.org/photos/polio-photos.asp.)

- **Common symptoms—symptoms depend on what part of the body is affected by infection**
  1. Ear infection—ear pain, fever, sleepiness
  2. Sinus infection—headache, face/teeth pain, fever, loss of appetite, fatigue
  3. Pneumonia—cough, fever, difficulty breathing, chest pain
  4. Bacteremia/sepsis—fever, chills, confusion, lethargy, high heart rate, shortness of breath, body pain
  5. Meningitis—headache, light sensitivity, confusion, fever, stiff neck

- **Complications**
  1. Middle ear infections
  2. Sinus infections
  3. Pneumonia
  4. Bacteremia (bloodstream infection) and sepsis (the body's response to an infection, which can cause organ failure, tissue damage, and death)
  5. Infection of the covering of the brain and spinal cord (called meningitis)
  6. Death—The young and the elderly are at greatest risk for invasive pneumococcal disease. 1 in 5 children with meningitis will die; 1 in 100 children with bacteremia will die[28]; and 5 to 7 in 100 people with pneumococcal pneumonia will die from their infection (this rate is estimated to be as high as 50% in those older than 65 years of age)[29]

- **Transmission/contagion**
  1. Transmission is via respiratory droplets.
  2. A person infected with pneumococcus is contagious until they are treated with antibiotics for 24 hours.

- **Vaccine information**
  1. The first pneumococcal polysaccharide vaccine was introduced in 1977. An improved version (PPSV23), containing 23 serotypes of pneumococcus, was licensed in 1983. The first pneumococcal conjugate vaccine was licensed in 2000 and improved in 2010 (PCV13), now containing 13 serotypes of pneumococcus.
  2. Both the polysaccharide and conjugate vaccines are killed virus vaccines.
  3. PCV13 is given at ages 2, 4, and 6 months, and at 12 to 15 months of age. It is also recommended once after 65 years of age or prior to 65 years of age in adults at greater risk of infection (those with immune suppression, for example). PPSV23 is recommended once for all adults of 65 years of age or older and those of 2 years of age and older with long-term health problems, immune suppression, asthma, tobacco use, etc.
  4. PPSV23 vaccine is about 50% to 80% effective in preventing invasive disease (blood infections and meningitis). The elderly and immune compromised don't mount as strong of a response but it is still recommended that they get the vaccine because they are at such high risk of severe consequences.

Continued

- **Impact of pneumococcal disease before vaccine was available[a]**
    1. Cases—Before pneumococcal vaccines for children in the United States, pneumococcus caused about 3000 cases of meningitis, 50,000 cases of bacteremia, and 500,000 cases of pneumonia.[30]
    2. Deaths–Before vaccine, there were approximately 1 million deaths annually worldwide from invasive pneumococcal disease.

- **Reduction in disease/complications after vaccine was available[a]**
    1. Cases—In 2012, there were an estimated 31,600 cases of invasive pneumococcal disease.
    2. Deaths—In 2012, there were an estimated 3300 deaths from invasive pneumococcal disease, many occurring in adults for whom routine pneumococcal vaccination was recommended.

---

[a]All data reflect US statistics unless otherwise indicated.

POLIOMYELITIS (FIGURE A14)

- **Common symptoms—72/100 people infected will *not* have symptoms**
  1. Headache
  2. Stomach pain
  3. Fever
  4. Nausea
  5. Fatigue
  6. Sore throat

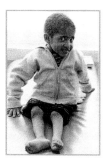

FIGURE A14
Boy with polio. (© *World Health Organization*. Found at http://www.immunize.org/photos/polio-photos.asp.)

- **Complications**
  1. Pins and needles feelings in the legs (called paresthesias)
  2. Infection of the covering of the brain and spinal cord (called meningitis)
  3. Inability to move parts of the body (called paralysis)—most commonly the arms and legs; paralysis of the breathing muscles can result in death
  4. 15 to 40 years after initial infection has resolved, new muscle pain, weakness, and paralysis (called postpolio syndrome [PPS]) can develop

- **Transmission/contagion**
  1. Transmission is through fecal (stool) contamination or, less often, through contact with respiratory droplets.
  2. Polio is highly contagious. Approximately 90% to 100% of unvaccinated household contacts of someone with polio will contract the infection.[31] It is contagious from 7 to 10 days before developing symptoms to 7 to 10 days after, though poliovirus can be excreted in stools for up to 6 weeks. It can contaminate food and water in unsanitary conditions. Those infected with polio who do not develop symptoms can still pass the illness to others.

- **Vaccine information**
  1. The inactivated polio vaccine (IPV) was introduced in 1955 with an enhanced version licensed in 1987. The oral poliovirus vaccine (OPV) was introduced in 1963.
  2. IPV is a killed virus vaccine. OPV is a live-attenuated (or weakened) virus vaccine and should not be used in those with a weakened immune system.[32] Owing to near elimination of polio in the United States with the only recent cases being linked to infection with vaccine-associated paralytic polio, use of the OPV vaccine was discontinued in 2000 with IPV now being used exclusively.
  3. The IPV vaccine is recommended at ages 2, 4, and 6 to 18 months, and again at 4 to 6 years of age.
  4. The polio vaccine is 99% to 100% effective after receiving at least three doses in the series.[33]

Continued

- **Impact of polio before vaccine was available**[a]
  1. Cases—Before the vaccine, there were approximately 25,000 cases of polio each year. In the 1916 epidemic, 27,000 people were paralyzed and 6000 died.
  2. Deaths—5% to 15% of patients with paralytic polio will die from their illness.

- **Reduction in disease/complications after vaccine was available**[a]
  1. Cases—As of 1979, there were only 10 cases of polio in the United States. There have been no cases originating in the United States since 1979.[34] Polio does still exist in other parts of the world, however. The last reported US case was in 1993 and was brought in by a traveler from another country.[35] With ease of travel, polio could be easily reintroduced if we don't maintain high levels of vaccination. There is hope for global eradication someday. Until then, we have to stay vigilant in our vaccination efforts.
  2. Deaths—There have been no reported deaths from polio in the United States in many years. However, rates of PPS are on the rise. Incidence in the United States of PPS in previous acute polio patients ranges from 22% to 68%.[36]

---

[a]All data reflect US statistics unless otherwise indicated.

ROTAVIRUS (FIGURE A15)

- **Common symptoms**
    1. Fever
    2. Vomiting
    3. Watery diarrhea
    4. Abdominal pain

- **Complications**
    1. Severe dehydration with its associated complications (kidney failure, heart arrhythmias, shock, etc.)
    2. Death

- **Transmission/contagion**
    1. Transmission is via the fecal-oral (stool-mouth) route and the virus can remain on surfaces for weeks if not properly sanitized.
    2. Rotavirus is contagious from 2 days before onset of symptoms until up to 10 days after symptoms resolve.[37] There are different types of rotavirus, so having had a prior infection does not necessarily prevent future infection (though subsequent infections are usually less severe).

- **Vaccine information**
    1. The rotavirus vaccine was licensed in 1998 but was withdrawn in 1999 because of an association with a type of bowel obstruction called intussusception. A newer and safer vaccine was introduced in 2006. A second brand was made available in 2008.
    2. The rotavirus vaccine is a live-attenuated (weakened) virus vaccine. It should not be given to those with a weakened immune system.
    3. The RotaTeq vaccine is given orally at ages 2, 4, and 6 months. The Rotarix is a two-dose series given at ages 2 and 4 months.[38]
    4. The vaccine is 85% to 98% effective against severe rotavirus disease and 74% to 87% effective against rotavirus of any severity through a child's first rotavirus season. It is also highly effective (96%) at decreasing rates of hospitalizations.

- **Impact of rotavirus before vaccine was available**[a]
    1. Cases—Prior to vaccine availability, rotavirus was responsible for approximately 3 million cases per year, more than 400,000 doctor visits, 200,000 emergency department visits, and up to 70,000 hospitalizations yearly.[38]
    2. Deaths—20 to 60 deaths occurred yearly, with infants and children most at risk.

- **Reduction in disease/complications after vaccine was available**[a]
    1. Cases—In children younger than 5 years of age, the incidence of rotavirus gastroenteritis after vaccine introduction was 16% to 45% lower than in the pre-vaccine era (depending on the year).[39] It was even more effective in reducing rotavirus hospitalizations (63%-94% decline seen).
    2. Deaths—Mexico was one of the first countries to receive the rotavirus vaccine in 2006[40] and studies of death rates in the pre- and post-vaccine eras show up to 41% reduction in mortality post-vaccine.

---

[a]All data reflect US statistics unless otherwise indicated.

RUBELLA (FIGURE A16)

- **Common symptoms—20% to 50% of people infected will have no symptoms**
  1. Fever
  2. Headache
  3. Mild pink eye
  4. Sore throat and swollen lymph nodes
  5. Cough and runny nose
  6. Followed by rash—typically starts on the face then spreads to the rest of the body, lasting about 3 days

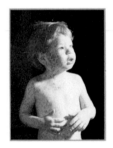

FIGURE A16
Child with rubella rash. (*Courtesy of Centers for Disease Control and Prevention*. http://www.immunize.org/photos/rubella-photos.asp.)

- **Complications**
  1. 70% of women who get rubella will develop painful, swollen joints (called arthritis)
  2. Brain infection (called encephalitis)
  3. Bleeding problems
  4. If contracted during pregnancy, there are higher rates of miscarriage and infant mortality after birth. The virus can also pass to the developing baby, causing a group of birth defects known as congenital rubella syndrome (CRS).
     a. Loss of vision and hearing, heart problems, liver or spleen damage, and intellectual disability

- **Transmission/contagion**
  1. Transmission is via respiratory droplets (coughing/sneezing) and from mother to fetus if contracted during pregnancy.
  2. It is contagious from 1 week before the rash appears to 1 week after.[41] Infants with CRS can shed the virus for up to 1 year.

- **Vaccine information**
  1. The rubella vaccine was licensed in 1969 and the currently used vaccine became available in 1979. It is administered in combination with the measles and mumps vaccines in the MMR vaccine.
  2. It is a live-attenuated virus vaccine and should not be given to those with compromised immune systems.
  3. The first dose is given at 12 to 15 months and the second dose at 4 to 6 years of age.
  4. The vaccine is highly effective. One dose offers up to 97% protection against rubella.[42]

- **Impact of rubella before vaccine was available[a]**
  1. Cases—From 1964 to 1965, there were approximately 12.5 million cases of rubella in the United States with 20,000 cases of CRS.[42]
  2. Deaths—During those same years, there were 2100 neonatal deaths and more than 11,000 abortions—some spontaneous and some elected (after learning of the 50% to 90% risk of CRS if the mother was infected in the first trimester).[43]

---

[a]All data reflect US statistics unless otherwise indicated

RUBELLA *(Continued)*

- **Reduction in disease/complications after vaccine was available[a]**
  1. Cases—From 2005 to 2011, there were a median of 11 cases per year. Endogenous transmission (originating in the United States) ended in 2004.[44] From 2004 to 2012, there were only six cases of CRS reported in the United States.
  2. Deaths—During those same years, there were a total of six deaths recorded by the Centers for Disease Control and Prevention.[3]

---

[a]All data reflect US statistics unless otherwise indicated

HERPES ZOSTER (SHINGLES) (FIGURE A17)

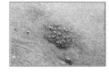

- **Common symptoms**
  1. Viral symptoms (fever, headache, malaise, upset stomach, chills, etc.)
  2. Itching/tingling
  3. Burning/pain
  4. Followed by development of a blistering rash along the distribution of a nerve, occurring on only one side of the body

- **Complications**
  1. Postherpetic neuralgia—a condition more common as we age where the pain of shingles (which can be severe and devastating) lasts years beyond resolution of the shingles rash
  2. Vision loss if shingles affects the nerves in and around the eye
  3. Rarely, shingles can lead to pneumonia, hearing loss, brain inflammation (called encephalitis), or death

- **Transmission/contagion**
  1. Shingles is not transmitted in the ways we think of with other infections. Shingles is a result of the chickenpox virus that lives on in our nerve roots even after the chickenpox illness has resolved. During stress or periods where the immune system is weakened, the virus can become active along a nerve and can result in an outbreak of shingles.
  2. Shingles is only contagious to those who have never had chickenpox or who have a significantly weakened immune system, and only then by coming into direct contact with fluid from the blisters. In these people, contact can result in an outbreak of chickenpox, not shingles. Shingles is not contagious before the blisters appear or after they have scabbed over. It can take up to 3 weeks for blisters to crust over.

- **Vaccine information**
  1. The Zostavax vaccine was licensed in 2006. Shingrix was licensed in 2017 and is now the preferred option.[45]
  2. The Zostavax vaccine is a live-attenuated (weakened) virus vaccine and should not be given to anyone whose immune system is compromised. The Shingrix vaccine is a killed virus vaccine and can be given to anyone.
  3. The Zostavax vaccine was recommended as a one-time injection starting at 60 years of age. Shingrix is a two-shot series (given at time 0 and then again 2-6 months later) and can be given as early as 50 years of age.
  4. The Zostavax vaccine is only about 51% effective in reducing rates of shingles and is about 66% effective in decreasing the incidence of postherpetic neuralgia. By 6 years after vaccination, protection from Zostavax declined to about 35%.[46] The Shingrix vaccine is closer to 90% to 97% effective, and immunity remains high at around 85%, 4 years out from vaccination.

- **Impact of herpes zoster before vaccine was available[a]**

  1. Cases—There are approximately 1 million cases annually in the United States. One in three people in the United States will develop shingles in their lifetime, 10% to 15% of those people will develop postherpetic neuralgia.[47] Shingles is an illness primarily of the elderly, however it does occur in children and young adults.
  2. Hospitalizations—1% to 4% of people with shingles will be hospitalized for complications.
  3. Deaths—There are approximately 96 deaths per year from herpes zoster.

- **Reduction in disease/complications after vaccine was available[a]**

  1. Cases—Rates of shingles are generally increasing over the decades, but rates of shingles in children have been declining since initiation of routine chickenpox vaccination.[48] Because the chickenpox vaccine is a live-attenuated virus vaccine, it can cause a latent (dormant) infection, which can later become reactive and cause shingles. However, shingles more commonly develops after infection with the wild-type virus that causes chickenpox than with the vaccine-strain virus.

---

[a]All data reflect US statistics unless otherwise indicated.

TETANUS (FIGURE A18)

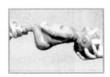

- **Common symptoms**
  1. Spasm of the jaw muscles (called "lockjaw")
  2. Painful muscle stiffness over the body
  3. Sudden involuntary muscle spasms, often abdominal
  4. Headache
  5. Fever and sweats
  6. Jerking or staring spells
  7. Rapid heart rate and changes in blood pressure

- **Complications**
  1. Broken bones (fractures) from severe muscle spasms
  2. Uncontrolled tightening of the vocal cords (called laryngospasm)
  3. Infections acquired during hospitalization
  4. Blood clots in the lungs that have traveled from other parts of the body (called a pulmonary embolism)
  5. Aspiration pneumonia
  6. Respiratory distress
  7. Death—today, 1 to 2 out of 10 people infected will die from their illness[49]

- **Transmission/contagion**
  1. Tetanus spores enter the body through injuries from objects contaminated with dirt, stool, or saliva—most commonly puncture wounds (metal, animal bites, etc), burns, and crush injuries.
  2. Tetanus is not contagious from person to person.

- **Vaccine information**
  1. Tetanus toxoid was first introduced in 1924 and became available in the United States in the 1940s.[50]
  2. It is a killed virus vaccine.
  3. The vaccine is recommended to be given at ages 2, 4, and 6 months, age 15 to 18 months, and at age 4 to 6 years. Immunity wanes and a booster is recommended every 10 years for life.
  4. The complete vaccine series has an estimated efficacy of 100%.

- **Impact of tetanus before vaccine was available[a]**
  1. Cases—In the late 1940s, there were approximately 500 to 600 cases of tetanus per year in the United States.[50]
  2. Deaths—Of those cases, there were an average of 472 deaths from tetanus reported.[51,52]

- **Reduction in disease/complications after vaccine was available[a]**
  1. Cases—Reported cases of tetanus have declined more than 95%.
  2. Deaths—Deaths from tetanus have decreased more than 99%.

---

[a]All data reflect US statistics unless otherwise indicated.

References

1. Centers for Disease Control and Prevention. Chickenpox (Varicella) – Monitoring the Impact of Varicella Vaccination. https://www.cdc.gov/chickenpox/surveillance/monitoring-varicella.html. Accessed January 17, 2019.

2. Centers for Disease Control and Prevention. Diphtheria – Clinicians. https://www.cdc.gov/diphtheria/clinicians.html. Accessed January 17, 2019.

3. Centers for Disease Control and Prevention. Appendix E. Reported cases and deaths from vaccine preventable diseases, United States. In: Atkinson W, Wolfe S, Hamborsky J, McIntyre L, eds. *Epidemiology and Prevention of Vaccine-Preventable Diseases.* 13th ed. Washington DC: Public Health Foundation; 2015.

4. Centers for Disease Control and Prevention. Haemophilus influenza B. In: Atkinson W, Wolfe S, Hamborsky J, McIntyre L, eds. *Epidemiology and Prevention of Vaccine-Preventable Diseases.* 13th ed. Washington DC: Public Health Foundation; 2015.

5. North Carolina Department of Health and Human Services. Diseases & Topics: Haemophilus Influenzae Infection. https://epi.publichealth.nc.gov/cd/diseases/hib.html. Updated May 23, 2018. Accessed January 19, 2019.

6. Immunization Coalition. Hepatitis A – Questions and Answers. www.immunize.org/Catg.d/p4204.pdf. Accessed January 17, 2019.

7. Centers for Disease Control and Prevention. Viral Hepatitis – Hepatitis B Questions and Answers for the Public. https://www.cdc.gov/hepatitis/hbv/bfaq.htm. Updated May 22, 2018. Accessed January 17, 2019.

8. Hepatitis B. Atkinson W, Wolfe S, Hamborsky J, McIntyre L, eds. Centers for Disease Control and Prevention. *Epidemiology and Prevention of Vaccine-Preventable Diseases.* 13th ed. Washington DC: Public Health Foundation; 2015.

9. National Cancer Institute. Human Papillomavirus (HPV) Vaccine. https://www.cancer.gov/about-cancer/causes-prevention/risk/infectious-agents/HPV-vaccine-fact-sheet. Accessed January 17, 2019.

10. Centers for Disease Control and Prevention. Human Papillomavirus (HPV) – Genital HPV Infection – Fact Sheet. https://www.cdc.gov/std/HPV/stdfact-HPV.htm. Accessed January 17, 2019.

11. Lee L, Garland SM. Human papillomavirus vaccination: the population impact. *F1000Res.* 2017;6:866. https://www.ncbi.nlm.nih.gov/pmc/articles/PMC5473416/. Accessed March 19, 2019

12. Doshi P. Trends in recorded influenza mortality: United States, 1900-2004. *Am J Public Health.* 2008;98(5):939-945.

13. Centers for Disease Control and Prevention. Influenza (flu) – Disease burden of Influenza. https://www.cdc.gov/flu/about/disease/burden.htm. Updated January 11, 2019. Accessed January 17, 2019.

14. Centers for Disease Control and Prevention. Measles (Rubeola) – Complications of Measles. March 3, 2017. https://www.cdc.gov/measles/about/complications.html. Accessed January 17, 2019.

15. Centers for Disease Control and Prevention. Measles (Rubeola) – Transmission of measles. https://www.cdc.gov/measles/about/transmission.html. Updated March 3, 2017. Accessed January 17, 2010.

16. Centers for Disease Control and Prevention. *Vaccines and Preventable Diseases – Measles, Mumps, and Rubella (MMR) Vaccination: What Everyone Should Know.* February 2, 2018. https://www.cdc.gov/vaccines/vpd/MMR/public/index.html. Accessed January 17, 2019

17. Centers for Disease Control and Prevention. Meningococcal disease. In: Atkinson W, Wolfe S, Hamborsky J, McIntyre L, eds. *Epidemiology and Prevention of Vaccine-Preventable Diseases.* 13th ed. Washington DC: Public Health Foundation; 2015.

18. Immunization Action Coalition. Meningococcal – Questions and Answers. www.immunize.org/Catg.d/p4210.pdf. Accessed January 17, 2019.

19. The College of Physicians of Philadelphia. Meningococcal Disease. https://www.historyofvaccines.org/content/articles/meningococcal-disease. Updated January 25, 2018. Accessed January 17, 2019.

20. Centers for Disease Control and Prevention. Meningococcal Disease – Surveillance. https://www.cdc.gov/meningococcal/surveillance/index.html. Updated November 21, 2018. Accessed January 17, 2019.

21. Centers for Disease Control and Prevention. Mumps – For Healthcare Providers. https://www.cdc.gov/mumps/hcp.html. Updated February 16, 2018. Accessed January 17, 2019.

22. The College of Physicians of Philadelphia. Mumps. https://www.historyofvaccines.org/content/articles/mumps. Updated January 25, 2018. Accessed January 17, 2019.

23. Cunha JP. Whooping Cough (Pertussis). eMedicineHealth. https://www.emedicinehealth.com/whooping_cough_pertussis/article_em.htm#self-care_at_home_for_whooping_cough. Accessed January 17, 2019.

24. Immunization Action Coalition. Pertussis (Whooping Cough): Questions and Answers. www.immunize.org/Catg.d/p4212.pdf. Accessed January 18, 2019.

25. Centers for Disease Control and Prevention. Pertussis (Whooping Cough) – Pertussis Frequently Asked Questions. https://www.cdc.gov/pertussis/about/faqs.html. Updated August 7, 2017. Accessed January 17, 2019.

26. Centers for Disease Control and Prevention. Pertussis. In: Atkinson W, Wolfe S, Hamborsky J, McIntyre L, eds. *Epidemiology and Prevention of Vaccine-Preventable Diseases*. 13th ed. Washington DC: Public Health Foundation; 2015.

27. Centers for Disease Control and Prevention. *2017 Final Pertussis Surveillance Report*. December 2018. https://www.cdc.gov/pertussis/downloads/pertuss-surv-report-2017.pdf. Accessed January 17, 2019.

28. Centers for Disease Control and Prevention. Pneumococcal Disease – Symptoms and Complications. https://www.cdc.gov/pneumococcal/about/symptoms-complications.html. Updated September 6, 2017. Accessed January 17, 2019.

29. Immunization Action Coalition. Pneumococcus – Questions and Answers. www.immunize.org/catg.d/p4213.pdf. Accessed January 17, 2019.

30. Tram PI, Madoff LC, Coombes B. Invasive pneumococcal disease after implementation of 13-valent conjugate vaccine. *Pediatrics*. 2014;134(2):210-217.

31. European Centre for Disease Prevention and Control. Disease Factsheet About Poliomyelitis. https://ecdc.europa.eu/en/poliomyelitis/facts. Updated July 11, 2018. Accessed January 17, 2019..

32. Centers for Disease Control and Prevention. Poliomyelitis. In: Atkinson W, Wolfe S, Hamborsky J, McIntyre L, eds. *Epidemiology and Prevention of Vaccine-Preventable Diseases*. 13th ed. Washington DC: Public Health Foundation; 2015.

33. Centers for Disease Control and Prevention. Vaccines and Preventable Diseases – Polio Vaccine Effectiveness and Duration Of Protection. https://www.cdc.gov/vaccines/vpd/polio/hcp/effectiveness-duration-protection.html. Updated May 4, 2018. Accessed January 17, 2019.

34. Immunization Action Coalition. *Polio Vaccine: What You Need to Know*. November 8, 2011. www.immunize.org/vis/ipv-00.pdf. Accessed January 17, 2019.

35. Centers for Disease Control and Prevention. Polio Elimination in the United States. https://www.cdc.gov/polio/us/. Accessed January 17, 2019.

36. Kedlaya D. Postpolio Syndrome. Medscape. https://emedicine.medscape.com/article/306920-overview#a5. Updated August 14, 2017. Accessed January 18, 2019.

37. Mayo Clinic. Rotavirus. https://www.mayoclinic.org/diseases-conditions/rotavirus/symptoms-causes/syc-20351300. Accessed January 17, 2019.

38. Immunization Action Coalition. Rotavirus: Questions and Answers. www.immunize.org/catg.d/p4217.pdf. Accessed January 18, 2019.

39. Centers for Disease Control and Prevention. *Rotavirus*. In: Payne DC, Parashar UD. *Manual for the Surveillance of Vaccine-Preventable Diseases*. Atlanta GA; 2018:Chap 13.

40. Richardson V, Hernandez-Pichardo J, Quintanar-Solares M, et al. Effect of rotavirus vaccination on death from childhood diarrhea in Mexico. *N Engl J Med*. 2010;362(4):299-305.

41. Centers for Disease Control and Prevention. Rubella (German Measles, Three-Day Measles) – Transmission. https://www.cdc.gov/rubella/about/transmission.html. Updated March 31, 2016. Accessed January 17, 2019.

42. Centers for Disease Control and Prevention. Rubella (German Measles, Three-Day Measles) – Rubella Vaccination. https://www.cdc.gov/rubella/vaccination.html. Updated July 11, 2016. Accessed January 17, 2019.

43. The College of Physicians of Philadelphia. Rubella. https://www.historyofvaccines.org/content/articles/rubella. Updated April 12, 2017. Accessed January 17, 2019.

44. Centers for Disease Control and Prevention. Rubella. In: Atkinson W, Wolfe S, Hamborsky J, McIntyre L, eds. *Epidemiology and Prevention of Vaccine-Preventable Diseases*. 13th ed. Washington DC: Public Health Foundation; 2015.

45. Centers for Disease Control and Prevention. Vaccines and Preventable Diseases – What Everyone Should Know About Zostavax. https://www.cdc.gov/vaccines/vpd/shingles/public/Zostavax/index.html. Updated June 18, 2018. Accessed January 17, 2019.

46. Zussman J, Young L. Zoster vaccine live for the prevention of shingles in the elderly patient. *Clin Interv Aging.* 2008;3(2):241-250.

47. Centers for Disease Control and Prevention. Shingles (Herpes Zoster) – Shingles Surveillance. https://www.cdc.gov/shingles/surveillance.html. Updated February 23, 2018. Accessed January 18, 2019.

48. Centers for Disease Control and Prevention. Shingles (Herpes Zoster) – Clinical Overview. https://www.cdc.gov/shingles/hcp/clinical-overview.html.

49. Centers for Disease Control and Prevention. Tetanus – Symptoms and Complications. https://www.cdc.gov/tetanus/about/symptoms-complications.html. Updated January 10, 2017. Accessed January 19, 2019.

50. Centers for Disease Control and Prevention. Tetanus. In: Atkinson W, Wolfe S, Hamborsky J, McIntyre L, eds. *Epidemiology and Prevention of Vaccine-Preventable Diseases.* 13th ed. Washington DC: Public Health Foundation; 2015.

51. Centers for Disease Control and Prevention; American Academy of Family Physicians; American Academy of Pediatrics. Tetanus: Also Known As Lockjaw. https://www.dshs.texas.gov/IDCU/disease/tetanus/Tetanus-fact-sheet.doc. Updated March 2011. Accessed January 17, 2019.

52. Roush SW, Murphy TV; Vaccine-Preventable Disease Table Working Group. Historical comparisons of morbidity and mortality for vaccine-preventable diseases in the United States. *JAMA.* 2007;298(18):2155-2163.

Fast Facts About Vaccines for Patients and Clinic Staff

GENERAL VACCINE INFORMATION

1. Vaccines are the single greatest public health success story we've ever seen.
2. Millions of lives and billions of dollars are saved worldwide because of vaccination.
3. Vaccine-preventable diseases have been reduced by 92% to 100% (depending on the illness) because of vaccines.
4. However, vaccine-preventable diseases are returning in large part because of misinformation about the safety and efficacy of vaccines, driven by a vocal anti-vaccine minority.
5. In recent years, there have been an increasing number of vaccine-preventable disease outbreaks across the country, including a mumps outbreak in Washington state; a measles outbreak in Minneapolis; a pertussis (whooping cough) outbreak in Southern Idaho; and current measles outbreaks in New York, brought back to the state by travelers to Israel; and in Washington state and Texas, among others. Other areas around the world have not been spared. Australia recently saw a case of diphtheria, a disease thought eradicated from that country; and in 2018, Europe saw tens of thousands of cases of measles in unvaccinated or under-vaccinated communities, leading to more than 70 deaths.
6. Vaccines are safe! The rates of harm from a vaccine are *significantly* lower than rates of harm from the illness itself. Serious events (such as stopping breathing, paralysis, etc) occurs only 1 to 2 times in 1 million people vaccinated.
7. Numerous studies show *no* connection between vaccines and autism.
8. Rates of autism have actually *increased* since thimerosal (an ethylmercury-containing preservative) was removed from all US-licensed vaccines (except multidose flu) in 2001.
9. For most vaccine-preventable illnesses, we are contagious some number of days *before* we see any symptoms. This is how these infections spread so easily.
10. It is important that vaccines be given on schedule to provide full immunity, decreasing the risk of disease outbreaks due to absent or incomplete immunity.
11. When we vaccinate ourselves and our children, we are also protecting others from vaccine-preventable disease—this is called *herd immunity* or *community immunity*.

12. Some people cannot get certain vaccines (people with compromised immune systems should not get live-attenuated vaccines, for example). They rely on herd immunity to keep them healthy.

13. Depending on the illness, more than 80% to 90% community vaccination is required in order to prevent disease outbreaks (for example, measles requires more than 95% herd immunity to prevent outbreaks). When rates of vaccination fall below these levels, we are all at risk.

14. There are fewer viral and bacterial proteins in the vaccines we give now than in those that were given in prior years—less than 200 in the 14 childhood vaccines given today compared with more than 3000 in the 7 vaccines given in 1980. Vaccines are not going to overwhelm our children's immune systems. They are exposed to many more proteins crawling around on the floor than they are ever exposed to in a series of vaccines.

15. As for the formaldehyde, aluminum, and other substances that are used in vaccine production, their presence in vaccines is *much* below risk levels. In the case of formaldehyde, we have more of this substance in our bodies naturally than we get in vaccines. And as for aluminum, babies get more aluminum from breastfeeding than they do in vaccines.

16. Killed virus vaccines contain *no* live/active viral proteins, so they *cannot* give you the illness they are meant to protect against.

17. Live-attenuated, or weakened, vaccines *could* cause illness in someone with a weakened immune system.

18. Mild to moderate redness, swelling, and pain at the injection site are common symptoms following vaccination. Even a low-grade fever can be within the realm of a "normal" response. When people feel under the weather after a vaccine, this is just their immune system revving up in response to the immunization.

19. It is important to continue vaccinating for illnesses that we no longer, or rarely, see in the United States (such as polio), because these vaccine-preventable illnesses are still present in other countries. These days, people travel between countries with ease and infection can readily be reintroduced if we don't maintain a high enough rate of vaccination.

INFLUENZA AND THE FLU VACCINE

1. Influenza ("the flu") is a respiratory infection (rarely causing nausea and vomiting in kids).

2. The "stomach flu" is not the flu and is, therefore, *not* prevented by the flu shot.

3. The flu shot is a killed virus vaccine. It cannot give you the flu.

4. The flu nasal spray is a live-attenuated vaccine. It could give the flu to someone with a weakened immune system.

5. It takes 2 weeks for the flu shot to work, so it is important to get the shot *before* flu season begins (typically October/November to April/May).

6. Egg allergy is no longer a contraindication to getting the flu shot. See the new guidelines or talk to your provider for specifics based on type of allergic reaction.

7. Even though the flu shot doesn't always prevent the flu (no vaccine is 100% effective), it significantly decreases the chance of dying of the flu.

8. Depending on the year, from 12,000 to 56,000 people die of the flu annually. In 2018, 80,000 people died of the flu; 185 were children.

9. Of those who die, greater than 80% were not vaccinated.

10. Although the flu does affect infants, the elderly, pregnant women, and the immune compromised more significantly, studies show that nearly 50% of kids who die of the flu were completely healthy to start.

11. Pregnant women should receive the flu shot to protect themselves and to pass protective antibodies to their newborn baby who cannot get the flu vaccine until age 6 months.
12. If a woman contracts the flu during pregnancy, rates of miscarriage and preterm labor increase.

WHOOPING COUGH AND THE PERTUSSIS VACCINE

1. Pertussis causes whooping cough, an illness that results in a prolonged cough in adults (commonly known as the 100-day cough). Whooping cough can kill babies.
2. The pertussis vaccine is only available in combination with the tetanus and diphtheria vaccines (DTaP and Tdap).
3. Protection from the vaccine and from a natural infection eventually wears off. It is possible to get pertussis again after natural infection.
4. In order to protect the infant, a Tdap vaccine is recommended to be given to the pregnant mother with *every* pregnancy, ideally between 27 and 36 weeks' gestation.
5. Anyone who will be around a newborn is recommended to have the Tdap vaccine as well.

MEASLES, MUMPS, AND RUBELLA AND THE MMR VACCINE

1. Even with medical advances, of children younger than 5 years of age who contract measles, 1 in 4 will need hospitalization, 1 in 1000 will develop brain inflammation that can cause permanent brain damage, and 1 to 2 in 1000 will die of the illness.
2. Mumps can cause brain inflammation, deafness, and inflammation of the ovaries and testes, which can contribute to infertility.
3. Rubella in pregnancy can commonly cause pregnancy loss or congenital rubella syndrome in the infant.
4. If you were born before 1957, you are presumed to have natural immunity to measles, mumps, and rubella (MMR).
5. You are considered immune to MMR if you have received two MMR vaccines.
6. If you are unsure of your immunity status, you could be tested for antibody levels or you could receive an MMR booster.
7. If there is an outbreak in your community, talk to your medical provider about what steps are necessary to keep you and your family safe.

ROTAVIRUS AND THE ROTAVIRUS VACCINE

1. Rotavirus is an intestinal virus transmitted through the fecal-oral (stool-mouth) route.
2. It is a common virus in day-care settings and spreads easily among children in groups.
3. Symptoms include high fever and watery diarrhea that can last up to a week.
4. If severe, diarrhea can result in dehydration, imbalance of electrolytes, and acid-base disturbances that can require hospitalization and could result in death.

HEPATITIS A AND THE HEPATITIS A VACCINE

1. Hepatitis A is a food-borne liver infection. It is common in other countries, but in the United States, it is usually transmitted by food handlers.
2. It does not cause chronic liver disease, like hepatitis B and C, but can cause severe acute illness with nausea, vomiting, diarrhea, dehydration, abdominal pain, and yellowing of the skin, urine, and stool (called jaundice). Symptoms usually last no longer than 2 months but occasionally will have an on-and-off-again pattern lasting up to 6 months. Rarely, it can cause liver failure, which can result in death.
3. There is no treatment for hepatitis A, other than supportive measures.

HEPATITIS B AND THE HEPATITIS B VACCINE

1. Hepatitis B is spread by blood and body fluids. Blood contact could be as simple as sharing a razor or toothbrush. We think of this as a sexually transmitted infection, but "body fluids" include tears and saliva. If a child gets a bite at day care, they can contract hepatitis B.
2. Hepatitis B is a virus that can cause liver failure and liver cancer if it becomes a chronic infection.
3. Of babies who contract hepatitis B in infancy, 9 out of 10 will go on to have chronic hepatitis B. This is why we give hepatitis B vaccine (HBV) in the routine pediatric schedule.

HAEMOPHILUS INFLUENZAE TYPE B AND THE HIB VACCINE

1. *Haemophilus influenzae* type B (Hib) infection, along with pneumococcal disease, is one of the most common causes of childhood and adult infections, including ear infections, bronchitis, and sinus infections.
2. Hib infections can become "invasive" and cause severe illness, such as meningitis, epiglottitis (swelling of the epiglottis causing breathing/swallowing trouble), pneumonia, cellulitis (skin infection), and septic arthritis (joint infections). These can be deadly despite appropriate treatment.

VARICELLA ZOSTER (CHICKENPOX) AND THE CHICKENPOX VACCINE

1. Chickenpox is a highly contagious virus that results in a blistering, itchy rash, malaise, and fever. It is contagious until no new blisters are developing, which means kids (and caregivers) can be out of school (and work) for weeks.
2. Complications can rarely develop, including bacterial skin infections, pneumonia, brain inflammation, and death (1 in 60,000 cases).
3. People who are immune compromised are at much higher risk of severe complications from chickenpox.
4. Chickenpox infection puts a person at lifetime risk of developing a severely painful rash called shingles (see "Herpes zoster" discussion below).

MENINGOCOCCAL DISEASE AND THE MenACWY AND MenB VACCINES

1. Meningococcal disease is a very serious infection that is spread most easily in close quarters (military barracks, college dorms, etc).
2. It can cause severe illness or death. Symptoms of brain infection, blood stream infection, shock, and multiorgan failure can come on rapidly, resulting in seizures, brain damage, loss of limbs, or death.
3. Death occurs in 10% to 15% even with proper medical treatment.
4. MenACWY vaccine is recommended for all kids of age 11 to 12 years with a booster 5 years later (before college).
5. MenB is currently optional for ages 16 to 18 years and is recommended for certain high-risk groups or in outbreak situations (check with your provider to see if you qualify).

HUMAN PAPILLOMAVIRUS AND THE HPV VACCINE

1. The human papillomavirus (HPV) causes a large majority of cervical, vaginal, vulvar, anal, rectal, penile, oral, and throat cancers, as well as genital warts.
2. HPV affects both girls *and* boys.
3. HPV is extremely common and takes *no* high-risk sexual activity to be exposed.
   a. In America, 79 million are currently infected.
   b. There are 14 million new infections each year.
   c. Nearly all of us will be exposed to HPV at some point in our sexual lives.
4. The HPV vaccine is one of our only cancer-prevention vaccines (hepatitis B is the other).
5. The HPV vaccine has been around since 2006 and is showing significant promise in decreasing genital warts and precancers.
6. It is better to give the HPV vaccine early for the following reasons:
   a. It only works as a prevention vaccine, not as treatment, so it is best to get the series completed *before* sexual activity begins.
   b. We mount a better immune response when we are young. It is likely to be relatively less effective the longer we wait to get the vaccine.
   c. If started before the age of 15 years, only two shots are needed. If started after the age of 15 years, three shots are required.
7. Studies show *no* earlier rates of markers of sexual activity (contraception prescriptions, rates of sexually transmitted infections, or pregnancies) in kids who receive the HPV vaccine than in those who don't. In fact, based on a recent Canadian study, sexual behaviors may be *safer* in kids who have received the vaccine.
8. Studies show *no* fertility problems associated with the HPV vaccine. However, contracting an HPV infection could result in procedures to treat precancer or cancer (biopsies, partial removal of the cervix, and hysterectomy), and these certainly can affect fertility and the ability to carry a pregnancy to term.
9. Studies show *no* increased rates of autoimmune diseases (such as lupus, rheumatoid arthritis, thyroid disease, and type 1 diabetes) after the HPV vaccine.
10. Teens are more likely to faint with any vaccine, but there is a slightly higher risk with the HPV vaccine. Make sure you administer the vaccine while the patient is sitting and monitor the patient for 10 to 15 minutes following each vaccine administration.

PNEUMOCOCCAL PNEUMONIA AND THE PCV13 AND PPSV23 VACCINES

1. Pneumococcal disease is one of the biggest killers of our infants and elderly patients.
2. Pneumococcal disease causes pneumonia but can also cause blood infections (bacteremia) and brain infections (meningitis).
3. The PCV13 vaccine is a routine part of pediatric vaccinations.
4. All adults older than 65 years of age, and select patients younger than 65 years of age, need a PCV13 and PPSV23 vaccine.
5. About one-third of patients getting a pneumonia vaccine will have more significant swelling and pain at the injection site. This is important for us to tell patients, so they know what to expect. It usually resolves within 48 hours.

TETANUS AND DIPHTHERIA AND THE TD OR Tdap VACCINES

1. Tetanus and diphtheria are severe and highly deadly diseases.
2. Children are routinely vaccinated against tetanus, diphtheria, and pertussis (DTaP vaccine).
3. Adults need vaccination against tetanus and diphtheria every 10 years as immunity from the vaccine wares off over time.

HERPES ZOSTER (SHINGLES) AND THE SHINGLES VACCINE

1. Shingles is a reactivation of the chickenpox virus that lives on in our nerves after chickenpox infection. Shingles often happens during periods of stress or illness when our immune system is down. It is only contagious to anyone who has never had chickenpox or to immune-compromised people if the lesions are touched. Shingles is an extremely painful condition, and the pain of shingles can last for years—this is called postherpetic neuralgia.
2. Shingles can happen repeatedly, so someone who has had shingles should still get the vaccine.
3. Zostavax is still available but is no longer routinely recommended as we have a more effective vaccine now on the market called Shingrix (recommended starting at the age of 50 years).
4. The manufacturer of Shingrix underestimated its popularity, and the vaccine is on national backorder. Vaccine supply is becoming available bit by bit, and it is likely easiest to find at pharmacies, even though they are having a hard time getting it in stock.
5. Shingrix is a killed virus vaccine, so it cannot cause shingles.
6. Shingrix is a two-shot series (the second dose is recommended 2 to 6 months after the first).
7. Have patients check with their insurance about coverage as it is quite expensive if they have to pay out of pocket (around $300).
8. Some people (one in six) have a more significant reaction (pain and swelling at injection site, fatigue, aches, feeling ill, low-grade fever). This typically lasts several days, then resolves. It is important to tell patients about this possible reaction, so they know what to expect.
9. Because it is a killed vaccine, it should be safe for people who are immune suppressed. However, it was not studied in this group. Patients who are immune suppressed should consider checking with the specialist managing their condition (rheumatologist, oncologist, etc.) before getting this vaccine.
10. It is advised to wait at least 8 weeks after getting a Zostavax vaccine to get Shingrix.
11. If someone has shingles, they need to wait until blisters are scabbed over before getting Shingrix.

Vaccine Topics Explained (Videos)

For a visual explanation of important topics in vaccination, check out the following videos:

HISTORY OF VACCINES

- Vaccines Today. A Brief History of Vaccination. Vaccines Today website. Published April 21, 2015.

HOW DO VACCINES WORK?

- Nova. Immunity and Vaccines Explained. PBS website. Published September 4, 2014.
- PBS SoCal. Why Vaccines Work. PBS SoCal website. Published July 21, 2015.

HOW VACCINES ARE MADE

- Desai R. Making flu vaccine each year. Khan Academy website. Published January 21, 2013. (this video is based on the 2012-2013 vaccine, but the concepts are similar across years.)
- Centers for Disease Control and Prevention (CDC). The Journey of Your Child's Vaccine. CDC channel on YouTube. Published September 14, 2018.

AN EXPLANATION OF HERD IMMUNITY

- Martyn A. Herd immunity and immunization. North Carolina School of Science and Mathematics website. Published October 27, 2016.

MEASLES EXPLAINED

- Bloomberg. Everything You Need to Know about Measles in 90 Seconds. Bloomberg website. Published February 5, 2015.
- ABC. A Brief History: Measles in America. ABC News website. Published January 9, 2019.

SUBACUTE SCLEROSING PANENCEPHALITIS—A DEADLY COMPLICATION OF MEASLES

- Oxford Vaccine Group. SSPE—A Serious Complication of Measles: Sarah Walton's Story. Vaccine Knowledge Project website. Published October 17, 2013.

THE EFFECT OF WHOOPING COUGH (PERTUSSIS) ON INFANTS

- Mayo Clinic. Infant Girl With Whooping Cough. Mayo Clinic channel on YouTube. Published October 7, 2013.

Evaluating Graphical Data

D

Sometimes it's easier to see how successful vaccines have been in reducing rates of illness and death by looking at disease trends graphically. The following pages include graphs and other representations of data that demonstrate the drop in illness and deaths that occurs after a vaccine is introduced. Though not showing graphs for every possible vaccine, I have picked those that best show the effectiveness of immunization. We will also see a graphical representation of the economic burden of vaccine-preventable disease, as well as the phases of vaccine development, which provides a visual snapshot of the processes involved in ensuring vaccine safety and effectiveness. Finally, we will offer a graphic that realistically reflects the incidence of vaccine-preventable disease versus the incidence of vaccine adverse events. Keep in mind that some graphs use world data while others are more specific to the United States.

But before we look at these graphs, let's talk about how to interpret vaccine-preventable disease graphical data. First, make sure to pay attention to what is being shown on the vertical axis as this may change your interpretation of the data being presented. For example, the reported *cases* of a disease will often be measured in the hundreds of thousands. *Deaths* will be either represented as the total number of deaths or as deaths per some number of the population. When deaths are reported as cases per 100,000 people, for example, we then have to consider the size of the population at the time the data were measured. In 1917, when the US population was 103,268,000, 2 deaths per 100,000 per year from polio would be 2065 lives lost in that year. Remember that the way the data are represented can color your interpretation.

Anti-vaccine websites prefer to use graphs showing deaths per 100,000 people because this visually looks a lot less impressive than showing the actual number of deaths or, even more impressive, the actual number of cases. They are counting on the fact that the reader isn't going to dig deeper into the meaning of the data being presented. They use graphs presented this way to suggest that deaths and, by extension, illness were decreasing before vaccines were introduced. We would expect deaths to have decreased to some degree before a vaccine was introduced because our health care and ability to treat disease have improved over time. What is most meaningful when looking at graphs, however, is the number of cases of a disease both before and after introduction of vaccines. If there are fewer cases, there will be fewer deaths. Simply put, if you don't have a disease, you can't die from it!

For example:

Here is a graph (**Figure A19-A**) showing *cases* of measles per hundred thousand. Let's look around the year 1952. The US Census Bureau lists the US population that year at 157.6 million. If we divide 157.6 million by 100,000, we get 1576. Looking at the peak on the graph at 1952, it looks to be around 425 cases per 100,000. If we multiply 1576 times 425, we get 669,800 cases of measles that year. That is a pretty impressive number. Then, when the measles vaccine was introduced in 1963, it is easy to see the significant drop in the number of cases that occurred.

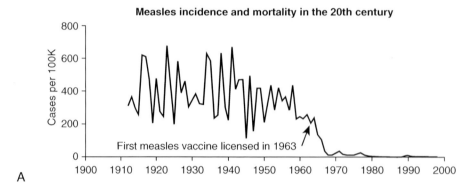

Measles incidence and mortality in the 20th century

A

FIGURE A19-A The visual impact of using cases per 100K to show reduction in disease following introduction of the measles vaccine in 1963. (A, Modified from Dr. Vincent Iannelli. When Was the Last Measles Death in the United States? https://vaxopedia.org/2018/04/15/when-was-the-last-measles-death-in-the-united-states/.)

Here is another depiction of the data (**Figure A19-B**), shown as *deaths* from measles per 100,000 people. This type of graph is commonly used on anti-vaccine websites. Such a representation of the data makes the effects of the measles, mumps, and rubella (MMR) vaccine look much less impressive. We know from examining the reported cases and deaths from vaccine-preventable disease[1] that the number of measles deaths in 1952 in the United States was 618. Interestingly, the cases listed are 683,077, which is very close to what we got by using our earlier graph to estimate. Using the data point on this graph, which is difficult to do because it looks so infinitesimally small, we can calculate an approximate number of deaths that year. I'm going to use a guesstimate value of 0.4 deaths per 100,000 people. If we take the population that year (157.6 million), divide by 100,000, which gives us 1576, then multiply by 0.4, we get a value of 630 deaths in 1952. Again, that is very close to what the actual census figures give us and is not an insignificant amount. It is more difficult to see the impact that the vaccine made on death rates when using the deaths per 100,000 graph, and that is exactly why anti-vaccine websites like to use it. It downplays the significance of the MMR vaccine benefit.

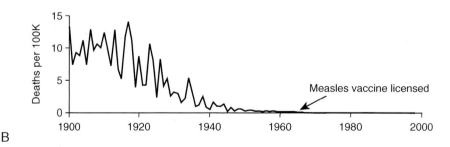

B

FIGURE A19-B The visual impact of using deaths per 100K to show reduction of disease following introduction of the measles vaccine. Anti-vaccine websites like to use deaths per 100k because the impact of vaccine introduction seems much lower with this representation of the data. (B, Modified from Dr. Vincent Iannelli. When Was the Last Measles Death in the United States? https://vaxopedia.org/2018/04/15/when-was-the-last-measles-death-in-the-united-states/.)

A different way to view the impact on illness and death rates would be to look at the absolute number of each and the drop in rates following introduction of the MMR vaccine, as is seen in **Figure A19-C**. If you compare the graph below to the deaths per 100,000 in the inset graph above, you can see how the difference in scale really impacts our impression of the data.

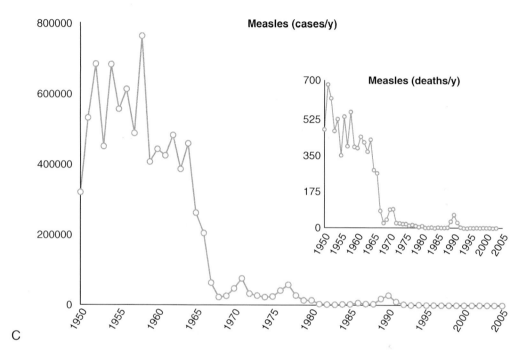

C

FIGURE A19-C Contrast Figures A19-A&B with Figure A19-C, which uses the actual number of cases and deaths to show the same information but in a much more impactful way.

When looking at graphs showing the effectiveness of vaccines, remember to examine the graphical data and sources carefully. Both can make a big difference in how we respond to the information being presented.

VACCINES WORK!

(A Visual Representation)

The development of vaccines is one of the greatest of all public health achievements. Since their introduction, the world has seen a remarkable reduction in rates of illness and death from vaccine-preventable disease (**Figures A20-A22**).

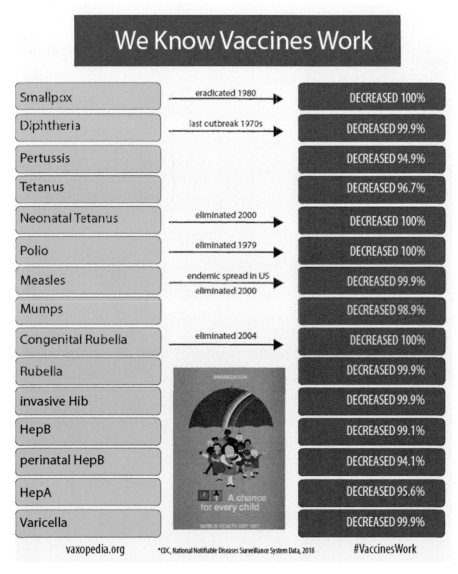

FIGURE A20 Although vaccination has done an outstanding job of controlling vaccine-preventable diseases, thanks to decreasing immunization rates in recent years, we have seen an increase in measles, mumps, and pertussis. (Reprinted with permission from Vaxopedia.org. https://vaxopedia.org/2019/02/24/we-know-vaccines-work/.)

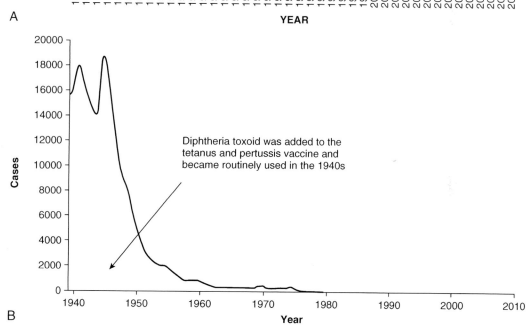

Varicella (Chickenpox) Cases 1972-2013

The varicella vaccine was introduced in 1995. There were 120,624 cases that year.

Diphtheria toxoid was added to the tetanus and pertussis vaccine and became routinely used in the 1940s

FIGURE A21 A, The rates of chickenpox, a highly contagious disease that results in prolonged time out of school for children and time off of work for parents, were significantly reduced following introduction of the varicella vaccine. B, Diphtheria, a terrible disease that killed from 5% to 20% of those infected, has been eliminated in our country, thanks to vaccines. (A, Reprinted with permission from ProCon.org. Varicella (Chickenpox) Cases, Deaths, and Vaccination Rates. https://vaccines.procon.org/view.additional-resource.php?resourceID=005925. B, Modified from Centers for Disease Control and Prevention. https://www.cdc.gov/vaccines/pubs/pinkbook/dip.html.)

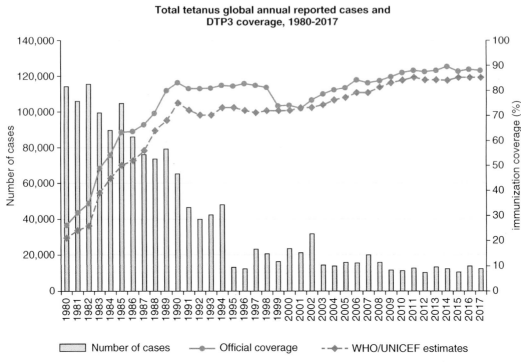

**Total tetanus global annual reported cases and
DTP3 coverage, 1980-2017**

Number of cases ⬜ Official coverage ● WHO/UNICEF estimates ◆

Source: WHO/IVB database, 2018
194 WHO Menber states.
Data as of September 2018

WHO

A

FIGURE A22-A Here, we see how rates of tetanus have decreased around the world as vaccine uptake has increased. (A, Reprinted from WHO/IVB Database. https://www.who.int/immunization/monitoring_surveillance/burden/vpd/surveillance_type/passive/tetanus/en/. Total tetanus global annual reported cases and DTP3 coverage, 1980-2017, Copyright (2018). Accessed April 10, 2019.)

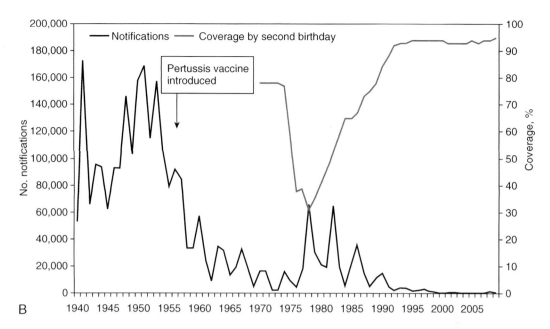

FIGURE A22-B This graph shows the number of pertussis cases reported (noted on the left vertical axis) among all ages and the percentage coverage with the pertussis vaccine among children less than 2 years of age (shown on the right vertical axis) in England and Wales between 1940 and 2009. The pertussis vaccine became available in the second half of the 1950s and a notable drop in cases was seen after introduction of the vaccine. Note the rise in pertussis cases that occurred in the 1970s when vaccination rates dropped. Vaccines work! (B, Modified from Campbell H, Amirthalingam G, Andrews N, et al. Accelerating control of pertussis in England and Wales. *Emerg Infect Dis.* 2012;18(1):38-47. doi:10.3201/eid1801.110784.)

HERD IMMUNITY

(A Visual Representation)

Herd immunity, or *community immunity*, occurs when a large enough percentage of a population is vaccinated against a disease, thereby protecting others in the community who cannot get the vaccine themselves (**Figure A23**).

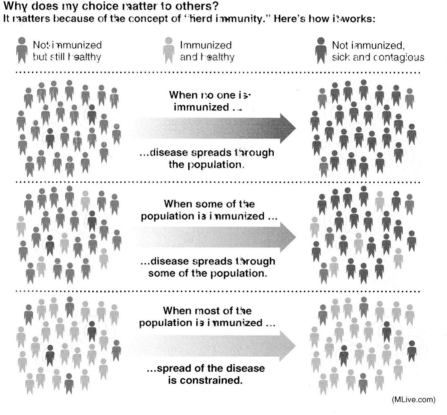

(MLive.com)

FIGURE A23 If not enough of the community is immunized, disease spreads with ease and all of us are at risk! (Reprinted with permission from Klingensmith M. How do vaccinations work? The science of immunizations. MLive. 10 Dec 2014. https://www.mlive.com/news/2014/12/how_do_vaccinations_work_the_s.html. Web. Accessed June 12, 2019.)

But does herd immunity really work? The graph below looks at the human papillomavirus (HPV) vaccine and its effectiveness against genital warts. The data come from Australia, a country that has instituted a nationwide HPV vaccination program (**Figure A24**).

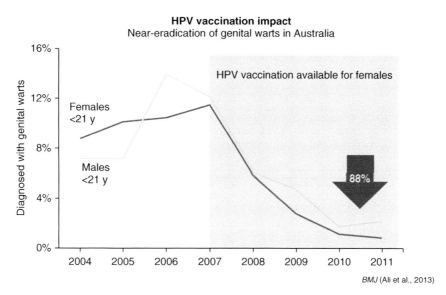

FIGURE A24 In the graph, we see that, after the human papillomavirus (HPV) vaccine was introduced in 2007 (originally only being offered to girls), the percentage of Australians diagnosed with genital warts dropped 88% by 2011. But this didn't only occur in girls, who were the target group for immunization. The HPV vaccination was not recommended to be given to boys until the year 2011. As you can see, the percentage of boys diagnosed with genital warts also decreased significantly and they weren't even being vaccinated. Vaccination of one group protected another. This is herd immunity in action! (HPV IQ at the UNC Gillings School of Global Public Health. https://www.hpviq.org/. Data from Hammad A, Basil D, Handan W, et al. Genital warts in young Australians five years into national human papillomavirus vaccination programme: National surveillance data. *BMJ*. 2013;346:f2032.)

HOW DO VACCINES WORK?

(A Visual Representation)

Trying to fight serious diseases without the aid of vaccines is like trying to defend our military troops against a surprise attack. As shown in the following graphic, vaccines allow our bodies to get a glimpse of what's coming and develop weapons against it so that when the full attack finally arrives, we are ready to defend ourselves and fight back, minimizing damage and losses (**Figure A25**).

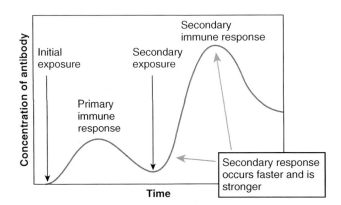

FIGURE A25 Vaccines give our bodies a chance to protect themselves against the attack of viruses and bacteria. When we are exposed to a live infection for the first time (first arrow), our bodies mount a primary immune response. This is a slow response, which produces lower levels of antibodies. The slow primary immune response can provide just enough time for a live infection to do some major damage, putting us at risk for complications such as pneumonia, brain inflammation, and even death. Luckily, we have an alternative in vaccines. Because they use killed or weakened forms of viruses or bacteria, vaccines can be used to trigger the primary response in a very safe and controlled way. This allows our bodies to develop antibodies, or memory cells, without putting us at risk for severe illness. That way, the next time we encounter that same virus or bacterium (second arrow), our memory cells can quickly mobilize and mount a much stronger attack, called the secondary immune response, which keeps us from getting sick. No amount of supplements or healthy eating can reduce the time it takes to mount a primary response and the only way to develop a secondary response is either through exposure to a safe and controlled vaccine or through risky infection with a live virus or bacterium. I'll take safe and controlled any day! (Modified from Open Stax. Anatomy and Physiology. https://cnx.org/resources/28eae4100180d232adf78a1e05faf19b23ee371f/2223_Primary_and_Secondary_Antibody_Respons_new.jpg. Download for free at http://cnx.org/contents/14fb4ad7-39a1-4eee-ab6e-3ef2482e3e22@15.5. CC-BY-SA-4.0.)

CONTAGION AND DEATH FROM VACCINE-PREVENTABLE DISEASES

(A Visual Representation)

Some think of vaccine-preventable diseases, such as measles and influenza, as "no big deal," but they have the potential to be *very* serious, even deadly (**Figure A26**).

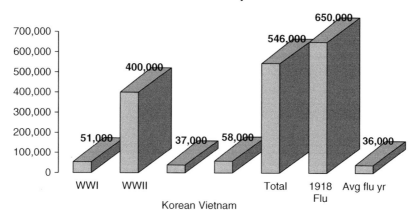

US deaths 20th century - flu and war

FIGURE A26 Influenza is the most deadly vaccine-preventable disease that we see in current times. This graph depicts the deaths from the major wars of the 20th century compared with deaths from influenza, both during the 1918 Spanish flu, which killed an estimated 50 million people worldwide (with some estimates higher), and during an average flu year in the United States. In 2018, 80,000 people lost their lives to the flu. Stated a different way, 1 out of every 4084 people in the United States died of flu in 2018. That is more loss of US life in 1 year than in all of the Vietnam War. Depending on the year, the flu shot does a pretty good job of preventing influenza. Some years are better than others. But it does an excellent job of keeping people from having very serious complications or dying of the flu. (Courtesy of College of St. Benedict and St. Johns' University. https://employees.csbsju.edu/hjakubowski/classes/Chem%20and%20Society/Influenza/1918%20Pandemic.htm.)

Why all the fuss over measles? Of those who contract measles, 1 in 4 will have to be hospitalized, 1 in 1000 will develop a brain inflammation that can cause permanent brain damage, and 1-2 in 1000 will die from the illness. If a person survives, about 1 in 10,000 will go on to develop a fatal degenerative disorder of the nervous system called subacute sclerosing panencephalitis. Moreover, measles is *highly* contagious (**Figure A27**).

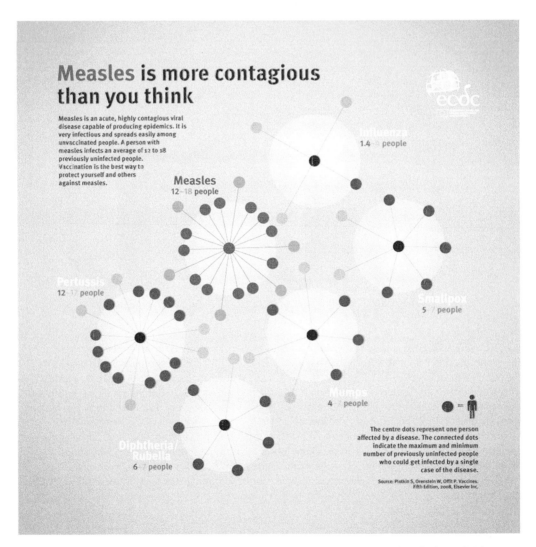

FIGURE A27 This image depicts the contagiousness of measles compared with that of other vaccine-preventable diseases. One sick person can infect up to 18 others, and, because the measles virus can linger in the air for about 2 hours, the infected person doesn't even have to be in the same room to pass the infection to someone else. Ninety percent of unvaccinated people who come into contact with a person with measles will come down with the illness. (Reprinted from the European Centre for Disease Prevention and Control. https://ecdc.europa.eu/en/publications-data/measles-more-contagious-you-think. Accessed June 10, 2019)

VACCINE-PREVENTABLE DISEASE IS EXTREMELY COSTLY

(A Visual Representation)

Every year, as a nation, we spend billions of dollars on the costs associated with treating vaccine-preventable diseases. There are doctor's visits, medicines, hospital bills, lost wages, lost productivity, and other factors that quickly build to negatively affect individual household budgets and serve to increase the cost of health care to all (**Figure A28**).

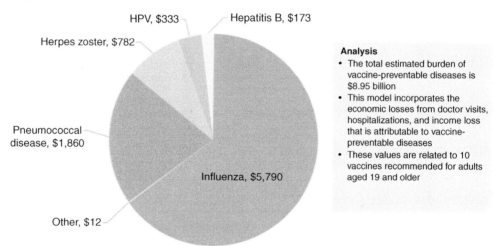

Low rate of vaccine uptake has led to an avoidable rise in costs for individuals and society

Annual economic burden of vaccine-preventable diseases, by pathogen, 2015

Millions of dollars

HPV, $333

Hepatitis B, $173

Herpes zoster, $782

Pneumococcal disease, $1,860

Influenza, $5,790

Other, $12

Analysis
- The total estimated burden of vaccine-preventable diseases is $8.95 billion
- This model incorporates the economic losses from doctor visits, hospitalizations, and income loss that is attributable to vaccine-preventable diseases
- These values are related to 10 vaccines recommended for adults aged 19 and older

FIGURE A28-A Vaccine-preventable diseases are extremely costly, not only to individuals, but to society as a whole. (A, Reprinted with permission from the National Journal. https://www.nationaljournal.com/media/media/2016/10/13/Screen-Shot-2016-10-13-at-2-48-37-PM.png. Accessed June 10, 2019.)

COST OF FLU

$10.4 billion / year
in direct medical expenses

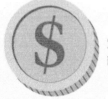

$15.3 billion / year
in loss of earnings

The flu causes U.S.
employees to miss

17
MILLION
workdays

Which is equivalent to
$7 billion / year
in sick days and
loss of productivity

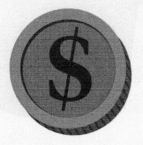

Loss of productivity
due to flu between 2017-2018
was more than **$21 billion**

Sources: Centers for Disease Control and Prevention (CDC)
Challenger, Gray, & Christmas, Inc.

healthline

B

FIGURE A28-B The cost of influenza in the 2017 to 2018 flu season was astronomical. Compare this to graph A, looking at the cost of all major vaccine-preventable diseases in 2015. Vaccine-preventable diseases are extremely costly in both dollars and lives. (B, With permission from Healthline Media, Inc. https://www.healthline.com/health/influenza/facts-and-statistics#6.)

VACCINE DEVELOPMENT

(A Visual Representation)

Vaccines undergo many years of rigorous testing before being released for general use. Studies looking at successively larger groups of participants seek to make sure that vaccines are effective and safe in their targeted populations (**Figure A29**).

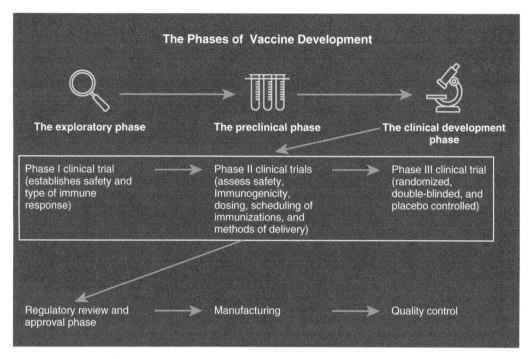

FIGURE A29 This graphic shows the phases of testing that occur in order to bring a vaccine to market and the postmarketing monitoring that continues after its release. Vaccines are closely monitored for any signals of safety or efficacy concerns.

WHAT ARE THE CHANCES?

(A Visual Representation)

We are, unfortunately, beginning to see climbing rates of vaccine-preventable disease across the world. However, if we never encounter a case of measles or mumps or pertussis ourselves, or see our loved ones afflicted, it's understandable how one might believe that the claimed risks of taking a vaccine are greater than the risks of the diseases themselves. In order to understand the safety of vaccines, the following graphic will help put the incidence of disease versus the incidence of adverse reactions to vaccines in perspective (**Figure A30**).

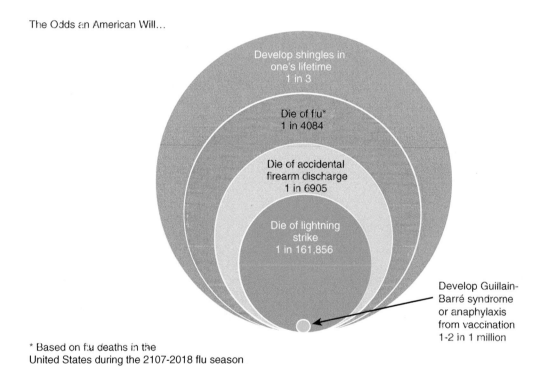

The Odds an American Will…

Develop shingles in one's lifetime
1 in 3

Die of flu*
1 in 4084

Die of accidental firearm discharge
1 in 6905

Die of lightning strike
1 in 161,856

Develop Guillain-Barré syndrome or anaphylaxis from vaccination
1-2 in 1 million

* Based on flu deaths in the United States during the 2107-2018 flu season

FIGURE A30 The risk of getting shingles in one's lifetime and the yearly risk of dying from influenza, for example, are significantly greater than other things that we think of as highly unlikely, such as dying by firearm injury or lightning strike. Moreover, the risk of a serious or life-threatening reaction to a vaccine in orders of magnitude is smaller still.[1-3]

Reference

1. Centers for Disease Control and Prevention; Hamborsky J, Kroger A, Wolfe C, eds. *Epidemiology and Prevention of Vaccine-Preventable Diseases*. 13th ed. Washington, DC: Public Health Foundation; 2015. Updated December 2016. Accessed December 13, 2018.
2. National Safety Council. What are the Odds of Dying From. Accessed December 13, 2018. https://www.nsc.org/work-safety/tools-resources/injury-facts/chart.
3. Miller ER, Moro PL, Cano M, et al. Deaths following vaccination: what does the evidence show? *Vaccine*. 2015;33(29):3288-3292.

E

Journal Articles Addressing Specific Vaccine Concerns

VACCINES AND AUTISM

1. Taylor LE, Swerdfeger AL, Eslick GD. Vaccines are not associated with autism: an evidence-based meta-analysis of case-control and cohort studies. *Vaccine.* 2014;32:3623-9. https://www.ncbi.nlm.nih.gov/pubmed/24814559.
    *   Summary: Meta-analysis of five case-control and five cohort studies, involving over 1.25 million children, shows no evidence of a link between vaccine receipt and risk of developing autism or autism spectrum disorder (ASD). This finding stands whether looking specifically at measles, mumps, and rubella (MMR) vaccines or cumulative mercury dosage and thimerosal exposure.

2. Smith MJ, Woods CR. On-time vaccine receipt in the first year does not adversely affect neuropsychological outcomes. *Pediatrics.* 2010;125(6):1134-41. https://pediatrics.aappublications.org/cgi/content/abstract/125/6/1134
    *   Summary: Looks at children vaccinated on schedule versus those with delayed or incomplete vaccination and the development of 42 different neuropsychological outcomes by ages 7 to 10 years. Results showed better performance in children vaccinated on schedule and no benefit to delaying vaccines.

MEASLES, MUMPS, AND RUBELLA VACCINE AND AUTISM

1. Jain A, Marshall J, Buikema A, et al. Autism occurrence by MMR vaccine status among US children with older siblings with and without autism. *JAMA.* 2015;313(5):1534-40. https://jamanetwork.com/journals/jama/fullarticle/2275444
    *   Summary: Authors found no association between MMR vaccine and ASD risk and no increased risk following one or two doses of MMR vaccine in children who had an older sibling with ASD.

2. Peltola H, Patja A, Leinikki P, et al. No evidence for MMR vaccine–associated inflammatory bowel disease or autism in 14-year prospective study. *Lancet.* 1998;351:1327-8. http://www.freenetpages.co.uk/hp/gingernut/lancet/Finland%20May%201998.pdf

   - Summary: Over a decade's attempt, involving study of 3 million adverse events, to detect all severe adverse events associated with MMR vaccine, researchers could find no data to support the hypothesis that MMR vaccine causes pervasive developmental disorder or inflammatory bowel disease.

THIMEROSAL (MERCURY) AND AUTISM

1. Doja A, Roberts W. Immunizations and autism: a review of the literature. *Can J Neurol Sci.* 2006;33(4):341-6. http://tinyurl.com/ddnqq7

   - Summary: No convincing evidence was found to support a link between autism and thimerosal, nor to support the use of chelation therapy in autism.

2. Hviid A, Stellfeld M, Wohlfahrt J, et al. Association between thimerosal-containing vaccine and autism. *JAMA.* 2003;290(13):1763-6. http://tinyurl.com/5rtzjd

   - Summary: Study of 467,000 children in Denmark compared rates of development of ASD in children receiving a vaccine containing thimerosal to those receiving a thimerosal-free version of the same vaccine. Results did not support a causal relationship between thimerosal and development of ASD.

NUMBER OF VACCINES AND AUTISM

1. Iqbal S, Barile JP, Thompson WW, et al. Number of antigens in early childhood vaccines and neuropsychological outcomes at age 7-10 years. *Pharmacoepidemiol Drug Saf.* 2013;22(12):1263-1270. https://www.ncbi.nlm.nih.gov/pubmed/23847024

   - Summary: There were no adverse associations between an increasing number of antigens received through vaccination at ages 7, 12, and 24 months and neuropsychological outcomes tested at age 7 to 10 years.

VACCINES AND THE IMMUNE SYSTEM

1. Glanz JM, Newcomer SR, Daley MF, et al. Association between estimated cumulative vaccine antigen exposure through the first 23 months of life and non–vaccine-targeted infections from 24 through 47 months of age. *JAMA.* 2018;319(9):906-913. https://jamanetwork.com/journals/Jama/fullarticle/2673970

   - Summary: There is no significant correlation between exposure to antigens through vaccines and risk of developing a non–vaccine-targeted infection (Translation: Vaccines don't make us sicker).

2. Nilsson L, Kjellman N, Björkstén B. A randomized controlled trial of the effect of pertussis vaccines on atopic disease. *Arch Pediatr Adolesc Med.* 1998;152:734-738. https://jamanetwork.com/journals/jamapediatrics/article-abstract/189740

   - Summary: No evidence found to support a significant increase in allergic manifestations following pertussis vaccination. There *was* an increased incidence of asthma following whooping cough infection.

VACCINES AND AUTOIMMUNE DISEASES

1. Stratton K, Ford A, Rusch E, et al. Adverse effects of vaccines: Evidence and causality. Institute of Medicine. The National Academy of Science. 2011. http://vaccine-safety-training.org/tl_files/vs/pdf/13164.pdf

   - Summary: Authors found evidence to reject a causal relationship between the MMR vaccine and type 1 diabetes; and the diphtheria, tetanus and pertussis vaccine and type 1 diabetes.

2. Genovese C, La Fauci V, Squeri A, et al. Human papillomavirus (HPV) vaccine and auto-immune diseases: Systematic review and meta-analysis of the literature. *J Prev Med Hyg.* 2018;59(3):E194-E199. https://www.ncbi.nlm.nih.gov/pmc/articles/PMC6196376/

   - Summary: Meta-analysis involving 243,289 in the vaccine group and 248,820 in the control group showed no relationship between the development of autoimmune diseases and HPV vaccination using the bivalent or quadrivalent vaccine.

3. Ascherio A, Zhang SM, Hernàn MA, et al. Hepatitis B vaccination and the risk of multiple sclerosis. *N Engl J Med.* 2001;344:327-332. https://www.ncbi.nlm.nih.gov/pubmed/11172163

   - Summary: A case-control study of two large groups of nurses involved in the Nurses' Health Study and Nurses' Health Study II showed no association between hepatitis B vaccination and the development of multiple sclerosis.

ADDITIONAL RESOURCES: FOR A MORE COMPLETE LIST OF STUDIES, PLEASE SEE THE FOLLOWING SITES

1. The American Academy of Pediatrics, HealthyChildren.org—https://www.healthychildren.org/English/safety-prevention/immunizations/Pages/Vaccine-Studies-Examine-the-Evidence.aspx
2. Immunization Action Coalition—http://www.immunize.org/catg.d/p4026.pdf

Navigating Information on the Internet and Social Media

These days it can be really difficult to tell reliable and trustworthy information from misleading and faulty information on the Internet. When making health decisions for yourself or your loved ones based on information found on the Web or social media, there are a few tricks you need to know to make sure that you aren't being led astray. Below you will find a check list that will help you in your reading and research.

1. _____ **Know your source.**

   - Look for articles published in reputable scientific journals. However, keep in mind that not all journals are created equal. Some open-access journals have less rigorous admission standards, and publication of minimally edited articles allows for the appearance of legitimacy when it is not always warranted.

   - Government-funded, not-for-profit, and university sites tend to be trustworthy.

     › Such as the Centers for Disease Control and Prevention, National Institutes of Health, the Mayo Clinic, etc.

   - Disease-specific sites are also typically reliable sources (with some exceptions).

     › These include sources, such as The American Cancer Society, The American Diabetes Association, and Autism Speaks.

   - Research the author. You can often find bios and critiques that will tell you if their work is considered mainstream or controversial.

     › Consider whether they have a background that allows them to speak with authority on the topic.

   - Check their references. Do their references come from legitimate sources?

     › If their references tend to link back to articles they wrote themselves or to journals or articles that have not followed rigorous research standards, move on.

2. _____ **Check the facts.**

- For articles written on blogs or in a newslike fashion, dig deeper into their claims. Just because someone says it, doesn't make it true. You can use various fact-checking sites to help in this endeavor.

  › Snopes.com
  › Politifact.com
  › *The Washington Post* Fact Checker
  › Factcheck.org, which includes a feature called SciCheck
  › NPR Fact Check
  › Univision's Detector de Mentiras (Spanish language)
  › Sciencebasedmedicine.org

3. _____ **Make sure your information is up-to-date.**

- Science is constantly changing, and we need to know whether the information we are working with is current.

  › Check the dates of the articles you are reading or the dates of the most recent update for the site you are working with.

4. _____ **Don't put all of your eggs in one research paper's basket.**

- Discovering scientific "truth" takes time and repeated testing. We can't rely on one study to give the whole picture.

  › If a study claims a particular finding, don't stop there. Read other studies on the same topic. Only if multiple studies come to the same conclusion, and the totality of evidence points in the same direction, can we put our faith in the finding.

5. _____ **Check for conflicts of interest**.

- As much as possible, we want to look for sources of information that are nonbiased.

  › If a site is trying to sell you something, there is more likely to be bias in their recommendations (for example, "Don't get vaccines! Instead, use this *amazing* supplement to boost your immunity. You can buy it on my site for the low price of $39.99!) If the site is trying to sell you something, it's time to move on.

6. _____ **If it sounds too good to be true, it probably is.**

- In desperation, we sometimes search for a miracle; that essential oil that will take away our anxiety or the ionized water treatment to cure cancer.

  › If there were a miracle cure for cancer, science wouldn't be hiding it from you.
  › If there were a miracle cure for anything, the pharmaceutical industry would be all over it and you wouldn't have to find it from an obscure online salesman.
  › If you are wondering if something you read online is legitimate, ask your doctor or clinician. They can help.

Index

Note: Page numbers followed by "f" indicate figures, "t" indicate tables and "b" indicate boxes.

A

AAFP Adolescent Immunization Awards. *See* American Academy of Family Physicians (AAFP) Adolescent Immunization Awards
AAP. *See* American Academy of Pediatrics (AAP)
ACCV. *See* Advisory Commission on Childhood Vaccines (ACCV)
ACIP. *See* Advisory Committee on Immunization Practices (ACIP)
Acknowledge concerns, Steer the conversation, and Know your facts (A.S.K.), 75–76, 75t
Adverse events following immunization (AEFI), 60, 62–63
Advisory Commission on Childhood Vaccines (ACCV), 61
Advisory Committee on Immunization Practices (ACIP), 60
  human papillomavirus (HPV), 139
  influenza, 136
Agency for Toxic Substances and Disease Registry (ATSDR), 101
Allergic reactions, 81, 85
Alternative Vaccine Schedule, 118
American Academy of Family Physicians (AAFP) Adolescent Immunization Awards, 181
American Academy of Pediatrics (AAP), 15, 120
Anaphylaxis, 85
Anti-abortion beliefs, 18
Anticipated Regret, 31
Antifertility agents, 19
Antimicrobial resistance, 184, 184b
Anti-vaccination messages, 32
Anti-vaccine claims, 99
Anti-vaccine community, 28, 35
  advantages and disadvantages, 45
  camp, 42–43
  children vaccination, 37–38
  claims, 38
  event/series of events, 36–37
  long-term trust, 45
  media/social media, 43–44, 43b
  organized movement, 40–41
  pro-vaccine movement, 44, 46
  religious/personal exemption, 44
  tactics, 39–40
  transition, 46
  vaccination efforts, 44–45
  vaccination rates, 39
  vaccine conversation, 47b–48b
  vaccine-hesitant patients, 46, 48–49
  vaccines safety, 41–42, 41t–42t
Anti-vaccine fallacies, 28, 28b
Anti-vaccine movement, 93, 115
  anti-abortion beliefs, 18
  antifertility agents, 19
  Catholic Health Ministry, 18
  cleanliness and purity, 14–15
  disease causation, atmospheric theory, 16
  effectiveness and safety of, 13, 14b
  Environmental Protection Agency, 17
  ethical dilemma, 18
  factors, 13, 14b
  government and industry, 17–18
  immunoglobulins, 19
  medical and public health efforts, 13
  personal liberties, 15–16
  physical and spiritual healing, 18
  pro-immunization messages, 20
  psychology of, 25–33
  religious concerns, 18–19, 20f
  science-based assessment, 21
  social media platforms, 21
  treatment and 'sanitary' methods, 17
  Tuskegee Experiment, 17
  Vaccination Act, 15
  vaccination rates, 19, 20f
Anti-vaccine sentiment, 8–9, 186
Appeal to Authority Fallacy, 28
Appeal to Pity Fallacy, 29
Armed Forces Epidemiological Board, 134
ASD. *See* Autism Spectrum Disorder (ASD)
A.S.K. *See* Acknowledge concerns, Steer the conversation, and Know your facts (A.S.K.)
Ask, Acknowledge, Advise (3-As) technique, 74–76, 75t

249

ATSDR. *See* Agency for Toxic Substances and Disease Registry (ATSDR)
Autism spectrum disorder (ASD), 28, 116, 243
  measles, 243–244
  mumps, 243–244
  number of vaccines, 244
  rubella, 243–244
  thimerosal (mercury), 244
Autistic enterocolitis, 92
Autoimmune disease, 117, 144, 245

B

Bacterial skin infection, 15
Bandwagon fallacy, 29, 31
Benzethonium chloride, 152
Big Pharma, 25, 106–107
1902 Biologics Control Act, 52
Bovine calf, 153
Bovine extract and casamino acid, 153
British General Medical Council Fitness to Practice Panel, 92

C

C.A.S.E approach. *See* Corroborate, About me, Science, Explain/Advise (C.A.S.E) approach
Catching flies
  Acknowledge concerns, Steer the conversation, and Know your facts (A.S.K.), 75–76, 75t
  Ask, Acknowledge, Advise (3-As) technique, 74–76, 75t
  caustic/acidic statements, 67
  Corroborate, About me, Science, Explain/Advise (C.A.S.E) approach, 73–74, 73t, 76
  Global Polio Eradication Initiative, 68
  health care costs, 68
  Independent Monitoring Board, 68
  MMR vaccine, 68
  National Institute of Mental Health, 67
  negative connotation, test results, 69
  PEW study, 68
  presumptive *vs.* participatory approach, 71–72
  scientific community, 69
  self-confidence, communication, 71
  Tdap immunization, 70b
  trial and error, 71
  vaccine-hesitant patient, 72
Catholic Health Ministry, 18
CDC's Autism and Developmental Disabilities Monitoring Network, 117
Centers for Disease Control and Prevention (CDC), 10, 53, 58, 60, 102, 178b
Chickenpox, 188, 188f
Childhood leukemia, 117
Childhood vaccinations
  Autism. *See also* Autism spectrum disorder (ASD)
    aluminum and formaldehyde, in vaccines, 117
    causes, 116
    features, 116
    in identical twins, 116
    measles, mumps, and rubella (MMR) vaccine, 116
      mercury exposure, 116–117
      in siblings, 116
      symptoms, 116
  chickenpox, 118
  double-blinded trial, 121
  hepatitis B virus (HBV), 119–120, 119f
  immune systems, 117
  pediatric dosing schedule, 120
  placebo-controlled trial, 120
  schedule for, 118
  sudden infant death syndrome (SIDS), 120, 121f
  vaccine-preventable diseases, 121
  Vaccines for Children (VFC) program, 121
Children and communities health, 96
Chronic fatigue, complex regional pain syndrome (CRPS), 144
Clinical Immunization Safety Assessment (CISA) Project, 60
Clinic vaccine champion, 179
Community immunity, 105
Confirmation bias, 30, 162
Corroborate, About me, Science, Explain/Advise (C.A.S.E) approach, 73–74, 73t, 76
Cowpox, 4

D

Department of Health and Human Services (DHHS) agencies, 53
Diphtheria, 5, 189, 189f
  and vaccine, 82–83, 224
Diphtheria, pertussis, and tetanus vaccine (DPT), 53
Disease resurgence, 96, 97b
Dunning-Kruger effect, 183

E

Egg (ovalbumin) protein, 154–155
EHR. *See* Electronic health record (EHR)
Electronic health record (EHR), 178, 180–181
Emergency Preparedness for Vaccine Safety, 60
Environmental Protection Agency, 17
Ethylenediaminetetracetic acid sodium (EDTA), 153

F

Fetal serum albumin/protein, 153
Financial conflict of interest, 94–95
Food and Drug Administration (FDA), 52, 60, 135

G

Gelatin, 153
Global Polio Eradication Initiative, 68
Government-purchased vaccines, 176
Graphical data evaluation
  chickenpox rates, 230, 231f
  disease reduction, 230, 230f
  effectiveness of, 229
  herd immunity
    disease spreads, 234, 234f
    human papillomavirus (HPV) vaccine, 235, 235f
  immune response, 236, 236f
  measles, 227–228, 228f
  MMR vaccine benefit, 228

shingles risk, 242, 242f
tetanus rates, 230, 232f–233f
vaccine development, 241, 241f
vaccine-preventable diseases
    annual economic burden, 239, 239f–240f
    contagion and death, 237–238, 237f–238f
Guillain-Barré syndrome (GBS), 108–109
Gulf War Syndrome, 103

H

Haemophilus Influenzae type B (HiB), 9, 190, 190f
    and vaccine, 83, 222
HBV. *See* Hepatitis B virus (HBV)
Health and Medicine Division (HMD), 86
Health and Medicine Division of the National Academies of
        Science, Engineering, and Medicine, 53
Health care services, 27
Health Resources and Services Administration (HRSA), 53, 61
Hepatitis A virus, 191, 191f
    and vaccine, 83, 222
Hepatitis B virus (HBV), 192, 192f
    "at risk" populations, 119, 119f
    cirrhosis, 120
    liver cancer, 120
    and vaccine, 83, 222
    virus transmission, 119
Herd immunity, 104–105, 219–220, 225
    disease spreads, 234, 234f
    human papillomavirus (HPV) vaccine, 235, 235f
Herpes zoster (shingles), 212–213, 212f
    and vaccine, 224
HMD. *See* Health and Medicine Division (HMD)
HPV. *See* Human papillomavirus (HPV)
HRSA. *See* Health Resources and Services Administration
        (HRSA)
Human papillomavirus (HPV), 118, 133–134, 145, 193f
    ACIP recommendations, 139
    cancers types, 140t, 1140
    complications, 193
    disease/complications, 194
    impact of, 194
    laryngeal papillomatosis, 137
    participatory approach, 139
    presumptive approach, 139
    sexually transmitted infection, 139. *See also* Sexually
        transmitted infection
    symptoms, 193
    transmission/contagion, 193
    vaccination programs, 138, 138f
    and vaccine, 223
    vaccine information, 83, 193–194
Human serum albumin, 153
Hygienic Laboratory of the Public Health and Marine
        Hospital Service, 52

I

Immune-compromised patients
    for asplenic patients, 127, 129b
    chronic illness, 127

influenza immunization, 127
    PCV13 and PPSV23 vaccines, 127
    pneumococcal vaccination schedule, 127, 128f
    suppressed immune systems, 126
Immune system, 244–245
Immune thrombocytopenic purpura, 85
Immunization Action Coalition, 61
Immunization Information Systems (IIS), 175, 176b
Immunization programs, 91
Immunization Safety Office, 60
Inactivated/killed virus vaccine, 100
Inactivated polio vaccine (IPV), 87
Independent Monitoring Board, 68
Influenza, 133, 134f, 145, 154–155, 195–196, 195f
    flu shot
        Advisory Committee on Immunization Practices
            (ACIP), 136
        allergy to eggs, 137
        "high-dose" flu vaccine, 135b
        hospitalizations limitation, 136
        immune-compromised patient, 136
        injectable influenza vaccine, 136
        pediatric flu deaths, 136
        retrospective studies, 135
        stomach flu, 136
    and flu vaccine, 1, 83–84, 220–221
    Food and Drug Administration (FDA), 135
    morbidity and mortality, 133
    subtypes A and B, 134
    US-licensed influenza vaccines, 135
Inoculation Theory, 32
Institute for Safe Medication Practices (ISMP),
        61–62
Institutional Review Board (IRB), 55, 96
Internet, 247–248
Investigational New Drug, 54
IPV. *See* Inactivated polio vaccine (IPV)

J

Japanese encephalitis vaccine, 84
Jewish dietary laws, 125

K

Kaiser Family Foundation study, 116

L

Liability issues, 185
Licensure costs, 56
Live-attenuated herpes zoster virus vaccine (Zostavax), 89,
        89b
Live-attenuated influenza vaccine (LAIV), 15, 83–84, 100,
        200

M

McCoy's research, 27
Measles, 155, 155b, 197–198, 197f, 225
    graphical data evaluation, 227–228, 228f
    "resets"/"disables" immune memory, 93, 93b
    and vaccine, 84–85, 221

Measles, mumps, and rubella (MMR) vaccine, 8, 10, 28, 91,
 117, 221
   data manipulation and fabrication, 95–96
   graphical data evaluation, 228
   pregnancy, vaccines, 122
   study participants, biased selection, 95
Media
   accountability, 161
   anti-science claims, 171
   anti-vaccine movement, 160, 160b, 166–169
   "balanced reporting," 160
   echo chamber, 162–163
   fact check, 170–171
   Internet, 161–162
   pseudoscience claims, 171
   social media impact, 161–162, 172
   source, 170
   tactics, 163, 164b–165b
   tropes, 163, 164b–165b
Medical Dictionary for Regulatory Activities, 63
MenB. *See* Serogroup B meningococcal vaccination (MenB)
Meningococcal meningitis, 199–200, 199f, 223
Meningococcal polysaccharide vaccine (MPSV4), 85
Meningococcal septicemia, 199–200, 199f
Minimum risk levels (MRLs), 101
Motivated Reasoning, 30
MPSV4. *See* Meningococcal polysaccharide vaccine
 (MPSV4)
Mumps, 201–202, 201f
   and vaccine, 86, 221

N

National Catholic Bioethics Center (NCBC), 124
National Center for Immunization and Respiratory Diseases,
 61
National Childhood Vaccine Injury Act (NCVIA), 53,
 61, 65
National Institute of Allergy and Infectious Diseases, 14b
National Institute of Mental Health, 67
National Institutes of Health (NIH), 52, 60–61
National Vaccine Information Center (NVIC), 162
National Vaccine Injury Compensation Program (NVICP),
 53, 56, 61, 65, 111
National Vaccine Program Office (NVPO), 53, 58
"Natural" infection, 118
Nonylphenol ethoxylate, 154

O

Omission bias, 31
Oral polio vaccine (OPV), 87
Organizational efficiencies, 175
Organizational interventions
   vaccine program
      acute care visit, 178
      adult vaccines, 180–181
      American Academy of Family Physicians (AAFP)
         Adolescent Immunization Awards, 181
      anti-vaccine sentiment, 179
      clinic vaccine champion, 179
         clinic-wide competitions, 179
         day-to-day clinical practice, 179, 179b
         educational resources, 177
         electronic health record (EHR), 178, 180–181
         government-purchased vaccines, 176
         immunization clinics, 181
         Immunization Information Systems (IIS), 175, 176b
         influenza vaccination, 180
         patient databases, 176–177
         primary care provider, 180
         Provider Enrollment Package, 176
         schedule updates, 180
         staff education, 177
         standing orders, 177, 177b
         vaccination rates, 181
         vaccine promotion, 178–179
         vaccine series, 178, 178b
         Vaccines for Children (VFC) program, 176, 176b
         "vital sign," 176
         wait times, 178

P

Package inserts (PIs), 111–112, 149
Parotitis, 86
Participatory approach, 71–72, 139
Paternalistic medicine, 71
Patients and clinic staff
   aluminum, 220
   community immunity, 219
   diphtheria and vaccine, 224
   formaldehyde, 220
   Haemophilus Influenzae type B and vaccine, 222
   hepatitis A and vaccine, 222
   hepatitis B and vaccine, 222
   herd immunity, 219–220
   herpes zoster (shingles) and vaccine, 224
   human papillomavirus (HPV), 223
   influenza and flu vaccine, 220–221
   live-attenuated vaccines, 220
   measles, 221
   meningococcal disease and vaccine, 223
   MMR vaccine, 221
   mumps, 221
   PCV13 vaccine, 224
   pertussis vaccine, 221
   pneumococcal pneumonia, 224
   PPSV23 vaccine, 224
   rotavirus and vaccine, 221
   rubella, 221
   tetanus and vaccine, 224
   vaccine-preventable diseases, 219
   varicella zoster (chickenpox) and vaccine, 222
   whooping cough, 221
Patients' vaccine doubts
   allergic reactions, 109
   aluminum in
      Agency for Toxic Substances and Disease Registry
         (ATSDR), 101
      Centers for Disease Control and Prevention (CDC), 102

facts, 101, 102b
immune response, 102b
minimum risk levels (MRLs), 101
anti-vaccine claims, 99
autoimmune diseases and cancer, 110–111
Big Pharma, 106–107
chemicals exposure, 104
common cold, 100
community health/illness impact, 108
doctors training, 112–113
formaldehyde in, 102–103
Guillain-Barré syndrome (GBS), 108–109
Gulf War Syndrome, 103
herd immunity, 104–105
hygiene and sanitation, 105–106
immune response, 99
inactivated/killed virus vaccine, 100
individual and population-level protection, 105
live-attenuated virus vaccine, 100
MTHFR gene mutation, 109–110
National Vaccine Injury Compensation Program, 111
organic foods, 106
package inserts (PIs), 111–112
polio, 108
squalene in, 103
subacute sclerosing panencephalitis (SSPE), 104
toxoid vaccines, 101
vaccination levels, 105
Vaccine Information Statement (VIS), 109
vaccine, types, 100, 101t
vitamin A supplementation, 105–106
in whooping cough, 106, 106f
Personal liberties, 15–16
Pertussis (whooping cough), 203–204, 203f
vaccine, 117, 221, 226
PEW Research Center, 27
Phenol, 152
2-Phenoxyethanol, 152
Pneumococcal conjugate vaccine (PCV13), 86, 224
Pneumococcal pneumonia, 9, 205–206, 205f
and vaccine, 224
Pneumococcal polysaccharide vaccine (PPSV23), 87, 224
Pneumococcal vaccination schedule, 127, 128f
Poliomyelitis, 207–208, 207f
Polio virus, 5, 52, 108
Polysorbate 20, 154
Polysorbate 80, 154
Post-Licensure Rapid Immunization Safety Monitoring (PRISM) program, 60
Postural orthostatic tachycardia syndrome (POTS), 144
Pregnancy, vaccines
flu shot during, 122–123
MMR vaccine, 122
pertussis vaccine, 122
Presumptive approach, 71–72, 139
Pro-immunization messages, 20
Provider Enrollment Package, 176

R
Rabies-human diploid cell (RAB-HDC) vaccine, 87
Rabies-purified chick embryo cell (RAB-PCEC) vaccine, 87
Recombinant human serum albumin, 153
Religious concerns, 18–19, 20f
aborted fetal tissue, 123–124
cow and pig tissues, vaccines, 124–125
God's will, 125–126
National Catholic Bioethics Center (NCBC), 124
philosophical exemptions, 123
Residual proteins, 154–155, 155b
Rotavirus, 87, 209, 209f
and vaccine, 221
Rubella, 122, 210–211, 210f
and vaccine, 88, 221
RV1 (Rotarix) vaccine, 87
RV5 (RotaTeq) vaccine, 87

S
School-based HPV vaccination program, 140–141
Search engine optimization (SEO), 161–162
Serogroup B meningococcal vaccination (MenB), 85
Sexually transmitted infection
at-risk teens, 141–142
autoimmune diseases, 144
cancer, 142–143
chronic fatigue, complex regional pain syndrome (CRPS), 144
for girls, 142
infertile girls, 143
postural orthostatic tachycardia syndrome (POTS), 144
prevention vaccine, 141
school-based HPV vaccination program, 140–141
vaccine-preventable diseases, 142
vaccine skeptics, 144
Shingrix, 89, 89b
Skin patch delivery system, 14b
Smallpox, 1, 3, 4f, 52
Anti-Vaccination Society of America, 16
Vaccination Act, 15–16
Social media, 185, 247–248
Social psychology
anti-vaccine *vs.* vaccine-hesitant patient, 26–27
bias
Anticipated Regret, 31
anti-vaccination messages, 32
attitudes and behavioral intentions, 33
"backfire effect," 30
bandwagon fallacy, 31
confirmation bias, 30
definition, 30
Inoculation Theory, 32
measles reduction, 31, 32f
Motivated Reasoning, 30
omission bias, 31
self-affirmation, 31
social and psychological factors, 33
Big Pharma, 25
education and self-sacrifice, 26

Social psychology *(Continued)*
  socioeconomic and political breakdown, 27–28
  vaccines and vaccine- preventable disease, 25
Sorbitan trioleate, 154
Sorbitol, 153
Spanish flu, 4–5
Subacute sclerosing panencephalitis (SSPE), 104, 226

T

Tetanus, 52, 214, 214f
  and vaccine, 88, 224
Thimerosal, 15, 93, 152
Toxoid vaccines, 101
Triton X-100, 154
Typhoid vaccine, 88

U

UK General Medical Council, 93
US-licensed influenza vaccines, 103, 135

V

Vaccination Act, 15
Vaccine Adverse Events Reporting System (VAERS), 51, 56,
    58, 144
  advantages, 64
  adverse events following immunization (AEFI), 62–63
  data, 62, 62b
  disadvantages, 64
  Medical Dictionary for Regulatory Activities, 63
  reactions to, 62
  reports, 63, 63b
  vaccine adverse reaction, 63
Vaccine-associated neurotrophic disease, 89
Vaccine-associated viscerotropic disease, 89
Vaccine development/licensure, United States, 5, 6t–7t
Vaccine development phases, 53, 54f
  approval phase, 56
  clinical development phase
    Institutional Review Board, 55
    Investigational New Drug, 54
    phase I clinical trials, 55
    phase II clinical trials, 55
    phase III clinical trials, 55, 55b
  exploratory phase, 54
  preclinical phase, 54
  production process, 56
  quality control, 56
  regulatory review, 56
Vaccine history, 1, 2b, 225
  Cutter Incident, 8
  degree of regulation, 7
  diphtheria antitoxin, 8
  polio vaccine production, 8
  syphilis, 8
  Tuskegee Experiment, 8
Vaccine Information Statement (VIS), 72, 80, 109
Vaccine ingredients
  adjuvants
    aluminum, 151–152

    CpG motifs, 152
    inactivated virus vaccines, 151
    MF59 (squalene oil), 152
    MPL (3-O- esacyl-4'-monophosphoryl lipid A),
      152
    QS-21, 152
    xanthan, 152
  buffers, 154
  emulsifiers, 154
  immunogenicity, 151
  latex, 155–156
  package inserts, 149
  preservatives, 152–153
  processing and purification
    antibiotics, 151
    inactivating agents, 151
    protein purifiers, 151
    vaccines production, 151
  residual proteins, 154–155
  stabilizers, 153
  taste improvers, 155
  viruses and bacteria growth
    growth media, 150–151
    human and animal cells, 150
    immune response, 150
Vaccine Injury Table, 61, 61b
Vaccine manufacturing process, 15
Vaccine-preventable disease, 1, 2b
  annual economic burden, 239, 239f–240f
  contagion and death, 237–238, 237f–238f
  cowpox, 4
  diphtheria, 5, 189, 189f
  Haemophilus Influenzae B (HiB), 190, 190f
  hepatitis A, 191, 191f
  hepatitis B, 192, 192f
  herpes zoster (shingles), 212–213, 212f
  human papillomavirus (HPV), 193f
    complications, 193
    disease/complications, 194
    impact of, 194
    symptoms, 193
    transmission/contagion, 193
    vaccine information, 193–194
  influenza vaccine, 1
  influenza virus, 5, 195–196, 195f
  inoculation methods, 3
  measles, 5, 197–198, 197f
  meningococcal disease, 199–200, 199f
  mumps, 201–202, 201f
  pertussis (whooping cough), 203–204, 203f
  pneumococcal disease, 205–206, 205f
  poliomyelitis, 207–208, 207f
  polio-virus, 5
  rotavirus, 209, 209f
  rubella, 210–211, 210f
  smallpox, 1, 3, 4f
  Spanish flu, 4–5
  statistics, 25
  tetanus, 214, 214f
  vaccination rates, 3

vaccine development/licensure, United States, 5, 6t–7t
"variolation," 3
varicella zoster virus (chickenpox), 188, 188f
Vaccine Research Center (VRC), 60
Vaccine risks
adverse reactions, 79
vs. adverse events, 85, 85b
rates, 82, 82t
allergic reactions, 81
diphtheria vaccine, 82–83
events, 79, 80f
Haemophilus influenzae type b (Hib), 83
hepatitis A, 83
hepatitis B, 83
human papillomavirus (HPV), 83
immune system, 81
inactivated polio vaccine (IPV), 87
influenza, 83–84
injection site, redness and swelling, 81
Japanese encephalitis, 84
limitations, 80
live-attenuated influenza vaccine (LAIV), 84
live-attenuated/weakened vaccines, 82
measles, 84–85
meningococcal polysaccharide vaccine (MPSV4), 85
mumps, 86
oral polio vaccine (OPV), 87
pain, 81
pertussis, 86
pneumococcal conjugate vaccine (PCV13), 86
pneumococcal polysaccharide vaccine (PPSV23), 87
rabies-human diploid cell (RAB-HDC), 87
rabies-purified chick embryo cell (RAB-PCEC), 87
rubella, 88
RV1 (Rotarix), 87
RV5 (RotaTeq), 87
Serogroup B meningococcal vaccination (MenB), 85
tetanus, 88
typhoid, 88
Vaccine Information Statement (VIS), 80
varicella (chickenpox), 88–89
yellow fever, 89
zoster (shingles), 89–90, 89b
Vaccine safety and efficacy
development phases. *See* Vaccine development phases

federally funded organizations, 58, 59f
Centers for Disease Control and Prevention (CDC), 58, 60
Food and Drug Administration (FDA), 60
Health Resources and Services Administration (HRSA), 61
National Institutes of Health (NIH), 60–61
National Vaccine Program Office (NVPO), 58
pharmaceutical companies, 51
pharmaceutical industry, 56–58
postlicensure monitoring, 51
privately funded organizations, 58, 59f
Immunization Action Coalition, 61
Institute for Safe Medication Practices (ISMP), 61 62
public health-related governmental programs, 51
regulation history
1902 Biologics Control Act, 52
National Childhood Vaccine Injury Act, 53
polio and Cutter Incident, 52
Vaccine Adverse Events Reporting System (VAERS), 51, 62–64
Vaccine Safety Datalink (VSD), 56, 58, 60
Vaccines for Children (VFC) program, 176, 176b
VAERS. *See* Vaccine Adverse Events Reporting System (VAERS)
Varicella zoster (chickenpox), 88–89, 188, 188f
and vaccine, 222
VIS. *See* Vaccine Information Statement (VIS)
Vitamin A supplementation, 105–106
VRC. *See* Vaccine Research Center (VRC)

W

Whooping cough, 203–204, 203f, 226
and vaccine, 221
WMA. *See* World Medical Association (WMA)
World Health Organization (WHO), 29, 29b, 103, 134
World Medical Association (WMA), 96

Y

Yeast protein, 155
Yellow fever vaccine, 89, 155

Z

Zoster (shingles) vaccine, 89–90, 89b